Understanding Prescription Drugs For Canadians

FOR

DUMMIES®

by Ian Blumer, MD, FRCPC
and Heather McDonald-Blumer, MD, FRCPC

BICENTENNIAL
1807
WILEY
2007
BICENTENNIAL

John Wiley & Sons Canada, Ltd.

Understanding Prescription Drugs For Canadians For Dummies®

Published by
John Wiley & Sons Canada, Ltd
6045 Freemont Boulevard
Mississauga, Ontario, L5R 4J3
www.wiley.com

Library and Archives Canada Cataloguing in Publication Data

Blumer, Ian
    Understanding prescription drugs for Canadians for dummies/Ian Blumer, Heather McDonald-Blumer.

Includes index.
ISBN 978-0-470-83835-8

    1. Drugs—Canada—Popular works. I. McDonald-Blumer, Heather II. Title.

RM301.15.B58 2007   615.1   C2007-901302-3

Printed in Canada

1 2 3 4 5 TRI 11 10 09 08 07

Distributed in Canada by John Wiley & Sons Canada, Ltd.

For general information on John Wiley & Sons Canada, Ltd., including all books published by Wiley Publishing, Inc., please call our warehouse, Tel 1-800-567-4797. For reseller information, including discounts and premium sales, please call our sales department, Tel 416-646-7992. For press review copies, author interviews, or other publicity information, please contact our marketing department, Tel 416-646-4584, Fax 416-236-4448.

For authorization to photocopy items for corporate, personal, or educational use, please contact in writing The Canadian Copyright Licensing Agency (Access Copyright). For an Access Copyright license, visit www.accesscopyright.ca or call toll free, 1-800-893-5777.

Figure Credit: Fig. 4-3: HumaPen Luxura is a trademark of Eli Lilly and Company and is used with permission.

Figure Credit: Fig. 6-1: Copyright © 2005 Massachusetts Medical Society. All rights reserved. Adapted with permission, 2007.

WILEY

About the Authors

Ian Blumer, MD, FRCPC, is an internal medicine specialist in Durham Region, Ontario. He is a graduate of Queen's University Medical School and is a Fellow of the Royal College of Physicians and Surgeons of Canada. Ian is the medical adviser to the adult program of the Charles H. Best Diabetes Centre and is a member of the executive of the Clinical and Scientific Section of the Canadian Diabetes Association. His previous books are *What Your Doctor Really Thinks* and *Diabetes For Canadians For Dummies* (co-written with Alan L. Rubin).

Heather McDonald-Blumer, MD, FRCPC, is a rheumatologist at Mount Sinai Hospital and University Health Network in Toronto, Ontario, and an assistant professor with the University of Toronto, where she also serves as Program Director for Rheumatology. Heather is a graduate of McMaster University School of Medicine. She has recently taken on the position of Chair, Specialty Committee in Rheumatology with the Royal College of Physicians and Surgeons of Canada.

Dedication

This book is dedicated, with all our love, to our children: Leslie, Brian, and Michael. It is also dedicated to their grandparents, Curt and Mary McDonald and Jack and Rhoda Blumer, without whose love, guidance, and DNA none of this would have been possible.

Authors' Acknowledgements

We would like to express our great thanks to Robert Hickey, our unflappable Wiley mentor and pillar of support. We consider ourselves lucky, indeed, to have had the opportunity to work with him. We also wish to express our appreciation to our editors Lisa Berland and Kelli Howey for their expert assistance. Lisa's ability to take an overwhelming breadth of information, toss it into the air and have it come out organized, synthesized, and readable can only be considered astonishing. Thanks also to our meticulous project coordinator, Pam Vokey.

Dr. Jean Gray, an esteemed physician and medical educator, can't be thanked enough for her insights and helpful tips.

We want to both thank and acknowledge Carolyn White (Heritage Market Pharmacy, Ajax, Ontario), a wonderful pharmacist and role model, for her invaluable advice. How lucky her patients are to have such a thoughtful and skilled pharmacist working with them.

The following people are to be thanked for their immensely helpful suggestions: Saied Asgarali, Tom Ashton, Natalie Baziuk, Stephen Betschel, Kelvin Chan, Hak Chiu, Shelley Diamond, Suha Eltayeb, Elaine Goldenberg, Michael Gordon, Jack Grainge, Bob Hyland, Richard Jay, Ralph Kern, Emad Khalil, Peter Lee, Joel Raskin, Mathew Sermer, Michael Silverman, Steve Smith, Jeff Stal, Sloane Waitzer, and Charles Wei. Thanks also to Sue Cavallucci of IMS Health Canada for the invaluable information she was able to share.

We have worked with hundreds upon hundreds of pharmacists and pharmacy technicians over the years and we never fail to be impressed by the care with which they dispense medication. We wish to publicly acknowledge their skills. Hear, hear!

We wouldn't pretend for one second that pharmaceutical companies create and sell drugs for purely magnanimous reasons. But we also wouldn't want to imagine for that same one second *not* having the fruits of their labours available to us. The thought of having no diuretic to help the elderly person with heart failure, no puffer to help the child with asthma, no insulin for the young adult with diabetes, no morphine for the dying person suffering from the pain of metastatic cancer; it's simply too horrific to consider. Yet sometimes, we think, perhaps it's all taken for granted. So without apology we take this opportunity to thank those people in the pharmaceutical industry who work to develop the important prescription medicines that we (doctors and patients alike) rely on.

Last, but not least, we would like to thank the patients with whom we have worked over the years. We can think of no greater honour than having the trust of those people who look to us to help them.

Publisher's Acknowledgements

We're proud of this book; please send us your comments at canadapt@wiley.com. Some of the people who helped bring this book to market include the following:

Acquisitions, Editorial, and Media Development

Editor: Robert Hickey

Developmental Editor: Lisa Berland

Copy Editor: Kelli Howey

Cover Photos: © Phanie/First Light

Cartoons: Rich Tennant, www.the5thwave.com

Wiley Bicentennial Logo: Richard J. Pacifico

Composition

Publishing Services Director: Karen Bryan

Publishing Services Manager: Ian Koo

Project Manager: Elizabeth McCurdy

Project Coordinators: Pamela Vokey, Adrienne Martinez

Layout and Graphics: Wiley Indianapolis Composition Services

Proofreaders: Aptara, John Greenough, Dwight Ramsey

Indexers: Belle Wong, Liisa Kelly, Colborne Communications

John Wiley & Sons Canada, Ltd

   Bill Zerter, Chief Operating Officer

   Jennifer Smith, Publisher, Professional and Trade Division

Publishing and Editorial for Consumer Dummies

   Diane Graves Steele, Vice President and Publisher, Consumer Dummies

   Joyce Pepple, Acquisitions Director, Consumer Dummies

   Kristin A. Cocks, Product Development Director, Consumer Dummies

   Michael Spring, Vice President and Publisher, Travel

   Suzanne Jannetta, Editorial Director, Travel

Publishing for Technology Dummies

   Andy Cummings, Vice President and Publisher, Dummies Technology/General User

Composition Services

   Gerry Fahey, Vice President of Production Services

   Debbie Stailey, Director of Composition Services

Contents at a Glance

Introduction..*1*

Part 1: A Healthy Look at Prescription Drugs........*7*

Chapter 1: Prescription Drugs and You...9
Chapter 2: Prescribing Knowledge...15
Chapter 3: Your Doctor, Your Pharmacist, and You............................31
Chapter 4: Making Sure Your Prescription Works for You 59

Part 11: Ailments A to Z *93*

Chapter 5: Ailments and Their Treatment 95

Part 111: Medications A to Z *169*

Chapter 6: All in the (Drug) Family 171

Part 1V: Common Concerns.................................*429*

Chapter 7: Side-Effects and Drug Interactions...................................431
Chapter 8: Prescription Drugs for Moms-to-Be,
      Kids, and Seniors 445
Chapter 9: Dealing with Emergencies and Hospitalizations 459
Chapter 10: Coping with the Costs of Prescription Drugs 471

Part V: The Part of Tens.....................................*477*

Chapter 11: Ten Changes We Hope to See in the
      World of Prescription Drug Therapy...479
Chapter 12: Ten Not-So-Trivial Facts about Prescription Drugs 485

Drug Index...*491*
General Index *518*

Table of Contents

Introduction *1*

About This Book 2
Conventions Used in This Book..............................3
What You Don't Have to Read 3
Foolish Assumptions 4
How This Book Is Organized....................................4
    Part I: A Healthy Look at Prescription Drugs 4
    Part II: Ailments A to Z 4
    Part III: Medications A to Z.................................4
    Part IV: Common Concerns 5
    Part V: The Part of Tens....................................5
Icons Used in This Book...5

Part 1: A Healthy Look at Prescription Drugs *7*

Chapter 1: Prescription Drugs and You 9

Prescription Drugs: The Basics.................................9
Your Doctor, Your Pharmacist, and You..................11
Treating What Ails You..12
Getting to Know Your Medicines 12
Addressing Your Concerns 13
Last(ing) Advice to Take from Chapter 1 14

Chapter 2: Prescribing Knowledge 15

How Drugs Work 16
    Entering the fray: How medicines
        get into our bodies 16
    The incredible journey: How a pill gets from your
        mouth to your brain, bones, and beyond................17
    How drugs affect your body's cells 20
    How your body rids itself of medication 21
What Is a Prescription Drug?....................................22
    The difference between over-the-counter
        drugs and prescription drugs 22
    The difference between behind-the-counter
        drugs and prescription drugs 24
    The difference between prescription drugs and
        complementary and alternative medicines............25

The Difference between a Brand-Name Drug
and a Generic Drug 26
    Brand-name drugs 26
    Generic drugs..26
    Choosing brand-name or generic drugs 27
The Non-Medicinal Ingredients in Oral Medications...........29

Chapter 3: Your Doctor, Your Pharmacist, and You 31
Prescribing Patience...31
Prescribing Prescription Drugs: Your Doctor's Role 33
    Why your doctor prescribed a drug 33
    What you need to tell your doctor 34
    How your doctor chooses your prescription drug 35
    What to make sure your doctor tells you....................39
Dispensing Prescription Drugs: Your Pharmacist's Role 41
    What your doctor needs to tell your pharmacist.......42
    What you need to tell your pharmacist 44
    What you need to make sure
        your pharmacist tells you..45
Consuming Prescription Drugs: Your Key Role....................49
    Understanding the prescription label........................49
    Noting the warning labels...51
    Understanding the package insert 52
    What to watch for with your medications..................53

**Chapter 4: Making Sure Your Prescription
Works for You 59**
Taking Your Medication: Practical Answers
for Common Questions 59
    What drugs am I taking? 60
    What dose am I supposed to take?..............................60
    How will I know whether I need to change doses?.....61
    How often should I take my medicine? 62
    What should I do if I miss a dose? 63
    Can I split the drug? 64
    Should I take my medicine with food? 67
    Are there things I should avoid
        when taking my medicine? 68
    Can I stop my prescription before it's finished?.........69
    Should I refill my prescription?...................................70
Head to Toe: Using Different Types
of Medication Properly..73
    Easy to swallow: Pills, capsules, and liquids 73
    In the eye of the beholder: Eye drops and ointments...74
    Hear, hear! Ear drops..75
    On the nose: Nose drops and sprays 76
    Hit me with your best shot: Inhalers............................77
    Getting it in the end: Suppositories and enemas........80
    For Women Only: Vaginal preparations 81

Rubbing it in: Lotions, creams,
        ointments, and patches.............................81
    Needling questions: Injections.....................82
Looking After Your Medication 83
    Storing your medication 84
    Dealing with leftover medication......................85
On the Road Again: Travelling with
    a Prescription Medicine 85
    Preparing for your trip...............................86
    Packing your prescription medicine 86
    Forgetting your prescription medicine at home........86
Why Your Prescription Drug Might Not Be Working 88
    Are you sure your medicine is not working?.............88
    Are you taking the right medicine? 89
    Are you on the right dose of the medicine? 90
    Are you taking the prescription properly? 91
    Is the medicine being absorbed into your body?.......91

Part II: Ailments A to Z *93*

Chapter 5: Ailments and Their Treatment. 95
Conventions We Use in This Chapter 95
Acne..96
Addison's Disease 97
Alcoholism 98
Allergies..98
Alzheimer's Disease 99
Anemia..100
    Iron deficiency 100
    Vitamin B12 deficiency..............................100
Angina...101
Anxiety Disorders 102
Arrhythmias...103
Arthritis..104
    Osteoarthritis......................................104
    Rheumatoid arthritis................................105
Asthma 106
Athlete's Foot 107
Attention-Deficit/Hyperactivity Disorder (ADHD) 108
Baldness 108
Bedwetting..109
Bipolar Disorder.......................................109
Blood Clots 110
Cancer 110
    Breast cancer 111
    Prostate cancer 111
Chlamydia...112
Chronic Obstructive Pulmonary Disease (COPD) 112
Claudication...113

Cold, Common...114
Cold Sores...114
Conjunctivitis 114
Contraception...115
Cough 115
Depression..116
Diabetes 117
        Insulin therapy...117
        Oral hypoglycemic agents 118
Diarrhea..119
Dizziness 119
Ear Infections..120
Eczema 121
Edema...121
Endocarditis Prophylaxis...122
Endometriosis 123
Epilepsy..123
Erectile Dysfunction 124
Fibromyalgia 125
Flatulence...125
Gastroenteritis 126
Gastro-esophageal Reflux Disease (GERD) 126
Glaucoma 127
Gonorrhea...127
Gout 128
Headaches...129
Heart Attack..130
Heart Failure 131
Hemorrhoids...132
Hepatitis, Viral..132
Herpes, Genital...133
Hirsutism..134
HIV/AIDS...135
Hyperprolactinemia (Enlarged Prostate).........................136
Hypertension...136
Hyperthyroidism..138
Hypothyroidism 139
Incontinence, Urinary..139
Infertility 140
Inflammatory Bowel Disease..140
Influenza...141
Insomnia...142
Irritable Bowel Syndrome 143
Kidney Failure...143
Kidney Stones...144
Libido, Reduced 145
Lipid Disorders (Abnormal Cholesterol
        and Triglyceride Levels) 146
Lupus..147
Menopause..148

Menstrual Cramps 148
Multiple Sclerosis..149
Muscle Cramps..149
Nausea and Vomiting......................................150
Obesity 150
Obsessive-Compulsive Disorder 151
Osteoporosis 151
Pain 152
Parkinson's Disease..152
Pneumonia 153
Polycystic Ovary Syndrome (PCOS) 154
Prostatis 154
Prostatism (Enlarged Prostate)........................155
Psoriasis...155
Restless Legs Syndrome..................................156
Rosacea 156
Schizophrenia...157
Shingles 157
Sinusitis 158
Smoking Cessation...159
Stroke...159
Syphilis 160
Throat Infections...161
Toenail Infections..161
Tremor, Essential 162
Tuberculosis 163
Ulcers, Peptic 163
Urinary Tract Infections...................................165
     Bladder infections 165
     Kidney infections 165
Vaginal Dryness..166
Vaginal Infections 166
Vitiligo 167
Warts, Genital 168
Warts, Skin 168

Part III: Medications A to Z *169*

Chapter 6: All in the (Drug) Family **171**

Conventions We Use in This Chapter 171
Prescription Drugs 101: A Primer 173
     Prescription drug use during pregnancy
       and breastfeeding 173
     Prescription drugs and children............................173
     Prescription drug interactions and side-effects 174
     Prescription drug choices 175
Alpha-adrenergic Agonists (Centrally Acting) 176
Alpha Blockers 178
Alpha-Reductase Inhibitors 182

Alzheimer's Disease Medicines 183
Aminosalicylates 186
Angiotensin Converting Enzyme (ACE) Inhibitors 189
Angiotensin Receptor Blockers (ARBs) 192
Anti-anxiety Medications 194
Anti-arrhythmics 199
Antibiotics..204
       Aminoglycosides...208
       Cephalosporins...210
       Fluoroquinolones..211
       Lincosamines 213
       Macrolides 216
       Nitroimidazoles..217
       Penicillins 219
       Sulfas 221
       Tetracyclines 222
Anticancer Drugs for Breast and Prostate Cancer.............224
Anticholinergics (for Overactive Bladder) 229
Anticoagulants 232
       Low molecular weight heparins............................235
Anticonvulsants 237
Antidepressants 249
Antifungal Agents...257
Antihistamines 261
Anti-obesity Drugs 264
Antiparkinsonian Drugs 267
Antiplatelet Agents 271
Antipsychotics 276
Antiretroviral Drugs...282
Antithyroid Agents..283
Antituberculosis Drugs 285
Antiviral Agents..287
Beta Blockers...290
Biologic Response Modifiers 295
Bisphosphonates 296
Calcium Channel Blockers 300
Cholesterol Absorption Inhibitors......................................304
Contraceptive Therapy 306
       Oral contraceptive therapies 307
       Medroxy-progesterone acetate (Depo-Provera).......309
       Levonorgestrel (Plan B) 311
Corticosteroids 312
       Nasal corticosteroids 316
       Ophthalmic (eye) corticosteroids.........................317
       Oral corticosteroids 319
       Otic (ear) corticosteroids.....................................322
       Rectal corticosteroids..324
       Topical corticosteroids...325
Diuretics 326
Dopamine Agonists...334

Gastrointestinal Tract Motility Modifiers
  and Related Drugs...337
Eye Drops to Treat Glaucoma...............................340
Fibrates (Fibric Acid Derivatives).........................347
Histamine (H1) Agonist.......................................349
Immunosuppressive Drugs..................................351
Inhaled Medicines to Treat Asthma and Chronic
  Obstructive Pulmonary Disease (COPD).............356
Insulin..365
Leukotriene Antagonists.....................................370
Lithium...371
Menopausal Hormone Therapy...........................374
Narcotic ("Opioid") Analgesics............................377
Nitrates..380
Nonsteroidal Anti-Inflammatory Drugs (NSAIDs)...384
Oral Hypoglycemic Agents..................................387
Phosphodiesterase Type 5 (PDE5) Inhibitors.......397
Proton Pump Inhibitors (PPIs)............................399
Retinoids..401
Selective Estrogen Receptor Modulators (SERMs)...404
Serotonin (5 HT) Receptor Agonists....................408
Skeletal Muscle Relaxants..................................411
Statins...413
Stimulants..416
Testosterone...418
Thyroid Hormones...421
Tricyclic Antidepressants (TCAs).........................423
Xanthine Oxidase Inhibitor.................................426

Part IV: Common Concerns.......................429

Chapter 7: Side-Effects and Drug Interactions 431

Understanding Side-Effects..................................431
  Allergic reactions...432
  Dose-related side-effects.................................433
  Side-effects from your drug acting
    where you'd rather it didn't...........................434
  Idiosyncratic reactions....................................436
  Drug intolerance..436
  Side-effects from non-medicinal ingredients.......437
How to Avoid Side-Effects...................................438
  Questions to ask your doctor
    before you leave the office.............................438
  Questions to ask your pharmacist
    before you leave the pharmacy.......................439
  Questions to ask yourself before
    you take your new medicine...........................439
What to Do If You Experience a Side-Effect...........440
Understanding Drug Interactions.........................441

Drug–drug interactions 441
Drug–food interactions 442
Drug–alcohol interactions 442
Drug–complementary and alternative
  medicine interactions 443
Drug–sunshine interactions 444

Chapter 8: Prescription Drugs for Moms-to-Be, Kids, and Seniors 445

Drug Safety for Women Who Are
  Pregnant or Breastfeeding 445
  Looking at whether a drug is safe when
    pregnant or breastfeeding 446
  What to do if you're taking a prescription
    drug and then find out you're pregnant 449
Drug Safety for Children 449
  Special issues regarding your child's use of
    stimulant medicines to treat Attention-Deficit/
    Hyperactivity Disorder (ADHD) 450
  How to help your child swallow a medicine 452
Drug Safety for Seniors 453
  Considering special risks for seniors 453
  Helpful ways for seniors to stay organized
    with their prescription medicines 454
  Watching out for special side-effects in seniors 457

Chapter 9: Dealing with Emergencies and Hospitalizations 459

Can It Wait? Deciding When You Require
  Emergency Medical Attention 459
Dealing with an Overdose 461
What to Do If You Run Out of Your
  Prescription Medicine 463
Your Prescription Drugs and Hospitalizations 464
  Your prescription drugs and the
    emergency department 464
  Your prescription drugs and the inpatient wards 466
  Your prescription drugs when you're
    discharged from hospital 468

Chapter 10: Coping with the Costs of Prescription Drugs. 471

How Your Doctor Can Help You Save Money 471
How Your Pharmacist Can Help You Save Money 473
How the Government Can Help You 474
How Your Private Health Insurer Can Help You 475
How the Pharmaceutical Industry Can Help You 475
Buying Prescription Drugs over the Internet 475

Part V: The Part of Tens....................*477*

Chapter 11: Ten Changes We Hope to See in the World of Prescription Drug Therapy 479

A Catastrophic Drug Plan...479
Drugs That Say What They Are...480
More Skepticism about New Drugs....................................480
Better Package Inserts and Information Sheets.................480
More Quality Time with Your Pharmacist 481
Better Medical News Reporting 481
More Certainty about a Drug's Effectiveness
    and Tolerability...482
Smarter Technology 482
Easier Ways to Know When It's Time
    to Take Your Medicine...483
Multipills 483
And a Final Fantasy... 484

Chapter 12: Ten Not-So-Trivial Facts about Prescription Drugs 485

How Many New Prescription Drugs Are
    Approved Each Year in Canada? 485
How Much Do Canadians Spend on Prescription Drugs? ...486
How Expensive Is It to Run a Drug Study?..........................486
How Often Do People Improperly Take
    Their Prescription Medicines? 487
What Are the Best-Selling Prescription Drugs in Canada? ...487
What Are the Best-Selling Prescription
    Drug Classes in Canada? 488
How Often Are Prescription Drugs Used
    for "Unapproved Indications"?.....................................488
How Many Pharmacists Are Practising in Canada?...........489
How Many Pharmacies Are in Canada?.............................489
How Much Medicine Is in a Pill?.......................................489

Drug Index *491*

General Index *518*

Introduction

● ●

A prescription drug is like a car. It can be a wonderful tool, allowing us to safely and effectively go about our business, and on the other hand it can be troublesome and hazardous, causing us difficulties, grief, and worse. And, like a car, a medicine is much more likely to keep us going in a healthy direction when we know how to use it properly, how to maintain it properly, and what things to watch for to alert us of developing problems (*before* the engine light comes on!).

In this book you won't learn how to drive a car, but you certainly will discover how to take your medicine for a spin (and minimize the likelihood your medicine will take *you* for a spin). In *Understanding Prescription Drugs For Canadians For Dummies* we look at all sides of the prescription drug spectrum, including what a medicine is, how a medicine can help you, and how a medicine can harm you (and how to minimize this risk).

We also address practical issues such as how to choose your pharmacist and how you can save money on your prescriptions, and we explore important issues such as the use of prescription drugs during pregnancy and breastfeeding. To help seniors deal with the often daunting challenge of contending with multiple medications, we provide tips to help you stay organized and safe with that often intimidating collection of pill bottles sitting on your shelf (which, by the way, may not be the best place to keep them, as we will discover).

Buying a new car is not everyone's favourite pastime, but whether we enjoy the experience or not it's certainly made a lot easier when we have some background information before we enter the dealership to kick a tire or two. So, too, with prescription medication — knowing that shiny, new, Ferrari-red (sorry, couldn't help it) capsule is the best choice for you is a key step before you drive it out of the pharmacy parking lot. To help you navigate this often confusing course, we discuss many of the most common ailments you may confront, with an emphasis on what the best choices are among the various prescription drugs available to treat these conditions.

A drug first used to treat high blood pressure ends up being used to treat baldness. A drug first used to treat high blood pressure ends up being used to treat excess hair growth. What a topsy turvy world of prescription drugs we live in! In *Understanding Prescription*

Drugs For Canadians For Dummies, whether you're having a bad hair day (or, as Ian is quickly discovering, a no-hair day) or not, we help to straighten out this tangled situation.

About This Book

Understanding Prescription Drugs For Canadians For Dummies is a reference tool and is not intended to be read from cover to cover (though of course you're welcome to do so if you like). It's designed to enable you to quickly find and use those key pieces of information you're looking for at any given time. We emphasize the practical and helpful to maximize the likelihood your prescription medication does what it should and minimize the likelihood it does what it shouldn't.

Although much of the information in this book applies to people of any age, we concentrate our attentions on adult users of prescription medicines. Particularly when it comes to issues such as drug doses, children have their own special needs that are outside the scope of this book.

For many ailments, lifestyle management and non-prescription drugs have important roles to play. *Understanding Prescription Drugs For Canadians For Dummies*, however, focuses — as you would expect from the title — on prescription drugs. In particular, as this book is designed to empower you to take your medicines safely and effectively, the overwhelming majority of drugs we mention are those you would be *giving yourself* rather than those given *to you* (for example, intravenous medicines given in an inpatient hospital setting). Not that those other medicines are unimportant for you to know about; they're just not what we address here.

This book was co-written by Ian (that would be me) and Heather (that would be me). In addition to having the same perspective on prescription drug therapy (we can't imagine co-writing this book otherwise!) we also have the same perspective on relationships — which likely accounts for the fact we've shared the same marriage certificate for more than 20 years.

We've bent over backward to make this book as accurate as humanly possible. If you identify what you believe to be an error, please let us know so we can be sure to correct it in future printings. We can be reached at `drugs@ianblumer.com`.

 This book is a guide and, we hope, a helpful tool to assist you in the safe and effective use of your prescription drugs. It does not in any way replace the care and advice you receive from your physician, pharmacist, and other members of your health care team.

We strongly recommend you consult with the appropriate members of your health care team regarding any and all matters pertaining to your prescription drugs.

Conventions Used in This Book

Although most prescription drugs are available throughout the world, sometimes a drug is called one name in one country and another name in another country. In this book, we always refer to the names used in Canada.

Because prescription drugs in Canada have one generic (scientific) name but can have many different trade names, we make a point of discussing drugs using their generic names. If you're unsure of your prescription medicine's generic name you can find it on the prescription label of the container your medicine came in. You can then quickly locate information on that drug in this book by looking up the name in the Drug Index.

Because so many medicines serve more than one purpose, we generally avoid referring to a specific drug in terms of its use. One current example of the rationale for this is the recent use of sildenafil (trade name Viagra) to treat high blood pressure in the arteries in the lung (a condition called *pulmonary hypertension*). We can picture the non-comprehending looks a man (or, especially, a woman!) might receive as he tells his friends he is "taking an erectile dysfunction pill to help my breathing." One could imagine how the drug, if anything, could have led to the amorous situation where he was rendered more short of breath, not less, but we digress...

When we discuss rules governing prescription drugs, we use those set down by the Government of Canada.

We use the words "drug" and "medicine" interchangeably and, unless specified otherwise, when we use either term we are always referring to *prescription* therapy.

What You Don't Have to Read

In this book, you'll find sections of text preceded by a "Technical stuff" icon, and you'll also find shaded sections we call sidebars. These two areas provide additional or supplementary information that round out topics, but are not essential reading. Feel free to skip these sections if you like; doing so will not prevent you from understanding everything else.

Foolish Assumptions

This book makes only one assumption: that you are in search of information about prescription drugs. Whether you've been taking prescription drugs since a Coke sold for five cents or just since yesterday (when we saw a can of Coke for sale in Paris for more than five dollars!), in this book you'll find what you need to know in order to safely and effectively take your medicines.

How This Book Is Organized

This book is divided into five parts. Each part looks at a different aspect of prescription drug therapy.

Part I: A Healthy Look at Prescription Drugs

This part looks at what prescription drugs are and how they differ from non-prescription medicines. We explore how medicines work and how you and your pharmacist and doctor can work together to ensure the best possible results from your therapy. We also look at warning labels, package inserts and information sheets, and what information they convey. And if even the notion of mistakenly inserting a suppository into, well, some place it doesn't belong makes you cringe, you won't want to miss the chapter on how to properly take your medicine.

Part II: Ailments A to Z

In this part we look at many of the most common ailments that are treated with prescription drugs. From acne to warts (okay we took some liberties with the title for this part, but what the heck, W is pretty darn close to Z), you'll find an overview of conditions that can affect you with a special emphasis on the preferred medicines available to help you.

Part III: Medications A to Z

This is where you'll find the details on well over 200 of the most commonly prescribed medications in Canada. We look at how a medicine works, how it can help you, what side-effects it may cause, important precautions to be aware of, when a medicine should not be taken, and how to most effectively take your drug. And, because we group medicines by the family to which they belong, if you're on a less commonly prescribed therapy you're still very likely to find your drug included in the tables in this section.

Part IV: Common Concerns

In this part we look at common concerns Canadians have about their prescription medicines. We discuss drug side-effects and interactions and how to help avoid them, we look at the costs of prescription medicines and ways to try to lessen their financial burden, we discuss drug therapy taken in special situations such as pregnancy, breastfeeding, and in the elderly, and we look at ways to help keep kids safe in households where prescription medicines are kept. We also look at drug emergencies and how to best handle them.

Part V: The Part of Tens

Here we get to "blue sky" our hopes for the future of prescription drug therapy including our fantasy of one day having a single Multipill to replace the fistful of drugs many people have to take. We also present ten not-so-trivial facts about prescription medicines.

Icons Used in This Book

We use seven icons in this book. The purpose of an icon is to let you know the general theme of the text immediately beside it. The icons we use (and their meanings) are:

This icon lets you know we're discussing critically important and therefore not-to-be missed information — it usually pertains to matters of safety.

This icon informs you we're sharing a practical piece of information that will make your life — well, at least as it pertains to your prescription medicine — easier.

Here we alert you to an especially important bit of information that is best not forgotten.

The "Technical stuff" icon advises you that we're discussing, ah, technical stuff. If you want to find out more about such things as the mechanism by which your medicine works, then read these sections. If that's not important to you, feel free to disregard passages marked with this icon.

When we use the "Ask your doctor" icon, we are mentioning a point we recommend you bring up with your physician.

When we use the "Ask your pharmacist" icon, we are mentioning a point we recommend you bring up with your pharmacist.

This icon indicates we're telling a story. Although the stories we tell are based on real events, we change some of the details as well as the names of the people involved (because, well, it's not for us to decide someone doesn't want to be anonymous).

Part I
A Healthy Look at Prescription Drugs

The 5th Wave   By Rich Tennant

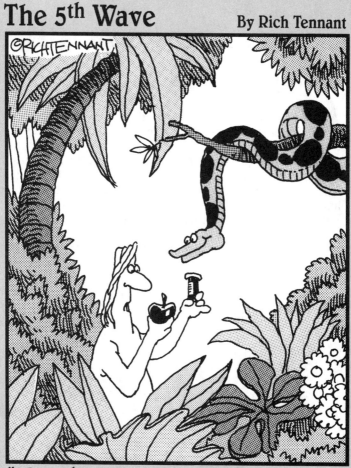

"Well, the label did say that I should take the medication with food..."

In this part . . .

We look at what prescription drugs are, how they differ from non-prescription medicines, how they work, and how they are taken. We discuss how you can work with your pharmacist and doctor to get the best possible results from your therapy. Lastly, we look at warning labels, package inserts, and information sheets and the information they convey — and, just as important, what critical information they may leave out.

Chapter 1

Prescription Drugs and You

● ●

In This Chapter

▶ Appreciating what prescription drugs can — and can't — do for you

▶ Understanding how you can work with your doctor and pharmacist

▶ Considering the best ways to treat what ails you

▶ Becoming familiar with your prescription drugs

▶ Making common concerns less concerning

▶ Checking out all your options

● ●

*I*f you're like most people we know, the only thing you'd rather do less than take a prescription drug is not take one when you should have. Or, to (woefully) paraphrase Prime Minister William Lyon Mackenzie King, "Prescription if necessary, but not necessarily prescription." Medicines are something never to take lightly, but thank goodness they are there to help us when we need them. And that reality of life is why we've created this book to assist you.

In *Understanding Prescription Drugs For Canadians For Dummies,* we look at how you can work with your physician and pharmacist to most safely and effectively manage your medicines. We discuss the best medicines to treat what ails you, and how they work. We look at how your medicines can help you, and how your medicines can harm you. We share, to quote Sergio Leone, the good, the bad, and the ugly — even if you've paid *handsomely* for that *ugly* medicine. (Speaking of which, one of the things we talk about is how you can pay less handsomely for your drugs: see Chapter 10.)

Prescription Drugs: The Basics

Prescription drugs are brilliant. They can reach every nook and cranny of your body to help you overcome infections, fight cancer, control diabetes, avoid heart attacks, and quell arthritis.

Prescription drugs are dumb. They often are unable to cure a disease, may cause unpleasant side-effects, frequently are costly, and typically are a nuisance to remember.

And how do Canadians deal with this paradox? Well, Canadians are clearly believers in prescription drugs, seeing as, in 2005, $20 billion was spent in this country on 400 million prescriptions. Yet, Canadians often are not very happy believers; at least judging by the comments ("Doctor, I feel like a walking drugstore") that physicians so often hear as their patients walk into the office, shopping bag full of medicines in hand.

And yes, having to take prescription medicines might make you feel hard done by. And if you feel that way, we don't blame you one little bit. But what wonderful health benefits so many people can get from these same medicines. So, sure — if you want to curse that bag full of drugs, we understand. But we also understand if you look at your medicines and say to yourself, "Hey, these medicines aren't an anchor pulling me down, they're a helping hand lifting me up." It's your call.

Prescription drugs may be yin and yang, good and bad, but whichever way we look at them we've got to, well, *look* at them. Swallowing a pill, putting on an ointment, or inserting a suppository isn't the end of the story — heck, it's not even the beginning. If you're going to safely and effectively take your medicine, you need to know some key things about it such as how to take your drug. Do you swallow it on an empty stomach, or take it with food? Do you need to avoid grapefruit (yes, grapefruit) or alcohol? What side-effects should you watch for? What should you do if side-effects occur?

Millions of Canadians benefit from taking prescription medicines. But many thousands of Canadians suffer from taking them. And some, tragically, even die from them. We've written *Understanding Prescription Drugs For Canadians For Dummies* to provide you with the information you need to do everything possible to benefit from your prescription medicines and to minimize the likelihood you'll be harmed by them.

You may well have enough on your plate, and feel that having to educate yourself about your medication is simply one more nuisance you don't have time for. Truth be told, however, effectively and safely taking prescription drugs requires a team effort, and the more people you have working together for the common goal of keeping you healthy, the more likely your goal will be reached. Hassle? You bet. Worthwhile? You bet!

Your Doctor, Your Pharmacist, and You

Understanding Prescription Drugs For Canadians For Dummies provides you with the tools to effectively work with your health care team. You'll discover the different roles that your doctor, your pharmacist, and you have in this partnership. You'll find out what to make sure your doctor tells you before you leave her office, and what to find out from your pharmacist before you walk away from the counter (such as who will provide refills for your medicine and, for that matter, how you'll know if you even need a refill). Who do you need to call if you're having side-effects from your drug? How should you store your medicine? In the first four chapters, we address these topics and more, including how you can help your health care providers avoid making prescribing and dispensing errors.

Your doctor and your pharmacist not only care *for* you, but also care *about* you. (And if they don't, change health care providers, and fast!) Caring about you means they'll be thrilled if you work with them in the cause of safe drug-taking. We'd bet dollars to donuts your pharmacist checks, double-checks, and possibly even triple-checks your prescription medicine before he hands it to you. (We're so sure, we'd even bet dollars to Timbits. Not that we've ever had Timbits, of course — we've especially never had the double chocolate ones ... you know, the glazed ones with the cake-like centre? *Hmm, mmm.*) So, if your doctor has written a prescription that clearly says "metoprolol" on it, you can be awfully certain your pharmacist will dispense "metoprolol" to you.

But what if the medicine you are prescribed has a name that is very similar to another, unrelated drug and your doctor's handwriting is stereotypically poor? Might the pharmacist misinterpret it? Well, stuff happens. For instance, clozapine has been mistakenly dispensed instead of olanzapine. Lamisil has been mistakenly dispensed instead of Lomotil. Losec has been mistakenly dispensed instead of Lasix. And the list goes on . . .

The likelihood of these sorts of errors is very small. But you can make the likelihood that much smaller by using the information in this book to inform yourself about your medicines. That way, if your doctor hands you a prescription for, say, Lasix to treat ankle swelling and you discover your pill bottle says the medicine is Losec, you'll be able to see if these are simply different names for the same medicine or if they are different drugs altogether (which, by the way, they are). With the help of this book, you can more readily recognize something that's amiss and know to get in touch with your doctor and pharmacist. Trust us — they (and you) will be thankful you did.

Treating What Ails You

Perhaps you've heard that, often, the best medicine is tincture of time; truth be told, it's only in the figurative sense that "time heals all wounds" (some, maybe, but definitely not all). If you have migraine headaches, angina, hypothyroidism, ulcerative colitis, rheumatoid arthritis, or one of myriad other medical maladies, you no doubt have already discovered how prescription drugs can help you.

However, in many circumstances prescription drugs are not required. Have some mild constipation? Maybe more fibre in your diet can help. Have a tension headache? Perhaps a couple of over-the-counter acetaminophen tablets would suffice. Stressed out from a bad day at the office? How fortunate for you that your partner gives such a great back rub!

So what about those many diseases requiring prescription medicines? In Chapter 5, we present "state of the art" treatment recommendations culled from many contemporary resources, including *clinical practice guidelines* (suggested therapies recommended by expert panels of physicians who specialize in a given field). By reading about your particular ailment, you'll be able to see what world authorities are recommending for your condition and get insights into why your doctor prescribed your medicine.

Getting to Know Your Medicines

A recurring theme in *Understanding Prescription Drugs For Canadians For Dummies* is the safe and effective use of prescription drugs. Indeed, it's the raison d'etre for this book, and the reason why we discuss general principles of healthy prescription drug use throughout the book. In Chapter 6 we look in detail at specific drugs: how they can help you, how they might harm you, how to take them, and how they carry out their work.

You may even discover certain things that your doctor and pharmacist hadn't necessarily mentioned to you. For example, suppose you're prescribed a drug such as ramipril (Altace), and after taking it you develop a cough. Looking up ramipril in Chapter 6, you quickly discover that a cough is a well-known side-effect. Aha! Rather than suffering for months, all the while attributing your cough to, say, sinusitis or allergies, now you can promptly get in touch with your doctor and have your medicine switched to another that doesn't cause this problem.

Just as Francis Bacon said many years ago, "Knowledge is power." *Understanding Prescription Drugs For Canadians For Dummies* provides you with this knowledge — and by doing so, empowers you as a consumer of prescription drugs. (And, speaking of famous quotes, you may be familiar with Henry Kissinger's saying, "Power is the great aphrodisiac." Whether you derive this additional benefit from the power this book bestows upon you we surely cannot say.)

Addressing Your Concerns

What would life be like without its many "ifs"? Certainly, when it comes to prescription drugs, "ifs" are all-important. For instance, *if* you have kidney disease, you need to avoid many drugs. And *if* you drink alcohol, you may have to stop because some drugs interact poorly with it. And *if* you are elderly you may be more sensitive to a number of medications and need to keep a special watch out for certain side-effects such as lightheadedness.

In *Understanding Prescription Drugs For Canadians For Dummies* we look at these and many other important "ifs":

- ✔ Taking several drugs? Find out how to protect yourself from drug interactions in Chapter 7.

- ✔ Children in your house? Chapter 8 shows you how to keep your drugs safely out of harm's way.

- ✔ Being discharged from hospital with a whole bunch of new prescriptions? Find out in Chapter 9 how to avoid the potentially catastrophic situation where old and new drugs get confused.

- ✔ Burdened by the high costs of some prescription drugs? Have a look at Chapter 10 for tips on how you may be able to lessen this financial load.

Last (ing) Advice to Take from Chapter 1

Most new medicines seem wonderful. And some live up to their billing. On the other hand, the world has seen the passing of drugs like cerivastatin (Baycol), which was withdrawn from the market because it could cause severe muscle injury; cisapride (Prepulsid), which is no longer sold because it could cause heart rhythm problems; and rofecoxib (Vioxx), which was removed from sale because of an increased risk of heart disease.

Establishing the true value and the true risks of a new prescription medicine may take several years. So unless you have a condition for which no already existing therapy is sufficient, we recommend you go with a drug that has a proven track record behind it. Put another way, don't be the first to try a new drug and don't be the last to stop taking an old one. When your doctor hands you a prescription, we suggest you ask her how long the drug has been around. If it's a new medicine, ask about the availability of older, tried and true drugs that would be equally good. The newest drug on the market may be the most expensive, but when it comes to safety and effectiveness, it's not necessarily the best.

Chapter 2

Prescribing Knowledge

● ●

In This Chapter

▶ Exploring how drugs work

▶ Sorting out how prescription drugs differ from non-prescription drugs

▶ Looking at the difference between generic and brand-name medicines

▶ Investigating the non-medicinal ingredients in your pills

● ●

*W*hen we started medical school way back when John Travolta first danced across the silver screen, the book Canadian doctors use to look up drug information (the *Compendium of Pharmaceuticals and Specialties*; thankfully abbreviated as *CPS*) was a few hundred pages long and had a font size similar to the text in this book. Now, 30 years later, the *CPS* is more than 2,500 pages long and has such small print that having a magnifying glass in hand isn't a bad idea.

The reason for this change is, of course, the explosive growth in the number and variety of prescription drugs available in Canada. Although they may differ in many ways, these medicines have some basic things in common. For example, they have to get into your body one way or another. And, if they are going to help you, they have to then act on your body in some way. In this chapter we look at how your prescription medicines carry out these tasks, and we also explore how prescription drugs differ from non-prescription drugs. Lastly, we discover how brand-name drugs differ from generic drugs. Before we begin this journey, however, we need to look at what exactly a drug is.

If you asked someone to define what a "drug" is, the response you'd get would vary quite a bit depending on the age of the person asked and their social background. But, truth be told, whether you're talking about street drugs (that is, drugs of the illicit kind), prescription drugs, naturopathic medicines, or over-the-counter products, they all share a common definition. Simply put, a drug is a substance (other than a food) that produces a change in some aspect of how your body functions.

How Drugs Work

For a drug to benefit you, it must first be introduced to you. Now, in this case a simple handshake just won't do. The kind of introduction we're talking about is much more intimate; indeed, for a medicine to work it has to enter your body, get to where it's needed, and then exert its effect on your body's cells. In this section we take a look at how all this happens.

Entering the fray: How medicines get into our bodies

Medicines can enter your body in a lot of ways. They can do this by being

- ✔ Put on the skin (in the form of a cream, ointment, or patch; so-called topical therapy).
- ✔ Put in the eyes (as an eye drop or ointment).
- ✔ Put in the ears (as an ear drop).
- ✔ Put in the nose (as a nose drop or nose spray).
- ✔ Swallowed (as a pill, tablet, capsule, or liquid).
- ✔ Sprayed (or placed) on or under the tongue.
- ✔ Sprayed into the throat (as a "puffer"), where the medicine mixes with air and travels down into the lungs.
- ✔ Placed in the rectum (as a suppository or an enema).
- ✔ Placed in the vagina (as a solid material that dissolves, or as a cream or foam).
- ✔ Placed into the penis (either through the opening — called the urethra — or injected directly into the side of the penis).
- ✔ Injected under the skin (a subcutaneous injection).
- ✔ Injected into the muscle (an intramuscular injection).
- ✔ Injected, by trained health care professionals, into a blood vessel (intravenous therapy), joint (intra-articular therapy), spinal fluid (intrathecal therapy), or other various and sundry parts of our anatomy.

After you apply or swallow or spray or insert or inject a drug (or take it by whatever means you are using — we talk about them all in Chapter 4), it has to then get to where it needs to work in order to help you. In the case of a skin cream, that journey can be very short. For example, you apply an anti-fungal cream to treat athlete's foot (we, ahem, kick this around in Chapter 5) directly to the area of infection, so it has to travel less than a millimetre. But when you take a medicine by mouth, the drug must take a much more complicated journey. Because the majority of medicines are taken orally, we devote the next section to looking in detail at this intricate trek.

The incredible journey: How a pill gets from your mouth to your brain, bones, and beyond

Because we're both physicians, perhaps it's not surprising we spend a fair bit of time discussing medical topics. And one of the things we often talk about is how we think prescription drugs are both incredibly brilliant and incredibly dumb. Modern medicines can kill off bacteria and cure pneumonia. Medicines can reduce inflammation and ease the suffering of people with arthritis. Certain drugs can treat heart disease and hypertension, dementia and dermatitis, Parkinson's and prostatitis. So why is it that researchers have not come up with an oral drug with the good sense to go where you want it and nowhere else? Is that asking so much? Well, we guess so, because virtually every oral medicine not only heads to the area of the body where it's needed, but also manages to visit most other places in the body at the same time.

Step one: From your mouth to your intestines

When you swallow a pill (or tablet, or capsule), it travels from your mouth, moves down your esophagus (the swallowing tube or "gullet"), and lands in your stomach. In your stomach, the pill is ground up by the mechanical action of the stomach and the stomach's acids. The extra stuff in the pill (like the coating that makes it easier to swallow, the dyes for colour, and the binding agents that keep the whole thing together) gets stripped away from the active ingredient and the whole concoction then gets propelled out of the stomach into the small intestine (see Figure 2-1). The small intestine (also called the "small bowel") is, basically, a long, coiled tube. The entire small intestine is about 20 feet (6.1 metres) long when stretched end to end (WARNING: do not try this at home!). Most medicines enter the bloodstream from the small intestine.

Step two: From your intestines to your blood

By the time the medicine you swallowed not long before makes its way into the small intestine, it looks so vastly different that you wouldn't even recognize it. At this point in its journey the medicine is in the form of molecules. Each pill contains millions of these molecules and each molecule is, in fact, the active ingredient that's going to help you (when it gets to its final destination — say, your prostate if you have prostatitis or your lungs if you have pneumonia). Each molecule is so tiny many millions of them could fit into the period at the end of this sentence.

These molecules now come into contact with the inside lining of the small intestine. This lining acts like a clever sponge. The medicine gets absorbed across the small intestine like water being absorbed into a sponge. Then, just as water can be applied to one side of a sponge and squeezed out the other side, the medicine that got absorbed from the inside of the intestine gets dropped out the other side, where it's caught by the blood vessels that are located there. It enters the blood vessels and floats on downstream along with the rest of your blood.

Frank's pressure was down, but so was something else

Medications — particularly those used to treat high blood pressure — can interfere with a man's sexual function, as Frank discovered. A little while ago, Frank, a 46-year-old accountant, came to see Ian because he was having problems with his blood pressure (hypertension). Ian recommended that Frank work with lifestyle treatment before resorting to a prescription medicine, and advised him to reduce his salt intake, try to shed some weight, and start to do more exercise. Frank worked quite diligently with these measures (he wasn't thrilled with the idea of taking pills and so had good incentive), but his pressure remained a problem and a prescription drug was needed. Ian prescribed hydrochlorothiazide, a typically quite effective diuretic used to control hypertension.

A month later, Frank returned to see Ian for a follow-up visit. "Hi Frank, how are things going?" Ian asked. "Not bad," Frank replied, a bit of hesitancy in his voice. Ian checked Frank's blood pressure and lo and behold it was much better. "Hey, great news," Ian said, "your pressure's down to target." Then, noticing Frank's less than enthusiastic demeanour, Ian asked if anything was wrong. Frank sighed, then said, "Well, doc, I don't know if it's coincidence or not, but ever since I started taking the hydrochlorothiazide, things are, well..." his voice trailed off. Ian read between the lines. "Frank, are you having problems with erectile dysfunction?" "Yes, I am," Frank immediately replied. Ian explained it was a not an uncommon side effect from the medicine. "But why," Frank reasonably asked, "would a medicine to make my body lose salt and lower my blood pressure cause sexual problems?" "Because," Ian replied, "*that* medicine doesn't have the good sense to just go to the kidneys to cause salt loss, it also goes to the brain and the blood vessels and the penis and pretty well everywhere else in your body. And in some places — like your kidneys — it helped you, but in other places it clearly did anything but."

Ian replaced the hydrochlorothiazide with a different medicine, and within a few days Frank's spirits, among other things, were up once again.

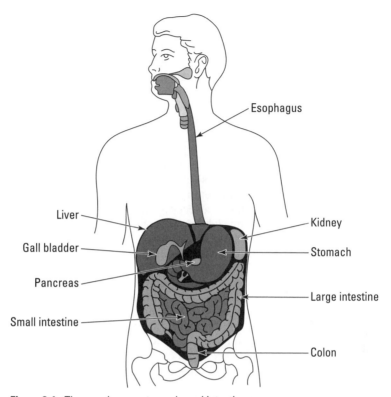

Figure 2-1: The esophagus, stomach, and intestines.

Labels: Esophagus, Liver, Gall bladder, Pancreas, Small intestine, Kidney, Stomach, Large intestine, Colon

Step three: From your blood to where it ails you

So now in the journey your medicine — in the form of millions of molecules — is swimming along in your bloodstream. Whether the medicine is doing a breaststroke or a backstroke we don't know, but what we can say with confidence is that if all the medicine does is hang around in your blood it's not going to help you (unless you are taking the medicine because of certain problems with the blood itself). Your medicine must get from the bloodstream into the unwell area.

Imagine you have diabetes and you've taken a pill — say, for example, glyburide — to help reduce your blood glucose levels. The glyburide has made its way from your mouth to your stomach to your small intestine and then into the bloodstream. Now the medicine must get from your bloodstream into your pancreas, where it stimulates the pancreas to make more insulin.

As the glyburide (in the current example) floats along in the bloodstream it passes by your muscles, your joints, your heart, your lungs, and so forth — but they all ignore it. Unlike the rude reception these other organs provided, when the glyburide passes through the blood vessels within your pancreas it finally is given a warm reception. Within the pancreas (and in other organs, too) there are numerous tiny cells upon whose surface are little pockets called *receptors*. Think of a receptor as being like a baseball glove and the drug molecule like a baseball. As the drug molecule passes by the receptor, the receptor, like an impeccable second baseman, grabs it, plucks it out of the bloodstream, and — performing flawlessly — hands it directly into the pancreas cell. And "you're out!" (Or "in," as the case may be.)

A drug would be attractive to the receptors in one organ (in our analogy, the pancreas) but not elsewhere because different organs generally have different receptors, and for a drug to be plucked from the bloodstream by a receptor the drug molecule and the receptor have to have the right fit. Just as your car key doesn't start your neighbour's car, a drug that fits into the receptors in your pancreas doesn't necessarily fit into the receptors in your kidneys.

Unfortunately, drugs can be pretty promiscuous. A drug molecule you take to treat a disease of the pancreas may be mighty attractive to receptors not only in the pancreas but also in some other organs. These other receptors may grab hold of the drug even though you don't want them to, which is part of the reason why drugs to treat a disease in one organ can lead to side-effects in another organ (we discuss side-effects in detail in Chapter 7).

How drugs affect your body's cells

When a medicine reaches the cells of your body where it's sup-posed to act, it must then influence these cells to do something. You can buy a magnificent red Ferrari, but if you can't start the engine that brand-new racing machine may just as well be a (very expensive and very beautiful!) doorstop. So, too, with your medi-cine: it can't just sit there and look pretty — it has to *do* something if it's going to help you.

How drugs work on a cellular level

After a drug attaches to a receptor on the outer surface of the cell membrane (the external lining of human cells), a series of chemical reactions within the cell are ini-tiated. The net result is that the amount and type of RNA (a substance manufactured from DNA within the cells) is altered, which in turn causes the cell to either manufac-ture more of a protein (a process called upregulation), less of a protein (downregulation), or different types of proteins. This change in the body's proteins then leads to the effect of a drug on the body.

A medicine can influence how your body's cells behave in several ways, including making a cell

- ✔ **Do more of something.** For example, clomiphene, a drug used to treat infertility, stimulates the ovaries to release eggs (ova). Repaglinide, a drug used to treat diabetes, stimulates the pancreas to make more insulin.

- ✔ **Do less of something.** Anti-inflammatory medicines (such as naproxen) cause inflammatory cells to slow down their actions. Anti-thyroid drugs (such as propylthiouracil) make the thyroid gland produce less hormone.

- ✔ **Die.** The word *antibiotic* comes from *anti* meaning "against" and *bios* meaning "life." Antibiotics cause cells to die, but fortunately the cells being targeted are germs such as bacteria, not our own healthy cells. Another example of drugs causing cells to die is cancer drugs, which typically work by causing the demise of cancer cells.

In Chapter 6 we discuss in detail how various drugs affect your body's cells.

How your body rids itself of medication

After your prescription medicine has done its job, it's time for it to pack up and leave your body. The organs most responsible for ridding your body of your medicines are your liver and your kidneys.

The liver is quite an amazing organ with many functions, one of which is to break down substances (including drugs) no longer needed in the body. Your liver helps you eliminate medicines in one of two ways:

- ✔ **Breaking them down directly.** The enzyme in the liver that's particularly important in performing this function is called Cytochrome P-450. Certain drugs — and even some foods — can affect how this enzyme works, leading to a potentially harmful accumulation of drugs within your body. (For the inside scoop on Cytochrome P-450, have a look at Chapter 4.)

- ✔ **Changing them into a form that can be passed through the kidneys into the urine.** Wow; talk about expensive urine!

Some drugs are passed directly into the urine by the kidneys without the liver having to do a demolition job first. If you have kidney failure and you're taking a medicine that's eliminated from the body in this way, your doctor needs to either have you take a lower dose than usual or avoid the drug completely.

Some drugs are excreted into breast milk. Although typically in minute quantities and not enough to cause harm to the breastfeeding infant, it's always best for a breastfeeding woman to check with her physician and pharmacist before she starts taking a prescription drug to make sure it's safe to breastfeed while on the medication (and, if it's not, to see whether she can take an alternative drug to enable breastfeeding to safely continue).

What Is a Prescription Drug?

Earlier in this chapter we define a drug as a substance (other than a food) producing a change in some aspect of how your body functions. A prescription drug differs from other types of drugs in one simple property: prescription drugs require a prescription! Typically, a drug requires a prescription if it has certain properties that make its use potentially dangerous and so, requires medical supervision.

Many drugs start off as prescription drugs and, after a number of years, become available without a prescription. This generally occurs only if a drug has been widely used and found to be very safe. Examples of this are common arthritis or pain remedies (such as ibuprofen), which were originally available only by prescription but are now available without a prescription and go by many different names.

The difference between over-the-counter drugs and prescription drugs

Talk about misnomers! When you go to the pharmacy and pick up some ASA (Aspirin) or acetaminophen (Tylenol), or a cold remedy or a nose spray, where do you typically find it — behind the pharmacist's counter, or freely available in the aisle? Right: you find it in the aisle. And when your friendly neighbourhood pharmacist hands your prescription drug to you, over what piece of furniture do they hand it? Right: over the counter. Well, then, it's settled. Prescription drugs are given over-the-counter, and over-the-counter drugs are ... not given over-the-counter. Phew! Yes, it's confusing. So we spend the rest of this section sorting these terms out.

An over-the-counter (commonly abbreviated OTC) drug is one for which you don't require a prescription from your doctor to buy. So, whether the OTC product is kept behind a counter, under a counter, on top of a counter, beside a counter, or 500 kilometres from the nearest counter, it's still called an over-the-counter drug. A better term for an OTC drug, but used pretty well only in government techno-speak, is a "self-selection" drug, which emphasizes the action of going to the pharmacy and choosing it from the shelf yourself.

Some drugs, like acetaminophen (Tylenol), have been sold over-the-counter from day one. Other products, like famotidine (Pepcid), started out as prescription drugs, but as time went by and they were found to be generally very safe. Health Canada (the Canadian governmental regulatory body in charge of such things) decided the drugs should be available without a prescription.

Just because an OTC product is an OTC product does not guarantee its safety. Just as you do with prescription drugs, you need to take OTC products properly per the package's instructions. For example, taking too much acetaminophen can cause fatal liver damage. Taking too much ASA can cause hearing problems. Taking too much calcium can cause kidney stones. Prudence remains the key word here regardless of whether a drug is classified as available only by prescription or over-the-counter.

Self-prescribing can lead to self-destruction

As tempting as it may be to play doctor and self-diagnose and self-treat, especially when the problem doesn't seem serious, this can be a dangerous game, indeed.

Shelley Campbell, a 30-year-old business executive, had come down with a sore throat so painful she could hardly swallow. Scheduled for a series of important meetings that day, she felt there was no way she could find time to see her doctor. "It's probably strep throat," she concluded — and, remembering her kids had been previously treated for this condition with penicillin — she searched for (and found) some left-over tablets in the medicine cabinet. She popped a couple of pills into her mouth and, moments later, found herself gasping for breath. She felt dizzy and fell to the floor. Luckily, her son heard her and called an ambulance, and the paramedics were able to quickly resuscitate her. She had had a severe allergic reaction to the penicillin.

"But doctor," she later said to the ER physician, "How could I have known I'd be allergic to penicillin? The only medicine I've ever had an allergic reaction to was Clavulin." "Shelley," the doctor replied, "Clavulin contains amoxicillin. And amoxicillin is a sister drug to penicillin. If you had an allergic reaction to one type of penicillin, there's a darn good chance you'd have a similar reaction to another member of the same family. You could have died doing what you did."

Shelley sheepishly looked at the doctor and said: "I guess you probably don't think it's so great I also kept some old pills lying around, eh?" "Well," the doctor replied, "You know the expression, 'a cat has nine lives?'" Shelley nodded. "Shelley," the doctor continued, firmly, but kindly, "you're not a cat."

Although a drug may be available as an over-the-counter product, often it can also be obtained by prescription. For most people this offers no advantage (and just additional cost because you have to pay the pharmacist's dispensing fee; a topic which we discuss in Chapter 10), but if you have a *private* drug plan, it may (depending on the plan) cover the cost of an OTC drug (and the dispensing fee) if your doctor first fills out a prescription for the drug.

Although we have been physicians since shortly after John Travolta traded his white suit for a mechanical bull (gee, without any manure around maybe he could have kept the suit), we're still frequently surprised when we find out that some powerful, potentially dangerous drugs that we prescribe are actually available *without* a prescription. Insulin is one such example — you can walk into any pharmacy in Canada and simply ask for it, no prescription necessary. A pharmacist, however, may not necessarily be comfortable giving out drugs like this without first seeing a prescription (which makes sense; she wants to be sure the drugs she dispenses are used safely).

You can find out if a drug requires a prescription by going to www.nocdatabase.ca (a Health Canada Web site). In the "Brand/Product Name" field, enter the name of your medicine and click "Search." If the drug is available only by prescription, the next screen says "Prescription Pharmaceutical" under "Product Type."

The difference between behind-the-counter drugs and prescription drugs

The term "behind-the-counter" is fairly new. It refers to non-prescription drugs that you can pick up in your pharmacy only after speaking to your pharmacist. Unlike the misnomer that is "over-the-counter," *behind-the-counter* really does mean behind the (pharmacist's) counter. The best-known examples of drugs in this group include the EpiPen (pre-filled syringes of epinephrine — also called adrenaline — for self-administration in the event of a severe allergic reaction, such as to peanuts or bee stings) and "Plan B," the emergency contraceptive more commonly called the morning-after pill.

A drug is categorized behind-the-counter if it needs to be sold with additional care. In the case of the morning-after pill, its behind-the-counter status offers pharmacists the opportunity not only to discuss important issues with their clients (such as possible side-effects to look out for) but also to also review things such as contraception and ways to avoid sexually transmitted diseases. This counselling is certainly well-intentioned (and, incidentally, is mandated by regulatory authorities), but we can envision circumstances where the purchaser may not be in a particularly receptive frame of mind for such a discussion.

The difference between prescription drugs and complementary and alternative medicines

A complementary and alternative medicine (CAM) is typically taken upon the advice of an alternative health care practitioner (such as a naturopath or homeopath) and does not require a prescription from a medical doctor. CAMs include certain herbs, vitamins (often in high dose), minerals, amino acids, and dietary supplements. Some of these — for example, minerals such as calcium — are also often recommended by your traditional physician.

Bear in mind that a CAM's "natural" status does not ensure its safety. Arsenic and poison mushrooms are natural, too, after all. Just as virtually any prescription drug can have significant side-effects, so can many complementary and alternative medicines. Whether you're taking prescription drugs or complementary and alternative medicines, prudence and care are always the most important ingredients!

How drugs are classified

Prescription drug sales are both federally and provincially regulated. Health Canada determines if a drug is going to be available by prescription. A national initiative of provincial pharmacy regulatory bodies known as the National Association of Pharmacy Regulatory Authorities (NAPRA) divides drugs into four categories:

✔ **Schedule I drugs** (prescription drugs)

✔ **Schedule II drugs** (non-prescription drugs sold behind-the-counter)

✔ **Schedule III drugs** (non-prescription drugs available for "self-selection" by the consumer but available for sale only within a pharmacy)

✔ **Unscheduled drugs** (medicines that may be sold outside of pharmacies including at grocery and convenience stores)

You can find more information on drug classification at NAPRA's Web site (www.napra.ca).

Certain CAMs can interact adversely with some prescription drugs, potentially leading to dangerous side-effects. If you're taking a CAM it's very important you bring it with you to show your regular medical doctor and pharmacist. By looking at both your prescription and non-prescription therapies these professionals can try to determine if they can be taken safely together. Sometimes this can be very difficult to determine, because many CAMs are categorized as "food supplements" and, as such, do not have all their active ingredients listed. Without knowing all of a CAM's contents (and their respective purity and potency), sometimes you're left in the dark.

The Difference between a Brand-Name Drug and a Generic Drug

Life (and the world of medicine) would be so much simpler if a drug had but one name...

Brand-name drugs

When a drug is first created, the pharmaceutical company (which has the patent on its creation, meaning no other company can manufacture or sell the particular drug) also gives its new drug a *brand* name. The company invariably then markets the drug under its brand name. It's not dissimilar to Kleenex (a brand name) and facial tissue (a generic name), or Vaseline (a brand name) and petroleum jelly (a — horrible! — generic name).

Generic drugs

Drug patents last 20 years in Canada, but the clock starts ticking from the day that a patent application is first filed, which may be many years before the drug is actually available in pharmacies. After a company's patent on a drug runs out, other companies can start to sell the same drug but must assign it a different trade name (that is, the drug is no longer patented but the trade name is, just as many companies can sell "facial tissue," but only Kimberly-Clark can sell "Kleenex"-brand facial tissue).

What companies tend to do is take the generic name for a drug and put a few letters in front of it to associate the name with their company. For example, Novopharm, a Canadian company that manufactures many generic drugs, typically puts the term "Novo-"

in front of the generic name, hence they sell Novo-Acebutolol, Novo-Atenol, Novo-Cefaclor, and so on. Another Canadian company, Apotex, makes the identical products but calls them Apo-Acebutolol, Apo-Atenol, and Apo-Cefaclor, respectively.

When a patent expires, it's typically said that the drug "has gone generic" (even though that's not perfectly accurate, because the drug always did have a generic name). Drugs sold under a generic name are of high quality and "just as good as the original."

Choosing brand-name or generic drugs

One main advantage exists in obtaining a generic drug rather than a brand-name drug. You save money! Drugs sold by generic manufacturers are invariably cheaper to buy than drugs sold under their trade name by their original manufacturer. (We discuss drug costs — including the huge costs of research and development of new drugs — in Chapter 10.) Incidentally, some trade-name drug manufacturers are getting into the generic game and selling their own drugs — after the patent expires — as generic drugs. It's the same drug as before, but with a new name on the bottle.

If a drug is available under both its original trade brand and a less expensive, generic version, your pharmacist is obliged to automatically supply you with the less expensive (generic) version *regardless* of what the drug name on the prescription says. If your doctor thinks that you'd be best served by having only one particular company's version of a prescription drug, she may write "No Substitution" on the prescription. In this case, your pharmacist gives you only the particular brand that your doctor has specified. Hardly ever, however, do we find this useful or necessary.

In rare instances, the amount of active ingredient absorbed into your body from a pill made by one company may differ slightly from the amount of active ingredient absorbed from a pill made by another company. This is seldom a problem, but occasionally it can be. For example, if you are taking L-thyroxine for hypothyroidism (we discuss this condition in Chapter 5) and your doctor finds in testing that your thyroid blood levels are varying, it could be that the thyroid medicine you're taking is sometimes made by one manufacturer and sometimes by another, and that the properties of the pill are slightly different.

In this case, we suggest that you ask your pharmacist to supply you with only one manufacturer's version of L-thyroxine (it doesn't matter *which* manufacturer, so long as you stick with just the one).

A drug by any other name

Every drug has a single *generic* name that is, basically, a scientific or official name, but — depending on the medicine in question — may be sold under one of several *brand* names. This fact understandably confused one of Heather's patients. Mrs. Rose Smith, a charming 85-year-old woman, was in to see Heather because of a sore knee. Mrs. Smith had a whole host of additional health problems and was taking a number of different medications for her various ailments. Her doctors always wanted to know what drugs she was on, so she always kept a list of them in her purse. What she wasn't quite as good at doing was keeping the list updated. When Heather asked Mrs. Smith what medicines she was taking, she dutifully pulled out the piece of paper. Heather scanned the list. "Oh, so you are still taking the Motrin, I see." Mrs. Smith took the list and looked at it. "No, I'm not on that anymore. It's been changed." Heather asked her if she knew what it was changed to. "Um, something similar. Apo-something. Or maybe it was Novo-something. No, wait, it was something Nu—." "Oh," Heather said, "so you're on something new then?" "No," Mrs. Smith replied, "Nu, not new." They both smiled, recognizing the *Who's On First* nature of their conversation.

Heather reached for the *CPS* (a very, very, big book listing all prescription drugs available in Canada). "Mrs. Smith, let's have a look at all the different drug names Motrin goes by and see if this helps. Motrin is one company's name for a medicine called ibuprofen. Other companies call it other names. It can be called Advil, Apo-Ibuprofen, Novo-Profen, and Nu-Ibuprofen, and you know what? They are all exactly the same thing. The active ingredient — the medicine — is the same in each of these products. Ibuprofen is the *generic* name and the other names are *brand* names." Mrs. Smith nodded. "Doctor," she said, "I'm taking *Nu*-Ibuprofen, which is the same as my *old* ibuprofen which is the same as my friend's Novo-Profen." "Exactly," Heather said. Mrs. Smith grinned widely. Then the old Abbott and Costello fan couldn't hold herself back: "But I don't know what I'm talkin' about!" Heather and Mrs. Smith simultaneously erupted in laughter.

One company's drug may also differ from another company's drug regarding non-medicinal ingredients, such as coatings and binders, and an individual may tolerate Company A's version of a drug better than Company B's version of the same medicine. If you find your stomach gets upset after taking an oral medicine, ask your pharmacist whether you may benefit from trying another company's version of the same product (if available); if he does think a change would help, he likely can order it in for you. We discuss coatings, binders and other non-medicinal ingredients in the next section.

Because companies differ in how they manufacture the same medicine, you may find that when your pharmacist dispenses a drug to you it differs in appearance depending on which manufacturer is her current supplier — this is not necessarily cause for concern, but it's prudent to double-check with your pharmacist that she's given you the correct drug in the correct dose.

The Non-Medicinal Ingredients in Oral Medications

Much of an oral medication may be made up of non-medicinal ingredients, of which hundreds upon hundreds of different types exist. General categories of non-medicinal ingredients include:

- **Lubricants** (for example, magnesium stearate). These make it easier for tablets to be extracted from the manufacturing machinery.

- **Dilutents** (for example, lactose). These add bulk.

- **Binding agents** (for example, gelatin) **and granulating agents** (for example, gum). These bind the different ingredients together to keep the dose intact until after it's swallowed. Binders also help control the rate at which the active ingredient is absorbed into the body from the gut.

- **Disintegrating agents** (for example, sodium bicarbonate). These help the tablet dissolve.

- **Coatings** (for example, sugar) **and transparent coverings.** These protect the dose from damage prior to use. They can also help control when the active ingredient is released from the dose.

- **Preservatives** (such as parabens and sulfites).

- **Dyes** (such as tartrazine).

- **Flavours and sweeteners** (to, well, make things more flavourful and sweeter).

- **Gluten** (to keep the active ingredient in suspension or used as a filler).

- **Peanut oil, soybean oil, soya lecithin** (to dissolve or suspend the active ingredient).

- **Alcohol** (in the form of ethanol). This may be used in oral liquid and topical medicines. Alcohol acts to dissolve the active ingredient and also serves as a preservative.

- **Miniature kitchen sink.** (Oops, got carried away.)

If you're allergic or intolerant to any of the substances in the preceding list, or to some other substance, check with your pharmacist before you leave the pharmacy to make sure that your medicine doesn't contain any non-medicinal ingredients making it unwise — or, frankly, unsafe — for you to take the drug.

Chapter 3

Your Doctor, Your Pharmacist, and You

. . . .

In This Chapter

▶ Understanding how your doctor makes the decision to write a prescription — or not

▶ Looking at how your doctor chooses your prescription drug, and exploring how you and your doctor can work effectively together

▶ Teaming up with your pharmacist for safer health care

▶ Understanding your responsibilities as a consumer of prescription drugs, including decoding warning labels and package inserts

. . . .

*T*he Latin saying "*Primum, non nocere*" expresses one of the fundamental medical precepts by which doctors practise. Roughly translated, this means "It's Wednesday afternoon and I tee off at 2 o'clock." No, wait, that's not right. (Well, it might be a precept for some doctors, but it's not the one we want to use here!) *Primum, non nocere* means "First, do no harm." Nowhere is this more true than when it comes to prescription drugs.

Of course, any prescription medicine you are given should *help* you, but most of all, it should not *harm* you. Regrettably, medical science is imprecise enough that to guarantee either of these things is impossible. Fortunately, you, your doctor, and your pharmacist can take certain steps to maximize the likelihood that your prescription drug works for you both safely and effectively. This chapter looks at these steps.

Prescribing Patience

Heather well remembers being told by her mother of the virtues of patience. (Ian, on the other hand, thinks his mother looked at her four wild boys and, shaking her head, didn't bother.) As it turns out, many doctors and patients can benefit from this old adage.

"Mr. Cooper, your blood pressure is too high," Ian said to his rather forlorn-looking patient. Mr. Cooper sat quietly, resignedly awaiting a prescription. "But," Ian went on, "I think we can manage it with lifestyle treatment." Mr. Cooper broke into a broad smile and said, "You mean I *don't* need to take a medicine?" Ian replied, "No — at least not for now. I think you should try other things first: a low-salt diet, going easy on the alcohol, exercising regularly — things like that." Mr. Cooper looked at Ian with a quizzical expression. "But, Dr. Blumer, I thought high blood pressure *always* required drug treatment!" To this, Ian was pleased to reply, "Not always, Mr. Cooper, not always..."

For a number of conditions, lifestyle therapy works just as well as (or, sometimes, even better than) prescription drug treatment. Examples include *mild* hypertension (as noted in the preceding anecdote) and measures to prevent osteoporosis (a calcium-rich and alcohol/caffeine/tobacco-poor diet along with weight-bearing exercise is excellent therapy).

For some other conditions, a doctor need only prescribe patience (both for their patients and themselves). Have a sore throat? Well, it could be strep throat, which would require an antibiotic, but it could just as easily be a viral infection that would go away on its own. Have sinusitis? Perhaps it's just a cold and will quickly be on its way without an antibiotic. Diarrhea? Most cases are gone in a day or two and antibiotics would be of no value (or even harmful).

If you have a symptom you are concerned about and you go to see your doctor expecting (and wanting) nothing more than reassurance, you may, on occasion, be surprised to be given a prescription. This is almost always because your doctor determines your problem cannot be managed without a medicine. Sometimes, however, a doctor believes a patient will be dissatisfied with reassurance alone and feels obliged to give a prescription.

This may sound silly or, frankly, even inappropriate, but Ian recalls a comment made by one of the best family physicians he ever met: "Ian, if I don't give a patient a prescription when they demand one, I am concerned when they *really* need one they won't seek medical attention." To avoid this circumstance, let your doctor know that reassurance alone, whenever appropriate, is just fine, thank you very much. We also recommend that physicians spend the extra time necessary to explain why a prescription drug isn't required.

Prescribing Prescription Drugs: Your Doctor's Role

We often say the best prescription is no prescription at all. What we mean is that if we can treat a patient with non-pharmaceutical measures alone, it makes our day. Nonetheless, for many health problems, prescription drugs are required.

Why your doctor prescribed a drug

Although the world of medicine can be extraordinarily complex, when we look at why a doctor prescribes a drug, it really comes down to a few basic reasons. We have a look at these now.

Treating you now so you don't get sick later

Do you care that your blood pressure is 160/110 when a normal value is closer to 120/80? Do you care that your LDL cholesterol is 4.5 whereas a normal value is closer to 2.5? We suspect that, should these abnormal values apply to you, you do indeed care. But the reason that you (and your doctor) care is not that high blood pressure or high cholesterol in and of themselves are going to make you feel sick (for, in fact, they rarely do) — it's that they put you at risk of *other* things, such as strokes and heart attacks.

Many prescription drugs are given to prevent something bad from happening later. Taking a pill day after day when you are feeling perfectly fine isn't fun, but it surely is less fun to be in a hospital bed after a stroke that could have been avoided by judicious use of a prescription drug to treat your high blood pressure.

Treating your ailment

The list of ailments that can be improved (typically) or cured (sometimes) by prescription drugs is virtually endless (although we do our best to tackle many of the most common diseases in Chapter 5). As we noted a moment ago, if you have a condition that can be managed without prescription drugs, that's wonderful. But when medicines are necessary, having them there to assist us is wonderful, too.

People used to suffer woefully from disabling migraine headaches, but modern medicines typically enable you to keep these in check. Bacterial meningitis, a uniformly fatal illness in times past, is now generally cured in short order. Early treatment of rheumatoid arthritis can now often prevent disabling joint deformities. The list goes on and on.

Oh, medical research still has a *terribly* long way to go — indeed, doctors have only very inadequate drug therapy for illnesses as innocuous as the common cold or as devastating as degenerative neurological diseases such as multiple sclerosis. Yet progress — though sometimes at an agonizingly slow pace and never as quickly as anyone would like — *is* being made. Every year physicians are given new tools to help people maintain or return to a state of good health.

What you need to tell your doctor

In this section, we look at certain key things you can tell your doctor to help him choose the right prescription drug for you.

Be sure to tell your doctor if you

- ✔ **Have drug allergies.** Make sure you mention *any* drug allergy you have experienced. Just because the drug you are being prescribed doesn't sound at all like a drug you previously reacted to does not necessarily mean they are different.

- ✔ **Have drug intolerances.** Make sure you mention *any* drug intolerances you have experienced. Drug intolerances are side-effects not due to allergies and most commonly show up as nausea, vomiting and/or diarrhea — although they can manifest in many other ways. (We discuss drug allergies and side-effects in detail in Chapter 7.)

- ✔ **Have other health problems.** Your family doctor may know your medical background very well, but other doctors you might see such as specialists, emergency room physicians, and walk-in-clinic doctors are not likely as familiar with your medical history, so making sure they know this information before they prescribe a drug for you is particularly important.

- ✔ **Take any other prescription drugs (and provide the names).** Many drugs have the potential to interact adversely with other drugs, so it's important for your doctor to review *all* your drugs any time they are prescribing a new medicine for you. We discuss this important topic in more detail below.

- ✔ **Take any non-prescription drugs (and provide the names).** A number of non-prescription drugs can interact with prescription drugs. One such example is St. John's wort, which has been used for depression but has been found to react poorly with *many* other medications. Let your doctor know whether you are taking *any* drug — prescription, herbal, homeopathic, naturopathic, or otherwise.

✔ **Can't afford a medication.** In almost all cases, your doctor can find an alternative, less-expensive drug for you.

✔ **Are unlikely to remember to take a drug multiple times per day.** If you know, based on past experience (or good self-insight), that you are not likely to remember to take a medicine that requires multiple doses per day (a pill at lunchtime is typically the most difficult one to remember), ask your doctor whether an appropriate drug exists requiring only once-daily dosing.

✔ **Have a hard time swallowing pills.** Some pills are humongous and, for some people, are hard to get down (even with Mary Poppins' spoonful of sugar!). If you have difficulty swallowing pills, let your doctor know so he can try to find a medicine for you that comes in a smaller size or can be split (we discuss pill splitting in Chapter 4).

✔ **Are planning on becoming pregnant, are pregnant or are breastfeeding.** Certain medications are more proven than others to be safe during pregnancy and breastfeeding; your doctor will make a point of choosing the safest possible drug for these circumstances. (There is the occasional drug which, taken by a man, can adversely affect his sperm. We recommend, if you are planning on becoming pregnant, that you ask your doctor if a drug that your male partner is taking might pose a problem. Of course, if you are male, you can ask yourself!)

How your doctor chooses your prescription drug

Quick: Do you know how many prescription drugs are available in Canada? Okay, time's up. More than *5,000* brand and generic versions of prescription drugs (including different dosages) exist. It's enough to make your head spin. With so many drugs to choose from, how in the world does a doctor decide which is the best one for you? We answer this question next.

As we point out in the preceding section, before your doctor decides which medicine you need, she must first be certain you actually need a medicine. After it has been determined that you do indeed require a prescription drug, your physician takes into account a whole host of different factors in deciding which drug is best for you.

Factors relating to the drug itself

One key factor in your doctor's choice of medicine for you is the specific properties of a given drug.

These are factors relating to the drug itself that your doctor needs to take into account when prescribing your medicine:

- **How effective a medicine is.** Hundreds of medicines may treat high blood pressure, for example, but some work really well and some work . . . not that well at all. Sometimes a drug's effectiveness is related to its specific properties, and in other circumstances one drug works better in some people than in others. (You may wonder why a drug that works poorly would ever be prescribed. Well, drugs that work poorly may still have a role as "third line" or "fourth line" therapy for people whose blood pressure has simply not sufficiently responded to typically better medicines. Even the backup goalie gets played sometimes.)

- **How often a drug needs to be taken.** In general, given the choice between two equally good drugs, a doctor will choose the drug that requires you to take fewer doses per day.

- **Whether your doctor has samples available to give you.** Doctors are often given samples of drugs by pharmaceutical companies. If your doctor has samples, she may well be able to provide these to you free of charge. (Bear in mind, though, that pharmaceutical companies typically provide samples only of drugs newly available in Canada, so they may not have the same "tried and true" track record of drugs that have been around for a while. Also, newly available drugs are typically more expensive than older drugs, so when your free samples run out, you may be in for some "sticker shock" if you need to get the medicine at a pharmacy.)

- **Whether the drug is complementary to others you are taking.** For example, to most effectively treat HIV/AIDS, combinations of drugs are used to take advantage of their complementary properties. A similar strategy is used to treat conditions such as high blood pressure, heart disease, diabetes, and many other ailments.

- **The drug's cost.** There may be a drug that would otherwise be the ideal choice for you, but that costs about the same as that Lamborghini our son Michael (okay, Ian too) keeps drooling over. Sometimes, the most expensive drug is the best — or only — one for the job. Many times, however, less expensive drugs work equally well. Given the choice between two or more equally good drugs, your doctor can prescribe the less expensive one.

✔ **How long a drug has been on the market.** One of our pet peeves is a very strong tendency in the world of medicine to always go with the newest drug on the block. Now, if no previous treatment was particularly good and a new, more effective drug comes along, then by all means prescribing this brand-new drug makes perfect sense. On the other hand, if we have at our disposal a drug that's been around for a long time and has proven itself to be both safe and effective, why not go with this one rather than a new drug that may well still have a whole bunch of unknowns about it? (A drug can be approved for use after being tested in only about a couple *thousand* people; drugs in use for a few years may have been taken by *millions* of people. As such, their safety profile and effectiveness is better understood.)

✔ **Whether the drug is available in combination with another drug.** The main advantage to combination drugs is that you get two medicines in one pill, so you have fewer things to swallow. (Prescription drugs very rarely contain more than two different medicines.) Combination medicines can be a combination of

- Two different but complementary medicines of the same general type (such as Moduret, which is a combination of two different diuretics that work slightly differently from one another and, taken together, have additive benefits).

- Two different but complementary medicines from two entirely different families of drugs (such as Avandamet, which is a combination of two entirely different drugs, both of which are helpful to reduce blood glucose levels).

- Two entirely different medicines used for entirely different purposes. An example is Caduet, a combination of a drug used to treat hypertension and another drug used to treat high cholesterol. The rationale behind this combination is that people who have one of these conditions often have the other and may need to be treated for both ailments.

One thing that's *not* important in deciding which drug to use is the strength (in terms of the number of milligrams contained in a pill/ tablet/capsule/what-have-you). You may be taking a 100-mg dose of Drug A (to treat high blood pressure, for example) and your neighbour may be taking a 1-mg dose of Drug B to treat the same condition. All other things being equal, the fact that your dose is one hundred times more (in terms of milligrams) is completely irrelevant. In other words, here's yet another case where size doesn't matter! (Having said that, the one exception would be when the size of a pill is so big it's hard for some people to swallow.)

Factors relating to you and your health

If it's true that "what's good for the goose is good for the gander," we guess the goose isn't taking birth control pills. Although most medicines work similarly well in most people (of either gender), a doctor must take into account factors relating to your particular health issues when selecting the best medicine *for you*. Your doctor needs to consider whether you

✔ **Have responded well to a drug in the past.** Some medicines, like antibiotics, are not taken indefinitely, so if you are in need of an antibiotic — depending on the nature of the infection requiring treatment — your doctor may elect to prescribe one that worked well for you in the past.

✔ **Are allergic to a type of medicine.** If you have had an allergic reaction to a drug, then clearly your doctor wants to avoid using that same (or a similar) drug for you again (as we look at in an anecdote in Chapter 2). Sometimes the situation is a bit more subtle. For example, sulfa is a key component of drugs from a number of different classes of medicines — it's easy to overlook that if you have reacted to, say, a sulfa antibiotic, you may react to a sulfa-based diuretic. We look in detail at drug allergy issues in Chapter 7.

✔ **Are intolerant to a family of medicines.** Some side-effects are common to all members of a family. For example, about 30 percent of people get a cough from drugs within the ACE ("*angiotensin converting enzyme*") inhibitor family. This group has nine members, so if you get a cough from one type, you will almost certainly get a cough from one of the other types. (We discuss ACE inhibitors in Chapter 6.)

✔ **Have other diseases or conditions.** If you have kidney failure, your doctor wants to avoid prescribing you a drug that's excreted (in its active form) by the kidney. If you have liver disease, your doctor wants to avoid prescribing you a drug that's metabolized by the liver. (We discuss the way your body rids itself of medications in Chapter 2.) Many other health conditions influence which drug you are prescribed, including whether you have stomach ulcers, malignant hyperthermia, or asthma — to name but a few.

✔ **Are taking other drugs.** Some medications interact with other medications. This can lead to dangerous side-effects. See "Watching for drug interactions" later in this chapter, and Chapter 7.

✔ **Are too young or too old for certain drugs.** Some drugs — like sedatives — are more likely to cause adverse effects if you are elderly. Similarly, some drugs are more likely to cause adverse effects in children.

✔ **Are planning on becoming pregnant, are pregnant, or are breastfeeding.** Some medications are more proven than others to be safe during pregnancy and breastfeeding; your doctor will make a point of choosing the safest possible drug for these circumstances. (The occasional drug exists that, taken by a man, can adversely affect his sperm. If you're planning on becoming pregnant, ask your doctor if a drug that your male partner is taking might pose a problem. Of course, if you are male, you can ask yourself!)

✔ **May respond better or worse based on your race.** Some evidence exists that certain drugs work more or less effectively in certain racial groups. These data are not known one way or the other for the overwhelming majority of drugs. Diuretics, for example, appear to be particularly good drugs to treat high blood pressure in people of African ancestry, whereas ACE inhibitors appear to be less effective in this group. The information is, however, somewhat tenuous and in any event both these classes of drugs often work nicely in people of any descent. (We discuss diuretics and ACE inhibitors in Chapter 6.)

As we look at these long lists, the most striking thing we notice is that all these factors need to be taken into consideration in the length of time it takes your doctor to reach for the pen and prescription pad (or sample cupboard). All the more reason to ensure that you work closely with your doctor and your pharmacist as a health care *team!*

What to make sure your doctor tells you

In order to maximize the likelihood that your new prescription drug works both effectively and safely, your doctor should tell you a few things before you leave the office, including:

✔ **The name of the medicine.** Oh sure, your prescription drug will work equally well whether you know its name or not. But it's going into your body, so what the heck — don't you want to know what it's called?

And while we're on the subject, if you know the correct pronunciation of your drug, it'll help you out when you see another health care professional — you'll be perceived as an informed consumer and treated with an extra measure of respect. Maybe this shouldn't be so, but, well, it is.

✔ **How many times per day you are to take the medicine.** This information is also on the label your pharmacist affixes to the bottle or the box your drug comes in.

✔ **The reason you are being asked to take the medicine (or, how this medicine may help you).** Many medicines are used to treat a wide variety of diseases. For example, a pill that lowers blood pressure can also be helpful for certain kidney problems. Your doctor should tell you the *specific* reason he is recommending that you take a prescription drug.

✔ **How you'll know the medicine is working.** Your doctor should tell you how you'll know whether your prescription drug is serving its function. Sometimes, it'll be easy for you to know whether your drug is working — for example, if you have less pain after you start taking an analgesic to treat a sore back. Sometimes, it'll be less apparent whether your medicine is working — for example, when you're taking a drug to treat high cholesterol (in which case a blood test would be required to see whether you're sufficiently responding).

✔ **How long it will take for you to respond to the medicine.** Some medications work very quickly. For example, if you take meperidine (Demerol), a very potent analgesic, to treat a bad headache, you can expect some relief within 20 to 30 minutes. On the other hand, if you were to take phenytoin (Dilantin) to prevent seizures, it may take days, weeks, or even months to see if you're benefitting depending on how often you were having seizures before you started the medication.

✔ **How long you should continue taking a medication.** If you're being treated for a chronic condition (such as congestive heart failure or rheumatoid arthritis), then in almost all cases your doctor will want you to continue the prescribed medication indefinitely. On the other hand, if you were prescribed a drug to treat a short-term, curable condition such as a throat infection, then you'll not likely be asked to continue the drug after the current prescription is used up. We discuss this in more detail in Chapter 4.

✔ **Who is to supply the "repeats" for your prescription drug.** If your family physician prescribed your drug, she will invariably be the one to write your repeat prescription when it comes due. On the other hand, if you obtained your prescription from a specialist and you won't be seeing the specialist on an ongoing basis, he should tell you whether you need to repeat your prescription and, if so, who is responsible for authorizing these repeats.

✔ **What the most *common* side-effects are.** Virtually every drug can have many different side-effects, but thankfully the great majority of these aren't serious. Your doctor should let you know what the most common side-effects are so you can watch for them. (We discuss side-effects in detail in Chapter 7.)

✔ **What the most *serious* side-effects are.** Although serious side-effects are rare, being alerted to what these may be is important. Your doctor should let you know what kinds of serious side-effects your prescription drug could cause — and the ways in which they may show up — so you can be especially vigilant.

✔ **What you should do in the event you get a side-effect.** The appropriate course of action may be something as simple as contacting your doctor when she is next in the office (typically what's done when you are having a relatively minor side-effect, such as abdominal bloating) to as major as immediately going to the emergency department (as you should if, for example, you start to vomit up blood).

If you have a question for your doctor about your prescription drug, don't hesitate to ask it (preferably, before you leave his office). He'll either answer it or, if it falls more within the domain of the pharmacist (see the section below), suggest that you ask your pharmacist. An *informed* consumer — that would be you! — is more likely to take medications properly, which translates into a higher likelihood of successful therapy.

The tear-out Cheat Sheet at the front of this book provides a helpful place to write in key pieces of information about your medicines. We recommend you take the Cheat Sheet with you when you see your doctor and your pharmacist and they can help you complete the sections pertaining to them (we discuss their roles in this chapter).

Dispensing Prescription Drugs: Your Pharmacist's Role

Thank heaven for pharmacists! The pharmacist is an invaluable member of your health care team and has a wealth of knowledge he can use to assist you *and* your physician. If you're taking a prescription drug, it's quite possible you see your pharmacist more than you see your physician (and maybe wait less when you do!). It's a shame, then, that sometimes pharmacists are simply looked at as "the person who fills the doctor's prescriptions." Pharmacists have so much more to offer — they can counsel, educate, monitor, support — and, most important of all, they can serve a crucial role in helping to make sure your drug is going to work safely for you.

The pharmacy technician

Your pharmacist may well be assisted by a *pharmacy technician*. These unheralded people — working under the pharmacist's supervision — provide invaluable assistance to the pharmacist by performing many labour-intensive roles including counting out doses and filling medicine containers, to name but a few. Unlike a pharmacist, the pharmacy technician cannot provide counselling to you.

What your doctor needs to tell your pharmacist

The information that physicians need to provide to pharmacists is contained within the prescription the doctor writes. The typical chain of events is that your doctor writes out the prescription and then either gives it to you to take to the pharmacist or sends it directly to the pharmacist by fax. (Occasionally, a doctor goes through a quaint but surprisingly efficient process, putting his ear to a phone and speaking directly to a real pharmacist!)

If your pharmacist is unclear on some aspect of the prescription's instructions, she'll contact the prescribing physician for clarification.

Figure 3-1 shows a typical prescription.

The components of a prescription are as follows:

- **Doctor's contact information:** Her name, address, phone and fax numbers.
- **Your information:** Your name and address.
- **Date:** The date the prescription was written.
- **Drug name:** The name of the drug being prescribed (the name may be written in its generic form or in one of the available trade names).
- **Dose:** The strength of each dose.
- **How it's taken:** The route by which the medicine is to be taken (the oral route is indicated by either the words "by mouth" or the initials *PO* — short for the Latin *per os*, which means "by mouth").
- **Frequency:** How often the drug is to be taken (*OD* — or *QD* — means once daily, *BID* means twice per day, *TID* means three times a day, *QID* means four times a day, and *HS* means at

bedtime). Because there have been cases where the abbreviation *OD* has been misinterpreted when a prescription is being filled, the trend nowadays is for doctors to write this out as "once daily."

✔ **Mitte:** How many doses the pharmacist is to dispense to you.

✔ **Repeat:** How many times the pharmacist is authorized to refill the prescription.

✔ **Prescribing physician's signature:** Your doctor's signature.

You've probably come across the symbol *Rx* either on a prescription or a pharmacy sign. In case you were wondering, it's an abbreviation for the Latin word *recipere,* or "recipe." Finally — a recipe that Ian knows how to prepare!

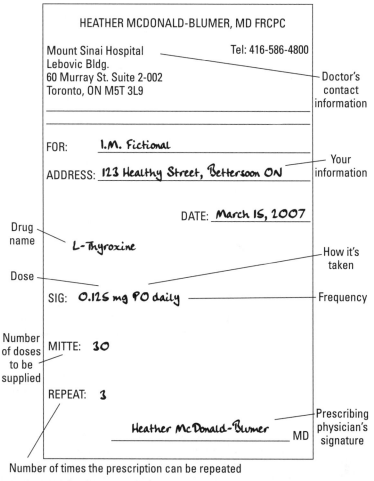

HEATHER MCDONALD-BLUMER, MD FRCPC

Mount Sinai Hospital
Lebovic Bldg.
60 Murray St. Suite 2-002
Toronto, ON M5T 3L9

Tel: 416-586-4800

Doctor's contact information

FOR: I.M. Fictional

ADDRESS: 123 Healthy Street, Bettersoon ON

Your information

DATE: March 15, 2007

Drug name
L-Thyroxine

How it's taken

Dose

SIG: 0.125 mg PO daily

Frequency

Number of doses to be supplied

MITTE: 30

REPEAT: 3

Heather McDonald-Blumer MD

Prescribing physician's signature

Number of times the prescription can be repeated

Figure 3-1: A Prescription.

What you need to tell your pharmacist

If you have a nice relationship with your pharmacist and spend a fair bit of time talking to her, then you're already familiar with the key things it's so helpful for you to share with this important player on your health care team. On the other hand, if you haven't yet had an opportunity to come to know your pharmacist, then consider our suggestions for things to tell her to ensure you're getting the best attention and care.

Tell your pharmacist *everything* you think could be important when it comes to your medications. As a minimum, however, we suggest that you let him know whether you

✔ **Can have your drug costs covered.** This would most commonly be through a provincial or territorial drug plan or private insurer. We discuss drug costs in detail in Chapter 10.

✔ **Are pregnant, are trying to get pregnant, or are breastfeeding.** Let your physician know this before he gives you a prescription so he can choose the safest possible drug in these circumstances, but in any event it can't hurt to have one more professional checking into the safety of a drug in these settings.

✔ **Have difficulty opening "child-proof" pill bottles.** Sometimes we think these could also be called "arthritis-proof" pill bottles given how tough it can be to twist off the lid on some of these containers. If you have arthritis or don't have biceps like Arnold Schwarzenegger, then be sure to ask your pharmacist whether she can package your pills in an easier-to-open container.

✔ **Are concerned that you might get your medicines confused.** Given the large number of different medicines some people are prescribed, it's no surprise they can't always remember which drug to take when. If you think you might get your drugs mixed up, be sure to ask your pharmacist whether she can put your prescription drugs in a specially designed dispenser (a *seven-day pill organizer*) that separates each dose for each day for an entire week. Most pharmacists do not charge extra for this service. (We discuss these packages in detail in Chapter 8.)

Do *not* leave the pharmacy if you're unsure how to take your medicine. It's simply too dangerous! People can get sick or even die from taking their prescription drugs the wrong way. Your pharmacist is there to help you and invariably takes both pleasure and

pride in doing just that. You're not inconveniencing her if you have questions — you are showing your respect for her considerable knowledge. And hey, you're paying her rent!

Your pharmacist is an expert when it comes to dispensing medications, and when it comes to deciphering some doctors' handwriting, pharmacists are often quite the detectives as well. They are, however, not mind-readers, and it's worth bearing in mind your pharmacist may not necessarily know the reason why a medication was prescribed for you. Many medications can be used for more than one purpose, and *your* specific purpose may not be noted on the prescription that your doctor gave you.

We encourage you to stay with one pharmacist for your pharmaceutical care where possible — they'll get to know you and can tailor their guidance to suit your individual needs. If you can't partner with a single pharmacist, at the very least try to stick with one pharmacy. All your prescription medicine records are then in one place, and any pharmacist helping you in that store can better keep an eye out for things such as potential drug interactions.

Pharmacists are highly trained and caring professionals who take pride in working closely with their clients. If, unfortunately, you're not getting the attention you deserve from your pharmacist, consider switching pharmacies. If you do, you have the right to ask your pharmacist to send your current prescription information to your new pharmacy.

What you need to make sure your pharmacist tells you

If you're simply getting a refill on a drug you've been taking for years, then the conversation you have with your pharmacist as you pick up your medicine is likely to be very brief. On the other hand, if you're getting a prescription filled for the first time, there's a whole bunch of information that your pharmacist should share with you.

About taking the drug

These are important points for your pharmacist to review with you concerning how you're to take your prescription drug:

- ✔ The name of your drug.
- ✔ How many times per day you are to take the medicine.
- ✔ What times you are to take the medicine.

✔ Whether you are to take the medicine with food or on an empty stomach. Some medicines are better absorbed into the body on an empty stomach. On the other hand, some drugs are less likely to upset your stomach or are better absorbed into the body if you take them with food.

✔ What you should do if you miss a dose.

✔ What you should do if you accidentally take an extra dose.

✔ Whether you can chew or split the medicine (if you have been prescribed a large pill and you might have difficulty swallowing it).

About storing the drug

These are important points for your pharmacist to review with you concerning how you are to store your prescription drug. She should tell you whether your medicine

✔ Needs to be stored away from light. This is true of many different drugs, including nitroglycerin.

✔ Must not be exposed to extremes of temperature. (Insulin, for example, is irreversibly damaged if subjected to very hot or very cold temperatures.)

✔ Must be kept refrigerated until used (more commonly a factor with medicines that are injected rather than taken orally).

About expiration dates and unused medicine

Important points for your pharmacist to review with you concerning expiration dates or unused medicine include:

✔ Whether your drug has an expiration date. Most of the time it's a moot point, because you're given a drug you'll take daily and use up quite promptly. Some drugs, however, you may take just on occasion (such as, for example, sumatriptan [Imitrex], which is taken to treat migraines). Quite a shame if you reach, in distress, for that seldom-used medicine only to find it has expired.

✔ What you should do with any expired or unused medicine. We recall the very formal, complicated ritual our parents followed years ago when faced with the predicament of dealing with leftover pills. Well, okay, it wasn't really complicated at all — they'd just dump them down the toilet. But that was then and this is now (when we know better). If you have extra medicine that needs to be discarded, your pharmacist can safely dispose of it for you.

About drug interactions

These are important points for your pharmacist to review with you concerning drug interactions. He should explain whether you should

✔ Avoid any foods or liquids altogether. Grapefruit juice, in particular, is notorious for interacting with prescription drugs. We discuss this further in Chapter 4.

✔ Be aware that another prescription drug you are taking might interact adversely with your new prescription drug. Your physician likely has looked into this before he gave you your prescription, but in reality few doctors and patients exist who have not benefited from a conscientious pharmacist discovering an overlooked and potentially harmful drug interaction. If this situation happens your pharmacist contacts your physician, who then determines whether an alternate drug is preferred.

✔ *Not* take the medicine within a few hours of taking an over-the-counter product. Physicians and pharmacists commonly overlook the issue of how your *non*-prescription drugs might interact adversely with your *prescription* drugs. This is particularly common with the use of iron or calcium. We discuss this further in Chapter 7.

✔ Avoid alcohol. Some prescription drugs cause some unpleasant side-effects if you consume alcohol while on the medicine (even if you don't take the alcohol at the same time as the drug). We look at this issue in detail in Chapter 7.

About side-effects

The following points are all issues that your doctor should discuss with you at the time she hands you your prescription (hence, we discuss them above; see "What to make sure your doctor tells you"). We mention them here again because we feel it's important that your pharmacist *also* share this information with you.

✔ What side-effects you need to be aware of. (If, instead of a conversation, you are simply given a pre-printed drug information sheet, look it over *before* you leave the pharmacy so you can direct any questions or uncertainties to the pharmacist right then and there. See "Understanding the package insert" later in this chapter.)

✔ The most *common* side-effects that this medicine can cause, and how common they are.

✔ The most *serious* side-effects that this medicine can cause, and how common they are.

✔ What you should do if you experience what might be a side-effect from this medicine.

ANECDOTE

Side-effects can occur, but how often?

Ian well recalls Donald Stephens, a 50-year-old man for whom he prescribed metformin to treat recently diagnosed diabetes. Although Ian had discussed possible side-effects with Mr. Stephens, he was still taken aback when Mr. Stephens showed up for his next visit with what seemed like a novel-length drug information sheet his pharmacist had given him. There, in *War and Peace* like detail, was a startlingly long list of horrible complications that the patient expected to experience from his new drug.

"Mr. Stephens, did the pharmacist tell you how *often* these bad things occur?" Ian asked. "No," Mr. Stephens said. "Not even whether these things occurred commonly or rarely?" Ian asked. "No," Mr. Stephens said again. "Well," Ian went on, "almost all of those horrible things listed on that sheet happen once in a blue moon. In fact, apart from some mild stomach upset or diarrhea, few people get *any* side-effects from metformin. It's important that you know what serious side-effects could *potentially* happen, but it's equally important that you know how *seldom* they happen."

Mr. Stephens looked at Ian for a moment before saying anything. "Doctor, can I be honest with you?" he asked. Ian nodded. "Well, I got so scared when I saw what was on that list I didn't even end up taking the pills." "You know," Ian replied, "I can't blame you. That sheet makes that drug look like the most dangerous thing since I gave my daughter my credit card." Mr. Stephens laughed as he smiled in relief. He then started on the medicine, was free of side-effects, and his diabetes control quickly improved.

Moral of the story: Context is all-important (and, for the record, just like the patient's metformin, Ian's daughter proved herself quite adept at safely using his credit card).

About allergies, intolerances, and non-medicinal ingredients

These are important points for your pharmacist to review with you concerning allergies, intolerances, and non-medicinal ingredients. He should check whether you

- ✔ Have an allergy to another medicine, which may indicate that you might also be allergic to this medicine. (We discuss drug allergies in Chapter 7.)

- ✔ Are intolerant to another medicine, which may indicate that you might also be intolerant to this medicine.

- ✔ Have celiac disease, in case the medicine contains gluten. (We discuss celiac disease in Chapter 5.)

- ✔ Have lactose intolerance, in case the medicine contains lactose.

- ✔ Are allergic to peanuts or soya, in case the medicine contains peanut oil, soybean oil, or soya lecithin.

✔ Are allergic to sulphites, tartrazine, or parabens, in case the medicine contains these ingredients.

✔ Have liver, kidney, or other serious health disorders, in case any of these health problems make it unsafe to take this medicine.

✔ Keep a Kosher or vegan diet, in case the medication contains any components that you want to avoid.

Consuming Prescription Drugs: Your Key Role

When it comes to consuming prescription drugs, you have to have a trusting relationship with your physician and your pharmacist. But you, the consumer, still have a crucial role to play. In this section we look at that role.

Understanding the prescription label

You may choose to skip the newspaper classifieds and you may pass on reading the latest entertainment magazine, but one thing that is truly a "must read" is the prescription label on your medication. Indeed, no prescription pill should go in one's mouth, no prescription cream on one's skin, no prescription drops in one's ears or eyes unless one has read the prescription label in detail.

Your prescription drug label typically looks something like Figure 3-2.

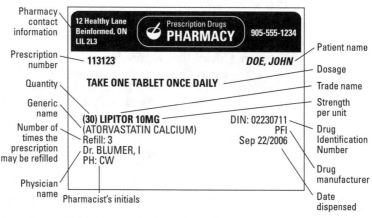

Figure 3-2: A prescription drug label.

The information described in the following list is almost always on every prescription drug label you receive, although the placement of the information on the label may vary.

- **Pharmacy contact information:** The name, address, and phone number of the pharmacy that dispensed the drug to you.

- **Prescription number:** The number that your pharmacy has assigned to your prescription. You can think of this as a tracking number. Each pharmacy keeps a running tab of each prescription it fills. If this number reads, for example, 1532, your prescription is the one thousand, five hundred thirty-second prescription that pharmacy has filled.

- **Patient name:** The person for whom the drug was prescribed. (If it isn't your name on the prescription label, it ain't your drug!)

- **Dosage:** How much of the drug is to be taken and how often. For example, the label might read: "Take one tablet daily" or "Take two tablets three times daily." If your prescription is for a dose of 180 mg and the pharmacist supplies you with 180-mg pills, then the label indicates you are to take one pill per dose. If the pharmacy had only the 90-mg pills in stock, then the label says to take two pills per dose. You need not be concerned, because in either case you'll receive 180 mg per dose.

- **Quantity:** The total number of pills/tablets/capsules (or other unit of medicine) in the container.

- **Trade name:** The trade name of the drug is the name that the pharmaceutical company decided to market the drug under.

- **Generic name:** The generic name of the drug is its scientific name.

- **Strength per unit:** The strength of each pill/tablet/capsule (or other unit of medicine) in the container.

- **DIN (Drug Identification Number):** The DIN is a number issued by a special branch of the Government of Canada (called the Therapeutic Products Directorate) after it has studied a drug and approved its use in Canada. (You can find out more about DINs at the Health Canada Web site: www.hc-sc.gc.ca.)

- **Refills:** The number of times your doctor has authorized the pharmacy to refill the prescription. (Sometimes the label, rather than saying "Repeat" or "Rep" or "Refill," says "Amount left" followed by the total number of doses your physician has authorized the pharmacist to dispense to you in the future.)

- **Physician name:** The name of the physician who prescribed the drug.

 ✔ **Date dispensed:** The date when the prescription was dispensed (filled).

 ✔ **Pharmacist:** The initials of the pharmacist who dispensed the prescription.

This list does not include the warning labels your pharmacist may also affix to the medication's container. We discuss these labels in the next section.

Some pharmacies can create prescription labels written in Braille, an invaluable service for people who are visually impaired and able to read Braille.

Noting the warning labels

We remember being struck by a comment David Rapoport, a Toronto family physician, made in the *Canadian Medical Association Journal:* "Sometimes when I reach for my prescription pad, I treat it like a loaded weapon." Every doctor writing a prescription needs to take this wisdom to heart. Every pharmacist filling a prescription needs to think about it, too. And every consumer of drugs should also mull this over. *Every drug that exists can cause harm.*

But, thank heaven, prescription drugs almost always do much more good than bad. And to keep the odds in your favour, just like driving a car, pedalling a bike, or, for that matter, crossing the street, when it comes to taking prescription drugs you need to heed certain warnings. Although your pharmacist undoubtedly will tell you these warnings when he gives you your medicine, he'll also likely affix stickers (called "warning labels") to your prescription container so you have an ongoing reminder.

A variety of warning labels exist, but some of the more commonly used ones may say something along the lines of:

 ✔ **"Warning: Do not exceed the dose prescribed by your physician. If difficulty in breathing persists, contact your physician immediately."** This label is affixed to asthma medicines to warn people that if an asthma attack is not settling with appropriate doses of the medicine, it's time to go to the hospital. Tragically, people have died because they did not follow this label's advice.

 ✔ **"Finish all this medication unless otherwise directed by the prescriber."** This label is typically used for antibiotics. If you have a bacterial infection and don't take your full complement of antibiotics, the infection is more likely to flare.

✔ **"Take with food."** Some medicines are gentler on the stomach or better absorbed into the body if taken with food. (We discuss this and the following topic in more detail in Chapter 4.)

✔ **"Take on an empty stomach."** Some medicines are absorbed more efficiently into the body if they are taken without food.

✔ **"You should avoid prolonged or excessive exposure to sunlight while taking this medication."** Some medicines make the skin more susceptible to sunburn.

✔ **"Do not eat grapefruit or drink grapefruit juice while taking this medication."** Grapefruit juice can affect the way a drug is processed in the body, which in turn can cause a drug to build up to dangerously high levels in your system. We discuss this topic in more detail in Chapter 4.

✔ **"Rinse mouth thoroughly after each use."** You'll typically find this label on steroid-containing puffers used to treat asthma or chronic bronchitis. Rinsing your mouth after using these medicines reduces your likelihood of getting an oral yeast infection as a side-effect from the drug.

✔ **"Before using salt substitutes, check with your physician or pharmacist."** You may see this label on certain types of drugs called potassium-sparing diuretics (such as spironolactone). These drugs cause the body to retain potassium. Salt substitutes are rich in potassium, and thus when consumed by someone who is also taking a potassium-sparing diuretic increase the risk of developing dangerously high levels of potassium in the blood.

✔ **"Do not crush."** Certain medicines have a coating to prevent irritation to the stomach. Other drugs are specially formulated so they are only slowly absorbed from the intestine into the blood. In either case, disrupting this coating (as would happen if you crushed the pill) would interfere with the action of the medicine.

Understanding the package insert

You may have noticed that your prescription drug from the pharmacy is sometimes accompanied by an information sheet. These may be supplied by the pharmacist, in which case they typically are stapled to or placed inside the bag containing your drug. Alternatively, they are supplied by the manufacturer of the drug, in which case the sheet (called a "package insert") can likely be found within the box containing your medication.

These package inserts vary significantly in format but generally provide, as a minimum, information regarding the following:

- ✔ The name and usual dose of your prescription drug.
- ✔ The condition the drug is typically used to treat.
- ✔ Side-effects you might experience.
- ✔ A comment on the safety of the drug if you are pregnant or breastfeeding.
- ✔ How you are to take the medicine.
- ✔ How to store your medicine.
- ✔ What other ingredients are in the pill/tablet/capsule.

Package inserts, though no doubt well intentioned, typically have a number of limitations, often being either too complex (or too simple) or too intimidating or too imbued with medicalese or what have you. As we mention earlier in this chapter, even the best package insert is not a replacement for a detailed chat with your physician and pharmacist. Nonetheless, keeping the insert on hand as a reference tool isn't a bad idea.

What to watch for with your medications

Drugs are funny things in some ways. A manufacturer makes them. Your doctor prescribes them. Your pharmacist dispenses them. And you take them. Simple enough. But how do you know that the drug is actually doing what it's supposed to? And how do you know when it's doing something it should not? This section looks at the key things you can watch for to make sure your drug is working safely and effectively.

Watching for effectiveness

For you (and your doctor) to know whether your medicine is working effectively, it's often helpful (depending on the particular drug in question) for you to keep tabs on certain measurements. For example, if you're taking a drug to treat high blood pressure, you can check your pressure regularly (either with your own blood pressure machine or using a machine available at your local pharmacy). When you see your doctor, you can show him the values you've obtained. This record helps your physician determine whether your medicine is working well or whether a change is required. (Another example would be in the case that you have diabetes. If you monitor your blood glucose measurements with a blood glucose meter, this record provides invaluable feedback for both you and your doctor regarding the effectiveness of your therapy.)

You can purchase a blood pressure machine at most drug stores and many department stores. If you do obtain a machine, be sure to take it with you to your doctor's office so that your doctor can assess its accuracy (by having you do your own measurement followed by the doctor performing a reading with her own equipment).

If you are prescribed a drug to control symptoms of a disease, then you can help your doctor help you by keeping tabs on whether the symptom being treated is getting better (or not) now that you've started taking your new prescription drug. For example, if you have arthritis and are prescribed a medicine to reduce joint pain, you can be an invaluable resource in your own health care if you let your doctor know whether your joint pains improve after you started taking your new prescription drug. Being treated for migraines? Let your doctor know whether you're having fewer headaches. Being treated for pneumonia? Let your doctor know whether your fever, cough, and sputum are lessening. Being treated for angina? Let your doctor know whether you are having fewer episodes of chest discomfort. And so on.

Watching for safety

Bad enough if a medicine is not helping you. Far worse for it to be actually hurting you.

Fortunately, the great majority of side-effects are not nearly so serious as to be life-threatening. Nevertheless, when your doctor prescribes a drug, make sure that she tells you what side-effects are common and what side-effects are serious and what you should do in the event any of these occur. This simple precaution could save your life! (We discuss drug side-effects in general in Chapter 7, and in Chapter 6 we discuss specific side-effects a given drug might cause.)

Taking all your prescribed drugs

One way you can help your physician help you is to always bring *all* of your medicines (prescription and otherwise and in their *original* containers) with you to every doctor's appointment. Even though you may find this (understandably) inconvenient, it allows your physician to be sure he has an accurate record of what medicines you are taking. This, in turn, helps your doctor not only to ensure you're taking the medicines you have been prescribed (see the anecdote, "Ah, so that's why I'm not feeling better!"), but also to avoid prescribing drugs for you that are redundant, inappropriate, or that could lead to adverse drug interactions.

Keeping a list of your drugs in your wallet or purse is helpful — so long as you keep it updated — but is still not *as* effective as bringing your medicines with you when you see the doctor. Even a list printed out for you by your pharmacist is not as good as actually taking your medicines along to your appointments. (The list shows what the pharmacist's records indicate you are to be taking, but that doesn't ensure they are what you are *actually* taking.)

If you don't have original medicine containers because your pharmacist sorts your medicines out for you into a seven-day pill organizer (as we explain in detail in Chapter 8), be sure to bring both it and copies of your prescription labels (the pharmacist usually affixes these to the back of the organizer, but may have just given you copies to carry) to your doctors' appointments.

Knowing what to watch for

Being an informed consumer will help you select a well-made car, a fuel-efficient furnace and nutritious foods. When it comes to prescription drug side-effects, being an informed consumer can help save your life.

Seymour Curtis had always been the picture of health — until, out of the blue one day, his heart started to beat so fiercely he thought it was going to jump right out of his chest. He became understandably alarmed and went to the emergency department, where he was diagnosed as having a heart rhythm problem called *atrial fibrillation.* Seymour consulted a cardiologist, who put Seymour on a drug called *amiodarone* (Cordarone) to control the problem. His doctor wisely cautioned him that this drug could lead to lung problems and that the first clue might be the development of shortness of breath.

Initially Seymour felt fine, but after being on the amiodarone for a few months he did indeed become breathless. He sought prompt medical attention and was quickly diagnosed as having lung inflammation due to the drug. He immediately stopped taking the drug, and the lung inflammation — and breathlessness — went away. Seymour was fortunate he had been made aware of what to watch for and that he did indeed watch for it. By keeping an eye out for side-effects and, when they occurred, promptly seeking medical attention, he staved off a potentially fatal lung complication.

ANECDOTE

Ah, so that's why I'm not feeling better!

You may be sure you can accurately rhyme off all your prescription drugs from memory. Your doctor may be sure she can find them all correctly listed in your chart. Your pharmacist may be sure he has an up-to-date record of your medicines on his computer. Yet nothing is as precise (or as safe) as actually sitting down with your health care provider and looking directly at all your medicines in their original containers, as Manuela learned.

Manuela's joints were "killing" her; indeed, her knuckles were so swollen it looked as if she had been in a fist fight. This wasn't, however, particularly likely seeing as she was a 72-year-old, frail grandmother with a flare of rheumatoid arthritis. Heather had seen her a few weeks before and had added prednisone to Manuela's other anti-arthritis medications.

"Dr. McDonald, I'm feeling so badly," Heather's patient plaintively told her. "I can tell," Heather replied, "you're clearly having lots of pain. You can hardly even move your fingers." Manuela nodded. "That's so disappointing," Heather said, then added, "I had been optimistic the medicine I prescribed last visit would help you. Can I look at your pill bottles? We'll see what we need to change." Manuela handed a Ziploc bag full of pill bottles to Heather. Heather took out one bottle at a time and carefully scrutinized each one.

After a while she asked her patient, "Are there any other medicines you're taking?" Manuela shook her head. "Hmm," Heather said. "But Manuela, the medicine I prescribed last visit isn't here." Manuela leaned forward and looked at the bottles assembled on the desk. "There it is," she said, as she pointed to a bottle with a label indicating its contents to be metoprolol, a medicine used primarily for high blood pressure. "I started taking that medicine the day I saw you." "But I didn't prescribe that drug for you," Heather said, "and, oh, wait, the label says it was prescribed by Dr. Silvera." Manuela looked puzzled for a moment. "But," Heather went on, "it was prescribed the same day I saw you." Now they were both confused. Could the pharmacist have made a mistake and accidentally given the patient the wrong medicine?

"Wait!" Manuela suddenly exclaimed, as she reached into her purse. A moment later she withdrew a carefully folded piece of paper; one that looked awfully familiar to them both. Neatly printed in Heather's meticulous handwriting was a prescription for prednisone. "Dr. McDonald, now I remember. I saw my family doctor the same day as you and my pressure was high so he gave me a new prescription. But when I went to the drugstore I forgot yours. No wonder why I'm not feeling any better." Manuela promptly went back to the drugstore, filled the prescription for prednisone, and soon thereafter was feeling much better. Moral of the story Part One: A prescription drug works only if you are taking it. Moral of the story Part Two: It's so, so easy to get confused or mixed-up about prescription drugs, especially when you're on a whole bunch of them.

Many of our patients tell us, "Doctor, my medicines are exactly the same as the last time I was here." Nonetheless, in our experience up to 50 (yes, 50!) percent of the time, some potentially important change in medications has indeed taken place. The *many* possible reasons for this discrepancy include patient factors (such as forgetting that some other doctor has made a change to one's therapy or, simply forgetting to take a medicine), physician factors (such as writing out a new prescription but inadvertently putting it inside the chart), and pharmacist factors (such as misreading a physician's handwriting and therefore dispensing a wrong medicine or a wrong dose — which, fortunately, occurs only rarely). For any of these situations, taking your pill bottles to your appointments can help prevent any (potentially dangerous) guesswork or assumptions regarding the exact details of your medications.

Sure, it may be a hassle to take your drugs with you to doctors' appointments time after time after time. But imagine how much more of a hassle it would be for you if you got seriously ill because of a drug error that could have been avoided!

Watching for drug interactions

Your doctor can look up whether the new drug she is prescribing for you might cause problems if taken with another drug you're on. Your pharmacist also can (and should) look this up. As yet another safeguard, you may want to look this information up yourself when you get home and before you take your first pill from that new prescription. Two excellent Web sites to check for drug interactions are www.drugdigest.org and www.epocrates.com.

Chapter 4

Making Sure Your Prescription Works for You

In This Chapter

▶ Taking your prescription drugs properly

▶ Understanding how to use the different forms your prescription drugs may come in

▶ Sorting out how to manage your medicines

▶ Travelling with your prescription medicines

▶ Recognizing when your medicines aren't working

*T*his past spring, as we got our sailboat ready for the forthcoming season, we opened up one of the cupboards and found quite the surprise. There, neatly lined up, were six cans of diet cola. Which wouldn't have been at all bad, except each can had exploded and its contents had splattered all over the place. What a mess! Note to all Canadian boaters: Storing canned soft drinks on a boat in the middle of winter is not a good thing to do. (Unless, of course, your boat is somewhere in the Caribbean!)

So what does our misadventure have to do with a book on prescription drugs? Simply this: medicines, like soft drinks, have to be stored properly. In this chapter we look at this and other important issues concerning your prescription drugs, including how to properly take them, how to travel with them, and how you can determine when they're not doing their intended job.

Taking Your Medication: Practical Answers for Common Questions

Some aspects of prescription drug therapy are highly complex and are the domain of biochemists, physiologists, and other laboratory scientists. We'll now spend the next 200 pages discussing in intricate detail these academic issues ... oh, wait, we hear our editor calling us. Oops, wrong plan. Okay, we have it right now: in this section we discuss practical answers to common questions concerning prescription drug therapy.

What drugs am I taking?

If you are the picture of health but come down with a relatively minor problem — say, a bladder infection — you'll likely be taking a grand total of one medication, in which case it's relatively easy for you to keep track of things. But many people are on five or more medications, and with each additional drug you take you have yet more stuff to try to remember.

So don't try to remember it all; do what Ian does and write everything down. The running joke in our household is that unless Ian writes something down, it won't happen. In fact, it's possible we used to have four kids, but because Ian forgot to write down that he was supposed to pick one of them up after school a few years ago we now have only three (which explains the extra bedroom).

 The Cheat Sheet at the front of this book is an ideal place for you to keep track of the name and other key information regarding your prescription medicine. Feel free to remove it from this book and keep it with you or put it in some handy place. (If you are taking more than one medication, you can enter the same type of information for your other drug[s] on similar sheets of your own creation.)

 It doesn't matter whether you know your drug by its generic name or its trade name. Should the need arise, you or your health care providers can easily look up the drug in this book or in most other health care materials by *either* name. (The Drug Index at the back of this book cross-references both names.) Bear in mind, though, that trade names for many drugs sold in Canada differ from trade names for those same drugs in other countries. (Generic names are more likely than trade names to be the same from country to country.) We discuss trade and generic names in more detail in Chapter 2.

What dose am I supposed to take?

The dose of a medicine is the amount you are to take each time it's due. (We talk about when to take the dose in the next section.) If it's a pill or tablet or capsule, the drug label tells you to take one, or two — or whatever the case may be. If it's a liquid, the label tells you to take a quantity either stated in millilitres or measured using teaspoons or tablespoons.

If the label on your liquid prescription medicine instructs you to take a certain number of teaspoons or tablespoons of the medicine, use a spoon (or other measuring apparatus) that *specifically states the volume* it contains. Don't rely on the assortment of differently sized "teaspoons" and "tablespoons" you may have in your cutlery drawer. These spoons may not hold a true teaspoon (5 mL) or tablespoon (15 mL) of fluid. As a result, if you use them to measure out your dose of liquid medicine, you could potentially take too large or too small a dose. Your kitchen *baking* spoons likely include 5-mL and 15-mL spoons as part of the collection. If not, you can purchase appropriately sized measuring devices at your pharmacy.

How will I know whether I need to change doses?

Quite commonly, your doctor will change the dose of a medicine as time goes by. This happens if she determines the original dose is either not strong enough or is too strong for you. In these cases, she will advise you of the recommended change — usually when you're in her office for a visit. If you still have medicine left from the original supply that your pharmacist dispensed to you, your doctor will likely ask you to take larger or smaller amounts from your existing supply.

Which is all perfectly fine — however, if your pharmacist does not know of this change in dose, when you obtain a refill of your prescription he will simply dispense the same amount of medicine he gave you the last time you were there. For this reason, it's important that whenever your doctor asks you to change the dose of your already dispensed medication, she should at the same time give you a new prescription (which has the new dose on it) for you to take to the pharmacy when you get your medicine refilled. Additionally — and importantly — if your doctor asks you to change the dose of your current supply of medicine, ask her to write the change on your medicine label (or write it on yourself).

You may discover, perhaps to your surprise, that your pharmacist can sometimes predict when your doctor has changed your dose. When you visit the pharmacy to obtain a refill on your prescription, your pharmacist may observe you're there earlier (or later) than expected based on the number of doses he previously dispensed to you. This alerts him that either your doctor has changed your dose or you (perhaps inadvertently) have not been taking the medicine as prescribed.

How often should I take my medicine?

Medicines can be taken on a variety of different schedules. Some are taken a number of times per day and others are taken only once a week (and some even less often). Some are taken at mealtimes, and some must be taken on an empty stomach. For your medicine to work both effectively and safely for you, it is essential you know how often you are supposed to take your medicine. The label on your prescription container tells you this information.

The number of times per day you need to take a medicine depends on how long the drug's effect lasts in the body. If a medicine loses its effect within a few hours, it needs to be taken several times per day. On the other hand, if a medicine's effect is long-lasting, then it needs to be taken less frequently.

Most commonly, medicines are taken according to one of the following schedules:

- ✓ **Daily:** If the prescription doesn't specify the time, you can generally feel confident taking your prescription drug at any time of the day or night (however, it is best to take it at a similar time day-to-day). Confirm this with your pharmacist, because some once-daily drugs do work best if taken at a certain time. (Simvastatin, for example, is a once-a-day, cholesterol-lowering medicine that works best if taken in the evening.) And, as you might expect, medications to help you sleep are taken at bedtime.

- ✓ **Twice daily:** Typically this means you should take your prescription drug in the morning and in the evening. However, depending on one's interpretation, "morning and evening" can be anywhere from 6 (or so) hours apart to more than 14 hours apart. This very big range could affect how your drug works, so it's important your pharmacist clarifies for you exactly what "twice daily" means.

- ✓ **Three times daily:** Your pharmacist should tell you if, for your particular prescription drug, this means a dose with each meal or a dose every eight hours or some other "three times daily" schedule.

- ✓ **Four times daily:** This means four times per day. As with the preceding point, your pharmacist needs to clarify for you whether this means a dose with each meal and at bedtime or a dose every six hours or some other "four times daily" schedule.

If you are a shift worker, the times you eat and the times you sleep may not be consistent. Speak to your pharmacist to find out the best times to take your medicines — especially for the days when your shift changes.

When your prescription says your medicine is to be taken a *specific number* of hours apart — for example, if it says "take one pill every six hours" — the timing of each dose is important, so more careful and precise spacing of each dose is strongly recommended. Again, ask your doctor or pharmacist if you are uncertain about the prescription instructions.

Some medicines — not many, mind you, but some — are taken on less typical schedules than those listed above. Some drugs are taken just once or twice per week, some just on weekdays (they must work very hard indeed, because they get a full two days' rest on the weekend!), and some just once per month.

Don't worry about a schedule for medications taken on an "as needed" basis (most analgesics, medicines used to treat a developing migraine headache, and drugs for erectile dysfunction, to name but a few). These you take only, well, as needed.

Occasionally, a prescription requires you to alternate between two different doses of the same medicine day-to-day. As you might imagine, this can be very confusing. ("Dear, did I take the blue pill yesterday or was it the purple pill? Must have been the blue one; no wait, the purple one. Oh heavens!") If one of the strengths happens to be an odd number (say, 0.175 mg) and the other an even number (say, 0.2 mg), then you might find it helpful to set up a schedule where you take the odd-numbered strength on the odd days of the month (the 1st, 3rd, 5th, 7th, and so on) and the even-numbered strength on the even days of the month (the 2nd, 4th, 6th, 8th, and so on). You needn't worry about those rare occasions where you end up taking the odd-numbered strength two days in a row (say, on the 31st of one month and the 1st of the following month); this will do you no harm. (Another option is to use a seven-day pill organizer. In Chapter 8, we discuss this and other helpful ways you can keep your medicines organized.)

What should 1 do if 1 miss a dose?

Remember in high school when you handed in that geography assignment a day late? Do you recall how appreciative you were when your teacher told you it was okay and not to worry about it? We do — and we remember it was such a relief to have a teacher who was so forgiving. Your medicines are almost always just as forgiving. In fact, the great majority of the time if you're late taking a dose it makes no difference whatsoever.

Unless you're specifically advised otherwise by your pharmacist, do *not* take a double dose when you're next due to take your medicine in an attempt to "catch up" for the missed dose.

Generally speaking:

- ✔ If you're up to two hours late taking your medicine, take it as soon as you remember.

- ✔ If you're closer to your next scheduled dose than the one you missed, skip the missed one and wait until your next dose is due.

One very important exception to these generalities occurs when you've missed a dose of your birth control pills. As we discuss in Chapter 6, if you miss *any* of your doses it's necessary to use another form of contraception (such as a condom). The length of time you'll need to continue with this alternative contraception depends on a number of factors, so ask your physician (or pharmacist) for advice specific to your circumstance.

To help you remember when your medicine is due, try to tie in some other activity to drug-taking. For example, if you have been prescribed a once-a-day drug, try keeping the medicine bottle on your bedside table beside your alarm clock (unless safety considerations — such as having children in the house — make doing so unwise). Also, if you tend to forget to take medicines, ask your physician if it's possible to prescribe a long-acting version of a medication (these require fewer doses per day than the regular version of a drug).

Everyone is fallible, and it's the rare person indeed who has never missed a dose of their medication. It's likely enough to happen (and enough exceptions to the guidelines noted above exist) that it's best to take a proactive approach: when you pick up your prescription, make a point of asking your pharmacist what to do in the event of a missed dose. Asking this question should make you feel wise, not foolish.

Can I split the drug?

In a few circumstances you may need to (or choose to) split a pill (or tablet) in half, including the following:

- ✔ **If you were supplied with pills whose strength is double what you need:** For example, the smallest-strength tablet of Lopressor brand of metoprolol is 50 mg, but your doctor may have advised you to take a 25-mg dose. Lopressor has a line down the middle (called a "score") that enables you to break the 50-mg tablet in half, thereby making you the proud owner of two 25-mg tablets.

✔ **If you want to save some money:** Some drugs cost the same regardless of the dose. So it can (literally) pay to buy a higher-strength pill, which you can then split in half. One good example is sildenafil (Viagra), which comes in three strengths (25 mg, 50 mg, and 100 mg) that all cost almost the same. So, if you've used the medicine and determined 50 mg works just fine for you, then you can save some money by getting the 100-mg tablets and breaking them in half. That way, for the same amount of money, you have twice the fun, err, number of doses.

✔ **If the pill is overly big:** Some pills are nice and small and go down the hatch just fine thank you very much. And some pills are so big they wouldn't fit through a hatch on the Queen Mary. If you have been prescribed such monster pills, breaking them in half makes them a lot easier to swallow.

If a pill is not scored (and, often, even if it is) you may find it a lot easier to break in half using a little tool called a *pill splitter* (see Figure 4-1). Your pharmacy likely has these for sale. Even better, some pharmacies will split your medicines for you free of charge.

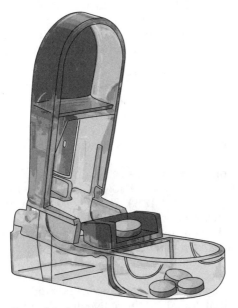

Figure 4-1: A pill splitter.

If you are unsure whether splitting a pill or other form of medicine is safe, ask your pharmacist. She either knows the answer or can find out for you. Don't split a medicine if

- ✓ **The medicine has an "enteric coating."** This type of coating is used primarily to make a medicine gentler on the stomach. If you split this type of pill, you expose the inner part of the pill and can no longer benefit from the coating. An example of this type of pill is coated ASA.

- ✓ **The medicine is contained within a capsule.** Capsules are almost always designed to be swallowed whole.

- ✓ **The medicine must be given in *very* precise amounts.** Some drugs require such extreme precision with their doses that even the smallest deviation may adversely affect how they work. Even if you're worthy of a gold medal in the not-yet-Olympic-sanctioned sport of pill-splitting, you won't always be able to be 100-percent precise with dividing a pill in exactly even halves. Accordingly, if you're on a medicine where even tiny deviations in doses are unsafe, then don't go for the split. Drugs within this group include (but are not limited to) medicines used to control disorders of the heart rhythm and medicines to prevent seizures.

- ✓ **The medicine is in the form of a patch.** Cutting a patch may affect how well it sticks to your skin and can also influence whether the right dose of medicine is absorbed by your body. Having said this, there *are* some patches you can safely split, so check with your pharmacist before you reach for the scissors.

- ✓ **The medicine is "time released."** Some medicines are designed to be slowly absorbed from the intestine into your bloodstream. The main advantage of this type of medicine is that it typically requires you to take fewer doses per day. If you split these medicines, the drug will be absorbed by your body more rapidly than it should.

One clue your medicine is time-released is the presence on the prescription label of a virtual alphabet soup of letters after the drug's name — examples are CD, CR, L, LA, SR, XC, or XL. However, the absence of any of these letters (or combination of letters) doesn't guarantee the medicine is not time-released, so it's best not to split a medicine without first checking with your pharmacist that it's safe do so. (Oh, and by the way, some time-released pills or capsules may be visible in your stool after the medicine they contained has been successfully absorbed by your body. What you're seeing is just the "vehicle" that contained the active drug. You can simply ignore it.)

Should I take my medicine with food?

Because many medicines are taken two or three times per day, often it's convenient to take a dose at mealtimes (typically at breakfast and at supper, for twice-daily medicines). This type of schedule works well for many medicines, but others can actually work less well when taken with food. We look at the important issue of medicines and foods in this section.

 Your pharmacist typically puts a warning label on your prescription container telling you whether you need to take your medicine on an empty stomach, or with food. If no warning label exists it likely makes no difference whether you take your medicine with food, but it's still always best to check with your pharmacist.

When to take a medicine with food

The most common reason for a drug to be taken with food is if consuming the medicine on an empty stomach is likely to cause *indigestion* (with symptoms such as heartburn, abdominal pain, and nausea). If you've been prescribed a medicine that tends to cause indigestion, your pharmacist likely affixes to your prescription container a "Take with food" warning label. Following this instruction will keep your stomach (and you) happier.

A far less common reason why you may need to take a drug with food is if the drug is better absorbed into your body when your stomach is not empty. An example of this type of drug is saquinavir.

When *not* to take a medicine with food

You need to take a medicine on an empty stomach if the presence of food in the stomach interferes with the body's ability to properly absorb the medicine. If your medicine isn't properly absorbed into your body, it can't help you. (Or, perhaps worse, the medicine may have unpredictable effects because the amount that does make its way into your blood varies in quantity from dose to dose.) Examples of medicines that should be taken on an empty stomach are ampicillin, captopril, and alendronate.

Some medicines are affected only by certain *types* of food within your stomach. For example, milk and dairy products can interfere with the absorption of L-thyroxine, and fruit juices can interfere with how your body handles certain antibiotics.

Generally speaking, your stomach is said to be "empty" first thing in the morning (assuming your last food intake was the evening before) or one to two hours before a meal. (However, in the case of our teenage sons "empty" happens 24/7 — at least judging by the number of times per day they raid the fridge!)

Are there things I should avoid when taking my medicine?

In the preceding section we look at whether you should take your medicine with food. In this section, we consider other things that can affect how your prescription drug works.

Over-the-counter drugs to avoid consuming at the same time as your prescription drug

Some over-the-counter medicines — including antacids, iron, and calcium supplements — should not be taken at the same time as certain prescription drugs because they may prevent your prescription drug from being properly absorbed into your body.

Because many over-the-counter drugs can affect prescription medicines, we recommend you ask your pharmacist for information specific to any you may be taking.

Foods to avoid at _any_ time if you are on certain prescription drugs

Earlier in this chapter we discuss how having food in your stomach can prevent some medicines from being properly absorbed into your body. However, some foods can affect how your prescription drug works even *after* the medicine has been absorbed. The most important examples include:

- ✔ **Grapefruit.** Many drugs are affected by the consumption of grapefruit or grapefruit juice. In some cases, consuming as little as 250 mL of grapefruit juice can affect the way a medicine works for up to three to seven days. Your pharmacist typically puts a warning label on your prescription drug package or bottle if the drug you have been prescribed is affected by grapefruit. Nevertheless, even if no such label exists on your drug package, it's wise to double-check with your pharmacist.

- ✔ **Green, leafy vegetables.** If you're taking a powerful blood thinner called warfarin (Coumadin), then it's very important the amount of vitamin K in your diet be fairly consistent from day to day. Vitamin K is found in green leafy vegetables such as spinach and cabbage, and is also found in abundant quantities in liver, broccoli, and brussels sprouts. Note that these foods are not forbidden if you're on warfarin; just be consistent with how much of them you eat. Overly variable amounts of vitamin K in your diet lead to inconsistent action of warfarin, which could make you prone to haemorrhaging or blood clots. We discuss warfarin in more detail in Chapter 6.

✔ **Alcohol** can interact adversely with many medications, in particular those that may cause sedation. Your pharmacist typically affixes a label to your medicine container informing you whether you should avoid alcohol. We recommend that you be extra cautious and ask your pharmacist anyway.

Can I stop my prescription before it's finished?

No, you can't stop taking your medicine before the prescription is used up, even if you start to feel better. Next question, please. Oh, wait a moment — we'll tell you about Doug first because his story explains the main reason not finishing your full prescription is a bad idea.

How grapefruit might affect your prescription drug

The interaction between grapefruit juice and certain oral medications was first noted in 1989. Medication taken orally passes through the stomach into the small intestine; from there it's absorbed into the bloodstream and is then carried to the liver. (We explain this process in Chapter 2.) Within the liver, the drug is exposed to a family of enzymes (collectively referred to as Cytochrome P-450), one of whose functions is to metabolize many incoming drugs, thereby partially deactivating them. One of these family members, known as CYP3A4, is responsible for metabolizing about 60 percent of orally taken drugs. Furanocoumarins and several other substances found in grapefruit and other similar citrus fruits inhibit the activity of CYP3A4 and thereby increase the amount of drug that stays active in the circulation. Having too much of a drug in your body can lead to side-effects and can be harmful.

Fruits having this effect on CYP3A4 include grapefruits and grapefruit juice (fresh or frozen), Seville oranges, limes and lime juice, tangelos, and pumellos.

Doug was feeling absolutely dreadful. He was congested and felt achy head to toe. Well, especially head. He went to see his family physician, who diagnosed his problem as sinusitis and gave him a prescription for a 10-day course of amoxicillin. Four days later, feeling much improved, he not unreasonably concluded the medicine had done its job and the worst was over — and he didn't complete the remaining six days' worth of medication. The next day went okay, but by the following day he started to feel stuffed up again — and within another 24 hours he was back to square one. Doug went back to his doctor and was re-prescribed a full, 10-day course of antibiotic. This time Doug completed the entire prescription and his sinusitis did not return.

Unless you're being treated with a medicine you're to take purely for symptom relief (such as acetaminophen with codeine for the treatment of a toothache), then by all means complete the entire prescription you've been given. In the case of Doug's sinusitis, he got sick again because the germs responsible for his infection were not completely killed off after only the first few days of his prescription; the darn critters required an entire 10 days of treatment to keep them at bay.

Should I refill my prescription?

We're thrilled you're reading this section. Why? Because inadvertently failing to get an important prescription refilled after the initial supply has run out is one of the most common, potentially serious errors we see with prescription drug therapy. You must know whether or not you're to continue taking your prescription medicine. In other words, are you supposed to go back to the pharmacy to have the prescription refilled after you've used up the medicine the pharmacist gave you? You can find out in three (complementary) ways:

- ✔ **Your doctor should tell you when she hands you your prescription.** Sometimes, however, doctors — including us, by the way — forget to do this. And sometimes, physicians inappropriately assume that if you're being treated for a chronic condition, you'll automatically know that therapy needs to be taken on an ongoing basis in order to be effective.

- ✔ **Your pharmacist should tell you when he hands you your medicine.** Like physicians, pharmacists sometimes forget to share this information so, as a failsafe mechanism, we recommend you follow the advice in the following bullet.

- ✔ **When your doctor hands you your prescription and/or when your pharmacist hands you your medicine,** ask them whether you're to refill the drug after you've finished taking the initial supply.

ANECDOTE

To renew or not to renew —
That is the question

If you are being treated with a medication to control a chronic condition, such as hypertension, stopping the medication will likely result in the ailment worsening as Craig discovered...

Despite Craig's efforts to control his hypertension with appropriate lifestyle therapy, his blood pressure had been progressively worsening. He had been resistant to the idea of taking medications to control it, but when his pressure reached 170/100 Craig agreed to begin prescription drug therapy. His physician, Dr. Jackson, started him on medication and a few weeks later they were both very pleased to see Craig's blood pressure had come down to 140/85.

A few months went by and Craig returned for his next appointment. To Dr. Jackson's dismay, Craig's blood pressure was back up to 170/100. "Craig," Dr. Jackson said, "those medicines aren't working well enough, so we're going to have to make some changes. Let's have a look at your pills, okay?" Craig looked at Dr. Jackson in surprise. "What pills, doctor? They're finished." "Finished?" Dr. Jackson replied with alarm. "What do you mean, 'finished'? You have to keep taking them or your pressure will climb back up."

Craig refilled his prescription and started taking his pills again, and his blood pressure promptly came down. Now, Craig was no fool — he was simply unaware. So was his physician, who hadn't pointed out the drugs were to be taken on an ongoing basis. Doctors often forget that even when something seems obvious to them it may be anything but to their patients, and sometimes they omit things that should indeed be said.

TIP

One strong clue that you're to continue your medicine after you've finished the initial supply is found right on the prescription label, where you find the word "Repeat" or "Refill" (or the abbreviation "Rep") followed by a number. If the number is anything other than zero, the odds are overwhelming your doctor intends for you to continue the medicine. If the number is zero, your doctor either doesn't want you to continue it *or* wants you to see him to have your condition reviewed before you take more medicine. It always pays to be cautious and contact your doctor if you're at all unclear about his plans for you.

Indulge us for a moment in a quick experiment. Turn to this book's table of contents and spend a moment scanning the list of diseases noted under Chapter 5. We'll wait right here until you get back.

Okay, you're back. Great! You probably noticed you've never heard of some of the illnesses on the list, but you likely have some passing familiarity with many of them. Now scan the list again, but this time pause for a moment to think about how many of those conditions are curable. Even if you're not a health care worker, you probably recognize that, sadly, modern medicine can cure very few of these conditions.

On the other hand, consider how wonderful it is that such effective therapies exist for the great majority of these illnesses. It wasn't all that long ago when physicians had virtually no treatments to offer, and these conditions could easily lead to prolonged suffering and, often, premature death. However, for many new therapies to keep a chronic condition in check there must be ongoing treatment. Until modern science can cure arthritis or emphysema or hypertension or high cholesterol or diabetes or what have you, most people with these conditions need to take medicines on an ongoing basis. If they stop the medicine, the condition being treated will typically act up.

Some drugs, such as many types of antidepressants and some heart drugs, should almost never be stopped suddenly, as doing so can cause dangerous symptoms.

So, unless your physician or pharmacist advises that your medicine is not to be repeated after the initial supply runs out, you can consider the likelihood you're to keep renewing the prescription very high indeed. The Cheat Sheet at the front of this book has a list of key things you need to know about your drugs, including a place to note whether you're to refill a prescribed medicine.

We have no idea whether this anecdote is true (let's be generous and call it apocryphal), but we love it so much we want to share it. The story goes that a while back, the CEO and founder of a huge chewing gum manufacturing company was flying between New York and Chicago when a fellow passenger said to him, "Your company is such a roaring success — heck, you dominate the market — so why bother to spend so much money on advertising?" The executive's response? "For the same reason the pilot of this plane bothers to spend money on fuel by keeping his engines on despite the fact we're already at 35,000 feet." And so it is with prescription drugs: if taking them is successfully controlling your chronic illness, stopping them is usually not the best thing to do.

Whenever you see your doctor, make a point of asking for new prescriptions for drugs which you're to continue but for which you have no repeats left (see the tip earlier in this section for a helpful way to find out how many repeats are left for your medicine). (Be aware, though, that a specialist is almost certainly comfortable re-prescribing only drugs falling within his specialty.)

Head to Toe: Using Different Types of Medication Properly

So you've recently found yourself getting this darn uncomfortable burning feeling when you pass your urine. Ouch. And you went to your doctor, who found you had a bladder infection. Okay, at least now you know what's wrong. And you got a prescription for an antibiotic pill. Ah, you can already envision the relief soon coming your way. You open the bottle, take out a pill, and sigh with anticipation as you crush the pill into a fine powder, mix it with a sprinkle of water, reach down, and ever-so-carefully rub it between your toes...

Okay, okay, we made that story up. And we know that you know an antibiotic pill to treat a bladder infection isn't going to help you if you rub it between your toes. The point is, for a medicine to *work* properly, it has to be *taken* properly — and that's what this section is all about.

Easy to swallow: Pills, capsules, and liquids

Lauren Bacall made it all seem so simple when she famously asked Humphrey Bogart whether he knew how to whistle: she told him all he needed to do was put his lips together and blow. And one would surely think swallowing must be equally straightforward. But, just as whistling does not come naturally to everyone, swallowing medicines doesn't either. Also, some special precautions are required when swallowing certain medicines.

Swallowing pills and capsules

To swallow most pills and capsules, you simply place them in your mouth, take a sip of water, and faster than you can say "Bob's your uncle," both the medicine and the water are on their way down your esophagus and heading into your stomach.

If you have a difficult time swallowing pills, be sure to ask your pharmacist whether your medicine can be split or crushed or chewed; doing any of these things likely make it much easier for you to swallow the drug. However, you might not be so lucky; earlier in this chapter we discuss reasons why some medicines must be swallowed whole (see "Can I split the drug?").

Swallowing liquid medicines

If you are prescribed a liquid medicine, remember these two important things:

✔ If the liquid is in the form of a *suspension* (that is, a liquid in which the medicine is present in tiny, non-dissolved particles), thoroughly shake the container so the contents are completely mixed together before you pour out your dose. (Your pharmacist will advise you if you need to shake your medicine.)

✔ Household teaspoons and tablespoons (unless they are "measuring spoons") do not necessarily hold a true teaspoon (5 mL) or tablespoon (15 mL) of liquid, so be sure to use a proper measuring device when pouring out your dose.

In the eye of the beholder: Eye drops and ointments

For many people, using eye drops and ointments is quite a challenge. In this section we provide the steps to follow to make this often difficult task somewhat easier.

You may find it preferable to have someone else put the eye drops or ointments in your eye for you.

Using eye drops

When you need to give yourself an eye drop, follow these steps:

1. Wash your hands with soap and water (to avoid transferring any germs from your hands to your eye medicine or to your eye).

2. Draw up the eye drop medicine from the container into the eye dropper. Make sure the end of the eye dropper does not touch the counter, as this might contaminate the dropper with germs. (For similar reasons, avoid having the eye dropper touch your face or your eye.)

3. Tilt your head backward and look up toward the ceiling.

4. With one hand, gently pull down the lower lid of the eye. With the other, hold the eye dropper.

5. Bring the eye dropper close to the eye without touching it. Approaching from the side is usually best. Resting your hand on your cheek helps keep the hand steady. When ready, squeeze the dropper gently to place the required number of drops into the eye. You may find it easiest to keep the eye closed for several minutes after putting the drops into the eye.

Using a mirror might make the above process easier.

Sometimes, it's recommended you put some gentle pressure on the inside corner of the eyelid after using drops so less of the medication travels through the tear duct and drains into the nose. This keeps the eye drop medicine in the eye longer so it has more time to do its job and also reduces the amount of medicine absorbed into your body (and so minimizes side-effects). Ask your doctor whether your particular condition requires this.

If you use contact lenses, be sure to remove them before using your eye drops and don't reinsert them for at least 15 minutes after your dose. (As we discuss in Chapter 6, many eye drops contain a preservative that can damage contact lenses.) Also, if you're using more than one type of eye drop, wait at least 5 minutes between using the different types.

Using eye ointments

The method to administer eye ointment is basically the same as with eye drops, except you need to squeeze a small ribbon of oint-ment into the pocket you have opened between the eye and the lower lid. Blink the eye for several minutes to spread the ointment across the eye. Ointments are a bit gooey, so it may take several minutes before you can see clearly again.

Hear, hear! Ear drops

Medication for your ears is usually supplied in the form of drops and comes in a small bottle with a pointed spout or a dropper.

Here's that to do when you need to give yourself an ear drop:

1. Wash your hands with soap and water (to avoid transfer-ring any germs from your hands to your ear medicine). Also wash the ear area with soap and water and then dry the area carefully.

2. Draw up the ear drop medicine from the container into the ear dropper. (This is not necessary if the medicine is in a container with its own spout.) Make sure the end of the ear dropper does not touch the counter, as this might contami-nate the dropper with germs. (For similar reasons, avoid having the ear dropper touch your ear canal itself.)

3. Tilt your head so the side that needs the medication is pointing upward.

4. Gently pull the ear up and slightly backward to straighten out the ear canal.

5. Hold the dropper near the opening of the ear.

6. Gently squeeze the dropper to expel the correct number of drops into your ear.

7. Keep the treated ear in the "ear up" position for about 5 minutes to enable the medication to work its way down into the far reaches of the ear canal.

If you're helping another person apply drops, the process is the same except for very young children, whose ear canals are of a different shape. For children under age three, gently pull the top of the ear down and back just before you expel the drops from the dropper into the ear. (Holding the mid portion rather than the uppermost portion of the ear makes this easier.) Holding the child on your lap is often useful — it's comforting for the child and provides easy control for you.

Your ear drop will feel more comfortable in your ear canal if the medicine is at room temperature when used.

On the nose: Nose drops and sprays

Whether you're blessed with a pert little button or equally blessed with a beautiful Jimmy Durante "schnozzola," following the steps in this section will help you take your nose drops and sprays effectively.

Using nose drops

When you need to give yourself a nose drop, do the following:

1. Before using your nose drops, gently blow your nose.

2. Wash your hands with soap and water (to avoid transferring any germs from your hands to your medicine).

3. Draw up the nose drop medicine from the container into the nose dropper. Make sure the end of the nose dropper does not touch the counter, as this might contaminate the dropper with germs. (For similar reasons, avoid having the nose dropper touch the inside of your nose.)

4. Lie down and tilt your head backward.

5. Hold the dropper just outside your nostril and then gently squeeze the dropper so the correct number of drops is administered.

6. Stay lying down for a minute or two to enable the drops to be absorbed.

Don't blow your nose right after using nose drops or that hard work you just went through will all be for nought (and we can safely say your facial tissue was not in need of nose drop medicine).

Using nose sprays

The procedure to follow for taking a nose spray differs depending on the particular spray being used. Read the instructions that come with your particular spray to find out the specifics. Here are the general steps to follow:

1. Prime or shake the nose spray container (the need for this depends on the specific medicine you have been prescribed).

2. Gently blow your nose to clear your nostrils.

3. Close one nostril by applying your finger to the outside of that part of your nose.

4. Tilt your head slightly forward and insert the tip of the nose spray container into your nostril. Make sure you keep the container upright.

5. Spray while breathing gently inward, keeping your mouth closed.

6. Breathe out through your mouth.

Hit me with your best shot: Inhalers

Inhalers (often called "puffers;" the fancy medical term is "metered dose inhaler") are plastic containers into which one inserts a small, metal, pressurized canister containing medicine (typically used for asthma and chronic bronchitis). When we talk about inhalers we are almost always referring to the combination of plastic container and metal canister. When the inhaler is activated, the medicine inside the canister is released as an aerosol (similar to the way spray deodorants work) and travels down into the lungs.

Inhalers are typically best administered using a spacer device, the most popular of which is called an "AeroChamber." A spacer device has two ends: one attaches to the inhaler, and the other you put in your mouth (see Figure 4-2).

Spacer devices are helpful for three main reasons:

✔ They make it easier to use the inhaler.

✔ They enable more of the inhaler medicine to get down into your lungs, which is where you want it to go (without a spacer device more of the medicine simply ends up being deposited in your mouth).

✔ They reduce the likelihood of getting a hoarse voice (hoarseness is a common side-effect from using an inhaler without a spacer device).

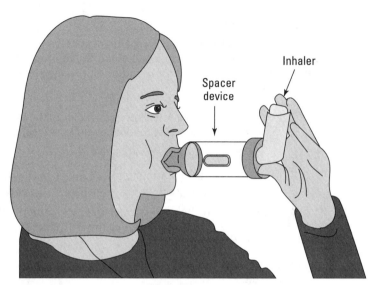

Figure 4-2: An inhaler and a spacer device.

Using an inhaler without a spacer device

When you need to give yourself an inhaler and are *not* using a spacer device, follow these steps:

1. Remove the protective cap from the inhaler's opening.

2. Shake the inhaler.

3. Hold the inhaler in your hand with your index finger on the top of the canister and your thumb on the under-side of the canister. Hold the inhaler a few centimetres (about the width of two to three fingers) from your lips.

4. Breathe out.

5. Press down on the top of the inhaler (which triggers the release of the medicine) just as you start to take a slow, deep breath in.

6. Hold your breath for 10 seconds, then exhale and breathe normally.

7. If you have been prescribed more than one dose ("puff"), wait a minute or so after the preceding dose before giving the next one.

8. If your inhaler is a steroid medicine, gargle and rinse your mouth after you've used it to reduce your likelihood of getting thrush (an oral yeast infection that can be caused by inhaled steroids).

Using an inhaler with a spacer device

Here are the steps to follow when you use an inhaler and you *are* using a spacer device:

1. Remove the protective cap from the inhaler's opening and attach the spacer device.

2. Shake the inhaler.

3. Put the mouthpiece end of the spacer device into your mouth and seal your lips securely around the mouthpiece.

4. Breathe out.

5. Press down on the top of the inhaler (which triggers the release of the medicine).

6. With the spacer device still in your mouth, take two to three slow, deep breaths. Some spacers have a whistle that sounds if you are breathing in too quickly. If you hear the whistle, slow down the speed at which you are breathing in.

7. If you have been prescribed more than one dose ("puff"), wait a minute or so after the preceding dose before giving the next one.

8. If your inhaler is a steroid medicine, gargle and rinse your mouth after you've used it to reduce your likelihood of getting thrush (an oral yeast infection that can be caused by inhaled steroids).

You can watch a video showing how puffers are to be used at www.umich.edu/~pharmacy/inhaler/im-mdi/index.html.

If the inhaler is being used on a young child, you can attach a small face mask to the end of the spacer device; the child then breathes through the face mask rather than inserting the spacer into her mouth. Children typically find this easier.

You don't want to be in need of your inhaler only to find it's empty. A simple — but not particularly accurate — way of determining how much medicine is left is to remove the canister from the plastic container and estimate its weight compared to when you obtained the new prescription from your pharmacist. A better technique is to ask your pharmacist what date you can expect to run out of medicine based on the prescribed dose and the size of the canister. Mark the date on your calendar (and, with a non-erasable marker, on the canister itself). As the date nears, be sure to pick up a refill from your pharmacy. Don't wait until the last minute; the date is only an *estimate* of when your puffer will run out. (This technique is of value only for puffers you use on a regular basis; it won't work for puffers you use intermittently.)

Recently, an increasing variety of new devices that use a dry powder have made their way onto the market. Some people find them easier to use than the traditional aerosol inhalers we describe above. Dry powder inhalers include the Aerolizer, the Diskus, the Handihaler, and the Turbuhaler. Each has its own technique for use, so if you're prescribed one of these newer devices we recommend you ask your pharmacist or physician to advise you how to administer it.

Another far less common way for inhaled medicines to be administered is by using a compressor that delivers a fine mist of medication though a mask. This topic is beyond the scope of this book, but more information is available from a variety of sources including the Asthma Society of Canada (www.asthma.ca).

Getting it in the end: Suppositories and enemas

In this section we look at the most effective way to administer suppositories and enemas.

Using suppositories

Here's what to do when you need to give yourself a suppository:

1. Wash your hands with soap and water.

2. Prepare the suppository. Feel the suppository while it's still in its wrapper. It should feel firm. If it feels soft, place the suppository — still in its wrapper — in cold water and it will become more solid and easier to use. If only half a suppository is prescribed, you can cut the suppository length-wise.

3. Insert the suppository. Lying down is easiest, on your side with your top leg drawn up toward your abdomen. Lubricate the end of the unwrapped suppository (a lubricant such as K-Y Jelly is preferred over one similar to Vaseline). Find the rectum (it's actually the "anus" you're finding, but heck, if you're brave enough to be exploring down there let's not get too technical, eh?), and gently push the suppository into the rectum (wearing a finger cot or disposable glove may make this easier for you) about 2 ½ centimetres (one inch) for adults, or 1 centimetre (one-half inch) for children.

4. Hold your buttocks closed for a few minutes and maintain a lying down posture for 15 minutes after inserting the suppository; this helps keep it in place.

Using enemas

When you need to give yourself an enema, follow these steps:

1. Remove the protective tip from the enema container (most enemas are supplied already prepared for you).

2. If the enema container nozzle tip is not pre-lubricated (they usually are), you can add a lubricant such as K-Y Jelly.

3. Insert the nozzle tip into the rectum, pointing the tip toward your navel (bellybutton). While this might cause a feeling of pressure, it should not be painful.

4. With the nozzle tip inserted, apply gentle pressure to the enema container until most of the contents of the container have been emptied (into the rectum).

5. Remain lying down (with the enema retained in your rectum) for the length of time your physician or pharmacist has recommended, then proceed to the bathroom to evacuate the materials from your rectum.

For Women Only: Vaginal preparations

Medications designed to be used in the vagina can be inserted by using a finger or by using a special applicator.

1. Wash your hands with soap and water.

2. Position yourself on your back with knees bent and spread apart.

3. Using either your finger or the applicator, insert the medicine (supplied either as a tablet, suppository, or *ovule*, which is a soft capsule), wide end first, into the innermost part of the vagina.

Creams, ointments, and gels are best inserted using the same position, but generally require use of an applicator.

Rubbing it in: Lotions, creams, ointments, and patches

In this section we look at the most effective way to administer topical drugs; that is, medicines such as lotions, creams, ointments, and patches you put on your skin.

Using lotions, creams, and ointments

Most lotions require shaking before you use them, but creams and ointments do not. These types of medication should be applied to clean, dry skin unless you have been directed otherwise. Usually, a thin layer of the medication is sufficient. (More is not necessarily better.) Avoid having the opening of the container touch the skin to help prevent the contents from getting contaminated.

Using patches

Patches should be applied to clean, dry skin. Avoid areas where there's an open wound (such as cuts and scrapes), excess skin buildup (calluses), lots of skin creases and folds, or where a patch is likely to get rubbed (such as under a waistband or bra strap). When possible avoid areas with lots of hair, to make the patch easier to remove later. Rotating the exact location of your patch keeps skin irritation to a minimum.

To apply the patch, peel off the protective backing and then, without touching the inside area where the medication is located, apply it smoothly on the skin. Hold the patch down for 15 seconds to ensure the adhesive is attached to the skin.

Needling questions: Injections

Self-administration of insulin comprises the great majority of injections Canadians give themselves. (That may change in the future as new ways of giving insulin emerge; for example, insulin given by inhaler is now approved for use in the United States, but not in Canada. Incidentally, the long-term safety of inhaled insulin is not yet known.)

Administering insulin

In Canada, insulin is typically injected using an insulin pen device. Insulin pen devices keep getting better and better, and the two newest devices on the Canadian market are truly wonderful. They are pictured in Figure 4-3.

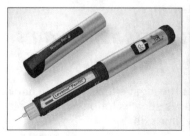 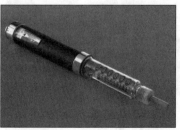

Figure 4-3: Novolin-Pen 4 and HumaPen Luxura.

The mechanics of the process differ depending on which insulin pen device you're using, whether it's one of the two models shown in Figure 4-3 or one of the older — but still very good — devices. Given these differences, and the reality that even small errors in insulin dosing can be hazardous, we strongly recommend you meet with a diabetes educator (or pharmacist with particular expertise in this area) to be taught how to use an insulin pen. This advice also applies if you're prescribed an old-style insulin syringe.

Regardless of which pen device (or syringe) you're using, avoid repeatedly injecting insulin into one small area of your body. Doing so leads to the development of collections of fat (called *lipohypertrophy*) in the area of the injections that over time can become larger than the size of a tennis ball. Moreover, insulin absorption from areas of lipohypertrophy is inconsistent and can cause erratic blood glucose control. Again, we very strongly recommend you meet with a diabetes educator to discuss insulin injection rotation techniques.

Administering epinephrine (adrenaline)

If you have severe allergies, your doctor may prescribe an emergency kit containing epinephrine for you to give yourself should the need arise. In Canada, several versions of this kit exist including the EpiPen or, for children, the EpiPen Jr. We recommend when you pick this up from your pharmacy that you sit down with the pharmacist and have them give you detailed advice about how you are to administer this.

A video demonstrating the use of an EpiPen is available at www.epipen.com/howtouse.aspx.

When you give yourself an injection of epinephrine you should, nonetheless, seek immediate medical attention. (Record the exact time the EpiPen was used, and inform the nurse or physician.)

Self-injected medication is being used increasingly frequently in the treatment of a variety of other conditions, including blood clots, some forms of arthritis, infertility, and cancer. If you're asked to perform these forms of specialized injection, ensure that your physician, pharmacist or another appropriately trained member of your health care team instructs you upon their use.

Looking After Your Medication

We grew up always knowing where the household medicines were kept — where else but the bathroom medicine cabinet? It was where most everyone kept their medicines. Little did we know the bathroom is one of the worst places to keep prescription drugs!

In this section, we discuss how to look after your medicines so
they can continue to look after you.

Storing your medication

Here are some important things to know about storing your
medicines:

- ✔ **Most medicines should be stored at room temperature.**
  Some exceptions — such as insulin — exist, where keeping
  them refrigerated is best. Just make sure refrigerated medicines don't freeze, as this may destroy their effectiveness.

- ✔ **Avoid excess humidity.** Excess humidity can reduce the
  potency of some medicines (and therein lies the reason for
  not storing your medicines in the bathroom; however, a bathroom that doesn't have a shower or bath is okay).

- ✔ **Keep your medicines in a separate location from those
  belonging to other members of your family.** Sharing a medicine cabinet is fine, but use different shelves for different
  family members.

- ✔ **If you have young children, store your medicines in a
  locked cabinet.** Even if your own children are all grown, you
  may be lucky enough to have your grandchildren visiting you,
  so storing your medicines safely away from their curious
  hands and minds remains crucial.

- ✔ **Avoid exposing some medicines to direct sunlight, which
  reduces their potency.**

You can discard the little wad of cotton from the top of your pill
bottle — it was placed there solely to prevent the pills from bounc-
ing around and breaking during shipping.

If you have a medicine you're not likely to use and thus won't
examine on a day-to-day basis, such as an EpiPen, mark the expiry
date on your calendar as a reminder to get it refilled when this
date nears.

We close out this section with a quick list of our absolute least
favourite places to store medicines:

- ✔ **In your car:** Too hot, too cold, too hard to get out of bed to
  trundle down to the car when you realize you forgot your
  pills there.

- ✔ **In your back pocket:** Well, this place actually isn't too bad so
  long as you don't mind never sitting down.

Dealing with leftover medication

A little while back, a no-doubt well intentioned inventor designed a plastic garbage bag that, upon being discarded, gradually breaks down into thousands of tiny fragments. It was proposed as an environmentally friendly option. Except all it ended up doing was changing one big piece of non-biodegradable plastic into thousands of little pieces of non-biodegradable plastic. Next idea...!

It used to be that leftover medication was simply flushed down the toilet, or thrown into the garbage. (Well, that is still often done.) But it has to end up somewhere, and medicine discarded in this way ends up in the water supply or landfill sites. Some evidence suggests even the low-level exposure to humans that ultimately results can be detrimental to our collective health. It's far better to dispose of any leftover medication in a safer way.

If you have medicines you won't be using (either because you don't need them anymore or because they are beyond their expiry date), your pharmacist is happy to assist you with discarding them. Just toss them in a bag and drop them off next time you're in the drugstore. The drugstore arranges for their safe disposal. (And while you're at it, grab the opportunity to go through your medicine cabinet and remove any outdated non-prescription drugs, too.)

 If you're using medication for which you give yourself injections, you can pick up a biohazard container from your pharmacy for collecting your used needles. When the container is full, simply seal it and drop it off at your pharmacy for safe disposal. (Not all pharmacies provide this service, so check with them beforehand.) In some cities the municipal biohazard station takes these, but you have to drop the sealed container off personally; it can't be left at the curbside with your garbage or recycling.

On the Road Again: Travelling with a Prescription Medicine

The clever person who came up with the jingle "Don't leave home without it" may just as easily have been talking about prescription drugs. If you are travelling, remembering to take your prescription medicines with you is surely the first step; *how* you take them with you is, as the famous American broadcaster Paul Harvey would say, "the rest of the story."

Preparing for your trip

Here are the most important prescription drug-related things for you to do in advance of your trip:

- ✔ Make sure you have a sufficient supply on hand to last for the duration of your trip (plus an extra few days — hey, there might be a snowstorm back home that forces you to suffer through an extra weekend on that Caribbean beach!).

- ✔ If you don't have enough, be sure to pick up a sufficient supply from your pharmacist before you leave.

- ✔ Keep your drugs in their original containers and make sure the prescription labels are affixed.

- ✔ If you use injectable drugs (for example, insulin) or lancets (for example, when you have diabetes and need to test your blood glucose levels), obtain a travel letter from your physician stating your need for these items to be with you at all times (that is, NOT kept in your checked luggage).

- ✔ If you use narcotic medication, obtain a travel letter from your physician stating the names of the medications you'll be carrying and, if possible, why you need them.

Packing your prescription medicine

If you're flying, it's best to always keep your prescription drugs with you, either on your person or in your carry-on luggage; not in your checked luggage. Airlines lose luggage (trust us; we know!).

If you're travelling by car through hot or cold climates and are carrying medicines that should not be subjected to extremes of temperature, remember not to leave them in the car for more than a brief period of time. (In particular, don't leave such drugs in your car overnight.)

When you get to your destination, put your medications in an appropriate location.

Forgetting your prescription medicine at home

If you arrive at your destination only to get a sickening feeling in the pit of your stomach as you frantically search through your belongings in a valiant but fruitless attempt to find your drugs — which, you eventually realize, are back home, nicely labelled and in their original containers but sitting on your dresser — don't despair. All is not lost!

The most reassuring thing about this situation is that very, very few ailments exist for which missing a dose or two of medication leads to disastrous consequences. Therefore, in most cases you have some time to scramble to find a solution to your predicament.

The easiest solution is often to have someone back home courier your drugs to you ASAP. If that's not feasible and you've travelled only within your province or territory, you can call your physician's office or home pharmacist and ask them to call or fax your prescription to the pharmacy nearest your current location.

If you've travelled within Canada but outside your home province or territory, you can still contact your physician or pharmacist and ask them to call (or fax) your prescription to the nearest pharmacy, but because this is outside their jurisdiction (physicians and pharmacists are governed by provincial/territorial regulations, not national regulations) the local pharmacy may not be able to help you. For example, if you're an Albertan visiting Ontario, your pharmacy in Alberta can fax your prescription to an Ontario pharmacist, who can fill the prescription only if in her professional judgment she believes you need the drug immediately.

It's unlikely a pharmacy would honour a prescription from outside the country, so if you've travelled outside Canada and are in need of a prescription you'll likely need to visit the nearest health care facility and explain your predicament to a physician. In most cases they'll be able to help you. Bear in mind, though, that although it may be relatively simple to obtain prescriptions for routine drugs — such as medicines for arthritis, hypertension, and so forth — physicians who do not know you may be understandably hesitant to issue a prescription for narcotics or other drugs often sold illegally on the street.

Some drugs you've obtained with a prescription are actually over-the-counter or behind-the-counter products in other areas. You may be able to replace some of your forgotten medicines simply by asking the pharmacist for them.

Your prescription drug may go by a different trade name in other countries. For example, in Canada Flomax is the trade name for tamsulosin, a drug used to treat an enlarged prostate. However, if you were prescribed Flomax in Italy, you'd be the proud owner of morniflumate, a drug used to treat inflammation. Generic names are much more likely to be the same from country to country, so if you ever need to have a forgotten prescription drug from Canada refilled elsewhere, be sure to ask for it by its generic, not trade name.

Why Your Prescription Drug Might Not Be Working

It can be so, so frustrating when things aren't working out the way they should. In this section we look at reasons why a prescription drug might not work the way it should, and suggest some ways you can be proactive in correcting the problem.

Are you sure your medicine is not working?

Before your physician can figure out *why* your drug is not working, she needs to first determine *whether* your drug is not working. It's all fairly straightforward if you're taking a medicine to treat a symptom. For example, if you're taking acetaminophen (Tylenol) to treat backache but your pain does not improve, then the medicine is probably not doing you much good. But what about medicines you're taking not to *treat* symptoms, but to *prevent* an illness or complication from an illness? How can you know whether a medicine is working in this type of situation?

Your prescription drug is probably *not* helping you if

- ✔ You're taking a medication to lower your blood pressure (an "anti-hypertensive agent") but your blood pressure has not improved.

- ✔ You're being treated with a medicine to lower your elevated blood glucose levels but your blood glucose levels haven't fallen.

- ✔ You've started a medication to improve your angina but your angina is as bad as ever.

On the other hand, consider a few examples where a prescription drug may well be working beautifully but you don't necessarily recognize it:

- ✔ You have coronary artery disease (we discuss this in Chapter 5) and are being treated with ASA. You feel no different on the ASA than you did before you started it. However, taking the ASA has helped you avoid having a heart attack.

- ✔ You have high cholesterol and have started simvastatin. You felt fine before and you feel fine now. However, your blood cholesterol level is now much lower and your risk of having a stroke is reduced.

These are but two examples of what could be a very lengthy list. As you can see, sometimes benefits from prescription drugs are not clear cut, and the *absence* of something may be the best indicator your medicine is in fact doing its job.

Are you taking the right medicine?

If you're not benefiting from your prescription (which may or may not be immediately apparent, as we discuss in the preceding section), one possible cause is that you're not taking the right medicine. This situation can exist when

✔ **You were diagnosed with (and are being treated for) condition A, but you actually have condition B.** Medicine is an imprecise science, and not infrequently the right diagnosis is not immediately hit upon. If you are not responding to treatment, get in touch with your doctor so she can re-evaluate her diagnosis and therapy. (In Chapter 3, we discuss ways you can help determine whether your medicine is working effectively for you.)

✔ **You were diagnosed correctly and are on the appropriate medicine for that condition, but aren't as responsive as others to that drug.** Nonetheless, things are not getting any better. It may simply be that a very effective medicine for your next door neighbour's irritable bowel syndrome (for example) may not be equally effective for *your* irritable bowel syndrome.

Many drugs have "non-response rates" as high as 30 percent (meaning three out of ten people will not respond to a given medication), and doctors are typically unable to predict which of their patients will be within this 30 percent. This makes prescribing drugs somewhat hit and miss. So, you may end up being switched from drug A to drug B to drug C until you finally end up on a medicine that works well for you. (The non-response rate will likely dramatically improve in the future as science develops more sophisticated ways to assess whether a given individual will respond favourably to a particular medicine.)

✔ **You were, quite literally, taking the wrong medication.** Hmmm, you sure do feel sleepy when you first awaken in the morning and force yourself to get out of bed. And the room is dark and your eyesight isn't quite what it used to be. So when you reach for that pill bottle you recently got, you don't happen to notice the label says Billy Smith — not a big deal, except that you happen to be Becky Smith and you just swallowed your husband's Viagra. You contact your physician and are reassured no harm is going to come to you, and the upshot is that you make sure the room is sufficiently well-lit for you to carefully read the prescription label before ever taking another pill!

Are you on the right dose of the medicine?

The great majority of medicines are manufactured in a variety of doses, for a simple reason: different people respond differently to different doses. So it could well be you've been prescribed an excellent medication, but you're not responding to it because the dose is insufficient to meet your needs. (We talk more about doses at the beginning of the chapter.)

Doctors often start a patient on a very small dose of a medication. It's typically better to be cautious and underdose a patient, later increasing the dose if the patient isn't responding, than to prescribe too strong a dose and find that the patient becomes ill because the dose was too much.

ANECDOTE

Never underestimate the importance of a decimal place

Because medication errors happen, it is important that you know what to watch for with your medication and that you bring your medicines with you to your appointments...

Jean-Paul was a 45-year-old man whom Ian diagnosed with thyroid cancer. Jean-Paul had his thyroid surgically removed, and was placed on thyroid pills. His thyroid levels were too low on a dose of 0.2 mg per day, so Ian wrote a prescription for a higher dose of 0.25 mg per day.

A couple of months later, Jean-Paul called Ian to say he was feeling very tired and achy. Ian was surprised by this unexpected turn of events and advised his patient to come in straight away. As Ian always does with his patients, he reminded Jean-Paul to bring his medicine in its original container with him to the visit. When Jean-Paul handed Ian his thyroid pill bottle, Ian gasped; the pills were *0.025* mg, not the prescribed *0.25* mg!

Ian checked the original prescription and found he had written it correctly; the pharmacist had accidentally dispensed the wrong dose. Fortunately, Jean-Paul had been wise enough to know to seek medical attention when he wasn't responding to the prescribed medicine as he thought he should. And more fortunately, there was no serious consequence from the mistake.

The morals of the story? One, if you know what a medicine is supposed to do you'll be more likely to know when it's *not* doing what it should (and thus you will know to seek medical attention). And two, *everyone* makes mistakes — even the most conscientious of pharmacists (and physicians) — so bringing your medicines with you to each and every appointment makes it much more likely the mistake will be detected if a prescription has been written or dispensed in error.

If you've been prescribed a medication in a low dose and your doctor subsequently increases the dose, don't automatically interpret this as indicative of a more severe problem. Often, it's simply a case of "one size doesn't fit all." You may wear size 9 shoes and your friend may wear size 10 shoes — your shoe size doesn't reflect the health of your feet, and your pill strength typically doesn't reflect the severity of your ailment.

Are you taking the prescription properly?

For your prescription medicine to work effectively, you need to take it properly. This may sound simple enough, but it actually involves a whole bunch of different steps. We discuss many of these steps elsewhere in this chapter, but here we highlight a few especially important points.

To benefit from your prescription drug, make sure of the following:

- ✔ You're taking the medicine prescribed for *you* (that is, *your* name is on the label).

- ✔ You're taking the medicine the number of times per day the label advises.

- ✔ You're taking the medicine in the dose prescribed for you.

- ✔ You're taking the medicine (if oral) with or without food depending on the instructions you got from your pharmacist.

- ✔ You're not splitting the medicine unless you've been specifically advised by your pharmacist or physician this will not interfere with the medicine's function.

- ✔ You're not taking an expired medicine. If your medicine came in a package marked with an expiry date, make sure that this date has not yet passed.

- ✔ You've stored the medicine properly to ensure that it hasn't gone bad because it was exposed to extremes of temperature, excess humidity, or excess sunlight.

Is the medicine being absorbed into your body?

In Chapter 2 we look at how oral medicines are absorbed into your body so they can then reach the part of you in need of help.

In some situations, a medicine may not be working because it's not being properly absorbed. Here are some examples of this:

- ✔ **Previous stomach surgery:** If you've had a portion of your stomach removed (for example, as treatment for ulcers) or bypassed (as may be done in the treatment of severe obesity), this can lead to ineffective absorption of many things including medicines.

- ✔ **Use of other, conflicting, medicines:** The absorption of some medicines, such as L-thyroxine, is impeded if you simultaneously ingest iron or calcium. This can be remedied, as we discuss in Chapter 6, by separating the timing of these medicines by a few hours or more.

- ✔ **Simultaneous ingestion of food:** Some medicines require you to take them on an empty stomach for proper absorption into your body.

- ✔ **Diseases of the small intestine:** If you have damage to your small intestine (which can be caused by many things including celiac disease or previous small intestine surgery), then a number of substances may not be absorbed into your body including nutrients from the foods you eat, vitamins, and, in this case, medicines.

If you're not able to absorb oral medicines because of a damaged bowel, you may need to take your drugs by another route, such as injection.

Part II
Ailments A to Z

The 5th Wave   By Rich Tennant

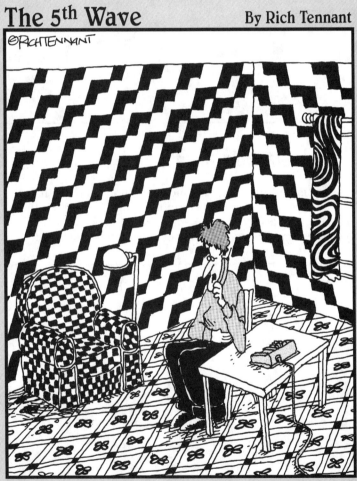

"I'd like to see the doctor as soon as possible.
It's the darnedest thing. I'm getting nauseous,
dizzy, and disoriented from this medication, too."

In this part . . .

*W*e look at some of the most common ailments that are treated with prescription drugs. We discuss the general approach to treating these conditions and point out those medicines that are most highly recommended.

Chapter 5

Ailments and Their Treatment

. . . .

In This Chapter

▶ Looking at common medical ailments

▶ Choosing the best medications for what ails you

. . . .

*I*n this chapter we look at the general approach to treating a wide variety of ailments. As you might imagine, many thousands of different diseases exist, so we have necessarily focused on those conditions most commonly affecting Canadians. We present a brief overview of an illness and then look at the medications available to help you deal with it.

Conventions We Use in This Chapter

Because this is a book on prescription drug therapy, we focus our attentions on medical, as opposed to surgical, treatments — which means you won't find a step-by-step guide here to taking out your appendix or removing your gallbladder.

The information we share is based on a number of sources, including, where available, "clinical practice guidelines" (recommendations made by leading experts in their fields). It is *very* important to recognize that in medicine few "rules" exist, and seldom is there an absolutely right or wrong way to treat a disease (indeed, for some ailments many different sets of guidelines exist, all recommending different things!).

It's also very important to be aware that the world of medicine is very rapidly changing and every day new research comes out pointing to new directions in therapy. So, if your doctor is treating you in a way that differs from what we discuss in this chapter, don't take it to mean he or she is providing you with inappropriate care.

For many health problems, lifestyle change and *non*-prescription drugs have important roles to play. *Understanding Prescription Drugs For Canadians For Dummies,* however, focuses — as you would expect from the title — on prescription drugs. We don't want you to interpret this to mean your non-prescription therapies are unimportant — they're simply not the focus of our attention in this book.

We use generic drug names in this chapter. (We talk about the difference between brand-name and generic drugs in Chapter 2.) You can find the generic name of your prescription drug on the label affixed to the container your medicine came in. You can also find the generic name for a drug in the cross-referenced Drug Index at the back of this book.

In this chapter, to make it easier for you to pick out the names of drugs and drug families we **bold** individual drug names and ***bold and italicize*** drug families. To avoid appearing, ahem, overly bold, we generally bold only the first occurrence of a term within a paragraph (or section).

In Chapter 6 we look in detail at many different drug families. We've set it up alphabetically so you can quickly find the drug family you want more information on. If you're unsure what family of drug your medicine belongs to, no worries, just flip to our handy-dandy Drug Index at the back of the book and it will point you to the right page(s).

Many ailments go by more than one name, so if you can't find the condition you're looking for have a look at the index, which can direct you to the appropriate place in this chapter.

Acne

Acne is a condition in which hormonal changes in the body lead to an excess production of skin oils, blocked pores, and an increase in the number of normal skin bacteria *(Propionibacterium acnes)*; collectively, these circumstances result in the development of pimples. Contrary to popular wisdom, acne is *not* caused by eating chocolate (phew!) or greasy food. Also, acne is not caused by "dirty" skin, so vigorous washing doesn't help — if anything, it makes things worse.

If you have acne that doesn't respond sufficiently well to routine hygiene and over-the-counter therapy (typically with **benzoyl peroxide**), prescription medication may be required. In this case most doctors will recommend a topical ***retinoid*** (**adapalene, tazarotene,** or **tretinoin**) and, when necessary, a topical ***antibiotic*** (most commonly **erythromycin** or **clindamycin**).

If, after a few months of therapy, this approach has not been successful, or if you have more severe acne, an oral *antibiotic* (usually **tetracycline** but sometimes **doxycycline**, **minocycline**, **erythromycin**, or **sulfamethoxazole/trimethoprim**) is often added. If this, too, has not helped you, then women may take certain types of *oral contraceptives* (**Alesse**, **Diane-35**, or **Tri-Cyclen**) or a medication such as **spironolactone** that blocks the action of male hormones. (Both men and women have male hormones, though women have far less.) In men, and in women for whom these latter medications have not been successful, **isotretinoin** (an oral *retinoid*) is used.

Oral retinoids (and possibly topical retinoids as well) can damage the fetus of a pregnant woman and therefore MUST NOT be taken if you're pregnant or if you're sexually active and not using sufficient contraception. If you're being considered for retinoid therapy, your doctor needs to discuss these issues in detail with you before you start taking the medicine.

Addison's Disease

Addison's disease is a condition, usually caused by *autoantibodies* (that is, antibodies that have attacked part of our own body), in which the *adrenal glands* (small glands located just above the kidneys) are irreparably damaged. As a result, your body becomes unable to manufacture essential hormones called *corticosteroids*. Two types of corticosteroids exist:

- ✔ **Glucocorticoids:** A deficiency leads to weight loss, fatigue, nausea, abdominal pain, and malaise (that is, you feel generally unwell).

- ✔ **Mineralocorticoids:** A deficiency leads to an imbalance of the body's sodium and potassium levels, which in turn can result in dehydration and, if severe, heart rhythm problems.

Addison's disease is treated by replacing your body's missing hormones with their equivalent in the form of pills. Missing *glucocorticoid* hormones are replaced with either **prednisone**, **dexamethasone**, or **hydrocortisone**, and missing *mineralocorticoid* hormones are replaced with **fludrocortisone**. Your doctor can determine the best dose of these medicines based on how you're feeling, what she finds (especially in terms of your blood pressure) when she examines you, and what your sodium and potassium levels are on a blood test.

If you have Addison's disease and you become ill with some other acute health problem such as an infection, you'll need to take a higher dose of your glucocorticoid medication until you're better. As a preventive measure, make sure you speak to your physician to find out how high a dose to take and for how long to take it, so you'll be prepared should such an event happen.

Alcoholism

Alcoholism (*alcohol dependence*) is a condition in which a person's drinking pattern leads to significant and recurring harm, both to him or herself and, often, to others. Alcohol dependence has no single cause, and it's often related to an interplay of genetic, psychological, physiological, and social factors.

Very few medications are available to treat alcohol dependence. **Disulfiram** (Antabuse) is occasionally prescribed. This medicine works by providing disincentive to drink — if you consume alcohol while taking this medicine you will feel dreadful, with flushing, nausea, vomiting, and a feeling of anxiety. Sometimes, **naltrexone** is prescribed. This drug works by reducing an alcohol-dependent person's drive to consume alcohol.

Allergies

The body has an amazing, exquisitely intricate, immune system that works to protect us from many things including germs. If you have allergies, however, your immune system has gotten its signals crossed and behaves inappropriately by reacting to substances (such as bee stings, peanuts, dust mites, animal dander, ragweed, and certain drugs) your body would normally tolerate.

Allergic reactions can range from relatively minor symptoms such as a stuffy nose or itchy eyes to severe problems such as breathing difficulties and shock. Severe allergy attacks are called *anaphylactic reactions.* The main substances in the body responsible for allergic reactions are histamine and — likely less familiar to you — prostaglandins and leukotrienes.

The most important part of therapy is to avoid exposure to things you're allergic to (these substances are called *allergens*). When that is either not possible or not sufficient, your doctor may recommend one or more of the following drugs (and/or "allergy shots"):

  ✔ *Antihistamines* are the most commonly used drugs.
    Antihistamines work, as you might imagine from the name,
    by combatting the effects of histamine.

  ✔ If an antihistamine is not sufficient and your main problem is
    with itchy, irritated eyes, your doctor may prescribe **sodium
    cromoglycate** eye drops. These work by preventing certain
    cells (*mast cells*) in your body from releasing histamine,
    prostaglandins, and leukotrienes.

  ✔ If these measures are not sufficient, *glucocorticoid* medica-
    tions are often required (these are given, depending on your
    particular situation, by one of many different routes including
    by inhaler, by nasal spray, as eye drops, or as pills).

If you're prone to severe allergic reactions, carry an emergency
epinephrine (*adrenaline*) kit with you at all times. (Epinephrine kits
go by several names including EpiPen and Twinject auto-injector.)
Also ask your doctor whether you should carry antihistamine
tablets with you.

Alzheimer's Disease

Alzheimer's disease is the most common type of dementia. *Dementia*
refers to a group of diseases that cause deterioration of your
memory and a loss of the processes enabling you to understand and
interpret the world around you. As a result, there's a decline in the
ability to function independently; this can progress to the point that
managing "activities of daily living" (routine activities such as personal care and navigating around your own home) becomes difficult.

The underlying cause(s) of Alzheimer's disease is unknown —
however, it has been discovered that affected individuals have a
buildup in the brain of a substance called *amyloid* and also have
low brain levels of an important chemical messenger called
acetylcholine. The uncovering of the latter fact has led to the discovery of new treatments, and in the future many more, better
therapies are certain to emerge.

Current therapies, unfortunately, have met with only limited success. For early Alzheimer's disease, *cholinesterase inhibitors* can
help. For more advanced disease, *NMDA receptor antagonists*
have been tried, but again, with only limited success.

Be aware that before a diagnosis of Alzheimer's disease is made,
it's important that your doctor exclude other causes of dementia
including strokes, low levels of vitamin B12, liver disease, and an
underfunctioning thyroid (*hypothyroidism*). Each of these conditions requires its own particular therapy.

Anemia

Many different types of anemia exist, and the treatment depends on the underlying cause. Here we look at two of the most common causes of anemia: iron deficiency and vitamin B12 deficiency.

Iron deficiency

In most cases, iron deficiency is easily diagnosed with a simple blood test. If you're low in iron, it's essential the cause be identified. If you're a *pre-menopausal* woman (that is, you still have periods), then you're prone to *iron-deficiency anemia* because, with each period, you're losing quite a bit of iron (blood is rich in iron). Because red meat has lots of iron, you also are prone to iron-deficiency anemia if you avoid this type of food source.

 If you're a man, or a woman who no longer menstruates, your doctor *must* exclude the possibility you're low in iron caused by hidden (*occult*) bleeding within your bowel (which can be caused by a number of causes including bowel cancer). If that's not the case, other causes (such as an inability to properly absorb iron from the gut) need to be looked at.

Iron therapy is typically given by mouth (often as **ferrous sulphate** or **ferrous gluconate**). If you're unable to tolerate oral iron or if it's not being absorbed into your body, you may be treated with iron injections.

 Oral iron therapy is a non-prescription medicine — however, if your drug costs are covered by an insurance plan, doctors typically are pleased to give you a prescription for the drug.

Vitamin B12 deficiency

Anemia caused by low vitamin B12 is usually diagnosed fairly easily with a blood test. If your doctor finds that you're low in vitamin B12, it's important to identify the cause. Although lack of vitamin B12 in the diet (most commonly seen if you're a strict vegetarian) can lead to anemia, more commonly it's a lack of absorption of vitamin B12 into the body that is responsible. This can be from a number of causes, including diseases of the gut (most commonly pernicious anemia) or a side-effect from a drug called **metformin** (an oral medicine used to treat diabetes and, sometimes, polycystic ovary syndrome).

It used to be thought the only way to effectively treat low vitamin B12 levels was by injections of the vitamin, typically given monthly by a doctor in his or her office. Doctors now know, however, that giving *high* doses (usually 1,000 to 2,000 micrograms per day) of *oral* **vitamin B12** may work well. Not all doctors are aware of this, so if you're advised you need vitamin B12 shots you might wish to ask your doctor whether you could try oral therapy first. (Oral vitamin B12 is available without a prescription.)

Angina

Angina is a feeling of discomfort — usually felt as a pressure or tightness in the area of the breastbone or left side of the chest — that occurs when the heart muscle is deprived of sufficient oxygen. This occurs if there is a narrowing of one or more arteries that feed blood to the heart muscle (a condition called *coronary artery disease*).

The treatment of angina (and coronary artery disease) is aimed at preventing episodes of chest discomfort, treating episodes when they do occur, and, most important of all, reducing the risk the condition will worsen and lead to a heart attack (*myocardial infarction* or, for short, MI). Angina is a temporary, reversible condition, whereas a myocardial infarction leaves a permanent scar on the heart.

The most important drugs to treat angina (and coronary artery disease) are:

- ✔ *Nitroglycerin.* Nitroglycerin given *sublingually* (that is, under the tongue) is used both to prevent attacks of angina and to treat an attack. Nitroglycerin given as a patch or taken orally (as a pill that is swallowed) is used only to prevent attacks. We discuss this in detail in Chapter 6.

- ✔ *Beta blockers.* Beta blockers both reduce the frequency of your angina and improve your exercise tolerance (that is, they enable you to do more activity before you get chest pain or discomfort).

- ✔ *Calcium channel blockers.* Calcium channel blockers are helpful in the prevention of angina attacks and in improving your exercise tolerance. They're especially useful if you're having (or are at high risk of having) side-effects from a beta blocker or if a beta blocker is not sufficiently helping you.

✔ **ASA or clopidogrel.** It's such a shame ASA is such a familiar drug. Why? Because, as Rodney Dangerfield would say, it "don't get no respect." ASA is possibly the single most powerful drug to prevent heart attacks. Yet, likely because it's such an old and widely available drug, it's importance is typically terribly underestimated. If you're unable to take ASA, then clopidogrel is a good alternative. Both these drugs are mild "blood thinners" and reduce the risk of a heart attack by helping to prevent a blood clot from forming in a coronary artery.

✔ *Angiotensin converting enzyme (ACE) inhibitors.* ACE inhibitors do not prevent angina, but do lower the risk that coronary artery disease will progress to a heart attack. ACE inhibitors serve many functions — including, in this case, protecting the circulation to the heart muscle.

✔ *Statins.* Like ACE inhibitors, statins do not prevent angina, but they lower the risk that coronary artery disease will progress to a heart attack. Statins work principally by reducing the level of LDL cholesterol (the so-called "bad cholesterol") in your body.

Of the medications in the preceding list, only sublingual nitroglycerin is effective at stopping your angina attack once it has begun; all the other medicines are taken for *preventive* purposes (to either prevent an angina attack from starting in the first place and/or to prevent a heart attack).

Anxiety Disorders

Although all of us may feel anxious at some point or another, it's only when the amount of worry is out of proportion to the cause that this becomes serious enough to be considered an "anxiety disorder." If you have this disorder, your amount of anxiety is higher, lasts longer (more than 6 months by strict definition), and disrupts your life more than is considered justified by logic. In addition to the "worry" component, people with an anxiety disorder typically feel extra tired, don't sleep well, feel depressed, and may have other symptoms such as muscle aching, palpitations, excess sweating, and an upset stomach. Also, those affected often don't see the relationship between their worries and their symptoms.

If you have an anxiety disorder, most of your treatment is likely focused on counselling and cognitive behaviour therapy. If medications are required, the drugs traditionally used have been **buspirone, benzodiazepines,** and *tricyclic antidepressants.* Nowadays, however, *selective serotonin reuptake inhibitors (SSRIs)* and *serotonin-norepinephrine reuptake inhibitors (SNRIs)* are being used increasingly often as they are less likely to cause side-effects.

Benzodiazepines, while helpful for *occasional* use, should not be used for long-term therapy as their potential to cause addiction is high.

Arrhythmias

An arrhythmia is a disorder of the heart rhythm. It's also one of the words we misspell the most! (Two *r*'s followed by a silent *h* — come on, how are we supposed to remember how to spell a word like that?)

 The heart has four chambers: two lower chambers called *ventricles,* and two upper chambers called *atria.* Problems with the rhythm of the ventricles are called *ventricular arrhythmias;* rhythm problems arising elsewhere in the heart are called *supraventricular arrhythmias.*

 You may also come across the term *dysrhythmia;* this is typically used interchangeably with arrhythmia.

The major types of arrhythmia and the ways they're treated include:

- ✔ **Extrasystoles.** An extrasystole is an extra (or *premature*) heartbeat. Everybody has these from time to time. Usually they do not cause symptoms — if you *do* have a symptom, it's typically felt as a fleeting "skip" or "thud" or "jump" in your chest. By the time you notice it, it's likely gone. Extrasystoles are not serious and almost never require drug treatment. (You may find reducing your caffeine or alcohol intake helps diminish them.)

- ✔ **Atrial fibrillation.** Our hearts are basically just pumps with fancy electrical circuitry. Atrial fibrillation is a condition wherein the normal electrical impulse within the atria that triggers a heartbeat has become disorganized and, rather than there being just a single impulse, a whole bunch of different impulses arise from a whole bunch of locations all at once. As a consequence, the heart rhythm becomes irregular and, often, overly rapid. It's not dissimilar to what would happen if your hall light were activated by a hundred different switches, each one operated by some mischievous elf randomly flicking the switch on and off.

  To slow down the heartbeat, certain **calcium channel blockers** (**diltiazem, verapamil**) or a **beta blocker** are used. Because it's typically less effective, **digoxin** is prescribed less often. Sometimes, **amiodarone** or other drugs may be used to try to restore (and maintain) a normal heart rhythm. (Another way to return the heart rhythm to normal is, in a carefully supervised, hospital setting, for a doctor to give your heart a special type of electrical shock; this is called a *cardioversion.*) Because atrial fibrillation can cause a stroke, the majority of people with atrial fibrillation should be treated with a strong **anticoagulant** ("blood thinner") called **warfarin.** Warfarin reduces the risk of a stroke.

✔ **Supraventricular tachycardia (SVT).** SVT is a suddenly onsetting, rapid, typically regular beating of the heart. It can make you feel dizzy, but is seldom life-threatening. Because an attack often goes away on its own, drug therapy may not be needed. If you're prone to frequent or severe attacks, your doctor may prescribe a *beta blocker,* **digoxin,** or a *calcium channel blocker* (**diltiazem** or **verapamil**) to be taken either daily or just when an attack occurs (the colourfully named "pill in the pocket" technique).

✔ **Ventricular tachycardia (VT).** VT is a serious, potentially life-threatening heart rhythm disorder. Nowadays it's often treated with an *implantable defibrillator,* which is a highly sophisticated device that is surgically placed in the chest. If VT occurs, the device corrects it by giving the heart a small shock. The most commonly used drug to prevent VT is **amiodarone.**

Arthritis

Many different forms of arthritis exist, each with its own specific characteristics. In this section, we discuss two of the most common types of arthritis: osteoarthritis, and rheumatoid arthritis.

Osteoarthritis

Osteoarthritis (OA) refers to joint damage usually caused by years of use of the joint ("wear and tear") or injury to it. The likelihood of developing OA increases as you age, and most of us eventually develop it to some degree. (And, lest you feel humans are being picked on, be advised that possible evidence of osteoarthritis has even been found in dinosaur fossils!) Other processes such as trauma (alas, Bobby Orr's early retirement) or the extra strain on the knees from obesity can be contributing factors. You're more likely to develop osteoarthritis if you have a family history of the condition.

The areas of the body most likely to be affected are the knees, hips, thumbs, and fingers. OA predominantly affects the cartilage in the joint — the part of the joint responsible for absorbing the "shock" of your day-to-day activities. As the cartilage gets progressively more damaged, the underlying bone begins to be injured. All of these factors contribute to the pain you feel if you have OA.

Osteoarthritis is treated by trying to minimize the strain put on joints, by, say, changing your activity patterns (avoiding kneeling, taking elevators and escalators instead of stairs, doing pool exercises instead of going to the gym), or by supporting the affected joints by using assistive devices such as braces, splints, canes, and walkers. Also helpful are *analgesics* (such as **acetaminophen**), which are used to ease the pain. If you don't get adequate relief from these therapies, using *nonsteroidal anti-inflammatory drugs (NSAIDs)* can be very helpful. Unfortunately, a drug to actually stop OA from developing or worsening is not yet available.

Rheumatoid arthritis

Rheumatoid arthritis (RA) is a disease affecting the joints in which they become painful, stiff, and swollen. Although doctors don't know why someone gets RA, we do know it is an *autoimmune disease* — meaning the immune system, which normally protects us, has become confused and has attacked part of our own body. Over time, rheumatoid arthritis can cause significant damage to the joints, and with this comes loss of normal joint function. Less often, RA affects other organs.

If you have RA, your doctor will likely prescribe drugs that reduce inflammation in the joints as quickly and completely as possible. *Nonsteroidal anti-inflammatory drugs (NSAIDs)* help to decrease pain and stiffness. Oral *corticosteroids,* though also very effective at improving these symptoms, are often avoided or used in the lowest possible dose because of their potential for significant side-effects.

The most important medications for long-term control of rheumatoid arthritis — and, in particular, for prevention of progressive joint damage — are *disease-modifying antirheumatic drugs (DMARDs)*, *immunosuppressive drugs*, and, most recently, *biologic response modifiers* (biologics). These three types of treatment can be used alone or in combination. Regardless of which of these latter drugs is used, most people with RA continue to take NSAIDs.

Asthma

The main features of asthma are shortness of breath, wheezing, and coughing. Over the past few years, asthma has become increasingly common in our society. The reasons why are not clear, but it may be because of higher levels of pollutants in the air.

Asthma is characterized by inflammation of the airways (the *bronchi*) in the lungs, which causes them to go into spasm — air trying to squeeze through the narrowed airways produces the characteristic wheezing sound. A number of things can trigger a flare of asthma (an asthma attack), including:

- Exposure to an *allergen* (substances that trigger allergy attacks in susceptible people), such as dust mites.

- Exposure to an irritant (such as smoke, car exhaust, or products — for example, some cleaning fluids — that have a strong smell).

- Respiratory infections.

- Exercising (which, in susceptible people causes a form of asthma called, surprise, *exercise-induced asthma*).

If you have very mild asthma, then drug treatment can be confined to using a *short-acting* **beta-2 agonist** inhaler, such as **salbutamol,** taken only when you need it (that is, only when you have wheezing). Beta-2 agonists work by helping to open the bronchial airways.

For more severe asthma — especially if you experience wheezing more than three days per week — you should also be treated with medications to *prevent* attacks:

- Initial treatment is usually with a **corticosteroid** inhaler such as **beclomethasone,** which works by reducing inflammation in the airways. If that doesn't work sufficiently well, adding a long-acting **beta-2 agonist** inhaler such as **salmeterol** is recommended.

- If that combination of treatments is not working, your doctor might try increasing the dose of the corticosteroid inhaler or, alternatively, adding a **leukotriene antagonist** such as **montelukast** — which sounds like it should be a mountain in the Himalayas but actually is a drug (discovered in Montreal hence the "mont" in montelukast!) that reduces bronchial inflammation and spasm caused by allergen exposure.

✔ If, despite these measures, your asthma is still problematic then your doctor will likely recommend an oral corticosteroid such as **prednisone.** Oral corticosteroids are very potent drugs and need to be used under close medical supervision. Oral corticosteroids are also used, on a short-term basis, to treat particularly bad (*acute*) asthma attacks.

A ***mast cell stabilizer* (sodium cromoglycate)** is sometimes used, particularly if your asthma tends to be made worse by exercise. Because they are not particularly effective, ***anticholinergic*** inhalers, such as **ipratropium,** are usually reserved for people who cannot tolerate beta-2 agonist inhalers because of side-effects such as palpitations and tremor. Finally, because of its limited benefit and significant risk of side-effects, **theophylline** medication is not used very often.

Almost all of the drugs mentioned in the preceding list (short-acting beta-2 agonists being the most significant exception) are used to *prevent* wheezing, not to treat it. So, if you're having an asthma attack, taking extra doses of these preventive therapies does you no good — and, indeed, simply delays your seeking appropriate emergency medical care. Additionally, if you're having an asthma attack and it's not responding to extra doses of your short-acting beta-2 agonist, you *must* seek emergency medical attention. Tragically, people having an asthma attack have died because they did not do go to hospital soon enough.

If your asthma is worse than usual and you're taking **Symbicort** — a combination of a medication that treats wheezing and a medication that helps prevent an attack — your doctor may *also* advise you to increase the dose of this medicine.

Athlete's Foot

Despite its name, you do not have to be an athlete to acquire athlete's foot. Athlete's foot (which goes by the fancy medical name *tinea pedis*) is a fungal infection of the skin on the feet — usually found between the toes. If left untreated, it can spread to affect the entire sole of the foot. Although it can affect anyone, you're more likely to acquire it if your feet (and the rest of you, therefore) hang around warm, moist environments such as swimming pools and locker rooms. You're also prone to athlete's foot if you participate in activities that tend to make your feet sweat.

The mainstay of treatment is with topical **antifungal agents.**
However, if your athlete's foot is particularly severe or if you have
an impaired immune system (by virtue of having another, serious
disease or because you're taking certain drugs that interfere with
functioning of the immune system), oral antifungal agents may be
necessary to get rid of the infection.

Attention-Deficit/Hyperactivity Disorder (ADHD)

ADHD is a disease, typically diagnosed in childhood, characterized
by difficulty paying attention, being overly active, and acting
impulsively. These symptoms often improve as the child gets older.
The cause(s) of ADHD is unknown.

Treatment of ADHD may include several different strategies including
behaviour therapy and/or medications. If prescription medication
is required, so-called **stimulant** drugs (usually **methylphenidate,**
but sometimes **dextroamphetamine**) are generally used first and
the substantial majority of children show improvement with this
therapy. A newer medicine, **atomoxetine,** has also been shown to
be effective, but there is much less experience with this medication and it's typically used only when stimulant medication has not
been successful or if concerns about side-effects from stimulants
exist. The great majority of children improve with one or another
of these medicines; however, good scientific studies regarding
long-term use of these treatments are not available. We discuss
ADHD in greater detail in Chapter 8.

Baldness

Although baldness can be caused by diseases and certain drugs,
far and away the most common cause is genetic. Men and women
can both be affected, but it's typically more obvious in males
because of their shorter hairstyles and a greater tendency for the
front part of the scalp to be involved.

Although doctors do not have very effective therapies, if you have
mild to moderate baldness you may see some benefit with use of
topical **minoxidil** (which can be used in either men or women) and
the *alpha-reductase inhibitor* finasteride — an oral medication
that may be helpful for men but is not effective for women (and,
indeed, can be dangerous for use by women of childbearing age, as
we discuss in Chapter 6). These medications are not of benefit if
you have severe baldness.

Bedwetting

Bedwetting (also called *enuresis*) is normal in young children and typically goes away by the time the child reaches 5 or 6. If it persists beyond that age, your doctor should determine whether your child has a problem with his or her urinary tract (that is, malfunction of the bladder, urethra, and so on) or if psychological factors may be present.

Drug therapy is not usually required — if it is needed, however, **desmopressin (DDAVP)** is often very effective. DDAVP is typically used only for brief periods, such as for sleepovers or overnight camps. Sometimes, *tricyclic antidepressants* such as **imipramine** are used; if so, very low doses are prescribed.

Bipolar Disorder

Bipolar disorder was previously known as *manic-depression* (and is sometimes referred to as *bipolar affective disorder*). People with this condition are prone to extremes of mood, with periods of severe depression and, conversely, episodes of extreme agitation (*mania*). During the former, people can feel so low they may consider suicide. During the latter, people can feel so "high" their thoughts and actions are scattered and no longer logical. In either situation, the symptoms may be so severe the person is unable to properly perform normal day-to-day activities. Bipolar disorder is thought to be caused by abnormalities in *neurotransmitters* (chemical messengers in the brain), but a detailed understanding of the mechanism remains to be sorted out.

Control of the acute symptoms is important so individuals are less likely to cause themselves physical harm. Long-term control is critical so individuals can get back to their normal activities.

- ✔ For acute control (to help stabilize your mood), the preferred drugs are *second generation ("atypical") antipsychotics,* **lithium,** and **valproic acid.**

- ✔ For long-term control (to prevent a flare of bipolar disorder), **lithium, valproic acid,** and **carbamazepine** are typically the preferred drugs. Other choices for long-term control include **lamotrigine** and *second generation ("atypical") antipsychotics*.

Blood Clots

Blood clots in our bodies are of two general types. Small blood clots within the arteries lead to strokes and heart attacks. (We discuss these conditions elsewhere in this chapter.) Larger blood clots within the veins are the subject of this section.

Phlebitis is a condition where there is a blood clot (a *thrombus*) within a vein (typically, within the leg). If a thrombus is located in one of the innermost veins within the leg it's called a *deep vein thrombosis* (DVT for short). A DVT may break off and travel through the veins until it gets lodged inside blood vessels in the lungs. This is called a *pulmonary embolism.* The two together are called a *pulmonary thromboembolism.*

Deep-vein thrombosis and pulmonary embolism are treated similarly. Most of the time, these conditions can be treated at home with the affected person giving him- or herself (or being given by a nurse) once- or twice-daily injections under the skin of a potent **anticoagulant** ("blood thinner") called **low molecular weight heparin.** Typically, this treatment would continue for a week or two.

You would also be treated with an anticoagulant called **warfarin,** which you would continue for a minimum of three to six months. Whereas low molecular weight heparin does not require much, if any, monitoring, warfarin requires frequent blood tests so your doctor can ensure you're taking the right dose. Too little and you will be prone to more clots; too much and you will be prone to bleeding.

Do not confuse deep vein thrombosis with *superficial* vein thrombosis, a far less serious condition that is treated very differently — usually with analgesics and **nonsteroidal anti-inflammatory drugs (NSAIDs).**

Cancer

Cancer develops when the normal, orderly, tightly controlled process of cells dividing (as virtually all the body's cells do) is replaced by uncontrolled cell division leading to more and more cells being present. These abnormal cells end up crowding out healthy cells, interfering with the normal functioning of the body. The name of the cancer is related to where the abnormal cells develop — hence, *lung cancer* is the presence of cancer cells originating in the lung, and *prostate cancer* is the presence of cancer cells originating in the prostate.

Many cancers require surgery, radiation therapy, and/or intravenous chemotherapy given in hospital. These therapies are beyond the scope of *Understanding Prescription Drugs For Canadians For Dummies*. In this section we discuss frequently prescribed *oral* drugs used to treat two of the most common cancers affecting Canadians: breast cancer and prostate cancer.

Breast cancer

The medication prescribed to treat breast cancer depends on the specific nature of the disease and, in particular, if the cancer is *estrogen receptor positive*. This means that the breast cancer comprises cells that are stimulated by the presence in the body of the hormone estrogen. This type of stimulation can make the cancer worse. The two most commonly used families of prescription drugs for breast cancer block estrogen:

- ✔ *Selective estrogen receptor modulators (SERMs)*: SERMs work by blocking estrogen from attaching to the estrogen receptors on the cancer cells. This, in turn, reduces the likelihood of the cancer cells growing. As such, if your breast cancer is estrogen receptor positive, your doctor may recommend you take a SERM (such as **tamoxifen**). (We discuss cell receptors in Chapter 2.)

- ✔ *Aromatase inhibitors*: Aromatase inhibitors work by blocking the production of estrogen. Thus, there is less stimulation of breast cancer cells to grow.

Prostate cancer

The goal of oral prescription drug therapy to treat prostate cancer is to block the effect of those hormones (especially testosterone) that stimulate the growth of prostate cancer cells. By decreasing the amount of testosterone the body makes or by blocking its stimulating effect on prostate cancer cells, prostate cancer can be slowed significantly both within the prostate itself and also in areas to which prostate cancer has metastasized (that is, spread).

The most commonly used of these therapies are *anti-androgens* (which work by blocking the effect of testosterone on prostate cancer cells) and *GnRH agonists* (which work by reducing testosterone levels in the body). As we discuss in Chapter 6, your doctor may advise you to take an anti-androgen for a few weeks *before* you start your GnRH agonist therapy, as this reduces the likelihood (and severity) of side-effects from the GnRH agonist.

Chlamydia

Chlamydia is a bacterial infection transmitted between partners during sexual activities (typically vaginal intercourse, but also during oral and anal sex). It may not necessarily cause symptoms, but if it does the most common ones are, in men, a discharge from the opening at the end of the penis (the *urethra*) and a burning discomfort when passing urine, and, in women, a vaginal discharge, burning discomfort when passing urine, and vaginal bleeding between periods.

If chlamydia is left untreated it can lead to infertility and/or arthritis, and allows the infection to be spread to other people. It should *not* be left untreated!

Chlamydia can be cured with oral antibiotic therapy. The preferred drugs are generally considered to be oral **azithromycin** and **doxycycline.** Azithromycin requires only one dose, whereas doxycline requires a week of therapy. Effective alternatives include certain *fluoroquinolones* **(ofloxacin, levofloxacin, moxifloxacin)** and **erythromycin.**

Chronic Obstructive Pulmonary Disease (COPD)

Chronic obstructive pulmonary disease is a lung disease in which the airways (the *bronchi*) and the air sacs (the *alveoli*) are damaged — usually, but not always, from smoking. COPD encompasses two related conditions: *chronic bronchitis* and *emphysema.* People with COPD typically experience shortness of breath (especially with exertion), coughing, excess phlegm (sputum), and wheezing.

The two most important prescription drugs to help you with your COPD are *beta-2 agonist* and *anticholinergic* inhalers. (We also talk about these drugs under "Asthma" in this chapter.) **Theophylline** medication may be used, but is typically of limited value. If you're prone to recurring *acute exacerbations* (during which you generally cough up large quantities of thick, green sputum and become more short of breath and wheezy than usual), using a *corticosteroid* inhaler on a daily basis is often a good idea as it will reduce the likelihood of such attacks.

Oral corticosteroids are helpful to treat an acute exacerbation of COPD and, in the lowest possible dose (to avoid side-effects), are sometimes used long-term.

Taking antibiotics — typically for about a week — is also helpful to treat a flare. The preferred antibiotics are **clarithromycin, azithromycin, cefuroxime,** a *fluoroquinolone,* **amoxicillin** (with or without **clavulanate**), **sulfamethoxazole/trimethoprim,** and **doxycycline.**

If your COPD has led to a low oxygen level in your blood, you will benefit from continuous use of supplemental oxygen, which can be supplied from big tanks (for use in the home) and fairly small, portable tanks (for use outside the home).

Quitting smoking is terribly important (we discuss this further in the "Smoking Cessation" section of this chapter). If you have COPD, be sure to get an annual flu shot from your doctor to reduce your risk of contracting influenza. Also, you should be given a pneumococcal vaccination to help protect you against pneumonia caused by a bacterium called *pneumococcus.*

Claudication

Claudication (also known as "intermittent claudication") is a condition wherein you experience an aching pain usually felt in one or both calves when you walk; the pain quickly eases when you rest. Claudication is caused by reduced blood flow (and, hence, reduced delivery of oxygen) to your calf muscles; this occurs when the blood vessels in the legs become narrowed by atherosclerosis ("hardening of the arteries"). When atherosclerosis affects the legs, the condition is called *peripheral vascular disease.*

The main treatments are lifestyle and, if the condition is very severe, surgery or angioplasty. (Angioplasty is a procedure where a balloon is placed into an artery and inflated to squeeze open the blockage; the balloon is then deflated and removed.) Drug therapy has a fairly limited role in relieving symptoms. However, importantly, if you have claudication you're at higher risk of stroke and heart attack — this risk can be reduced by taking certain medicines including **ASA** (or **clopidogrel**), a *statin,* and an *angiotensin converting enzyme (ACE) inhibitor.*

Cold, Common

The common cold has been recognized for millennia. It's most commonly caused by a virus called a *rhinovirus*.

The only reason to include an entry on the common cold in a book on prescription drugs is to let you know prescription drugs don't help you get rid of your cold. (We take a look at ways to distinguish the common cold from the more serious condition *influenza* in the "Influenza" section of this chapter.)

Cold Sores

Cold sores, those bothersome little red lesions occurring usually on the lip (and seeming to show up at the most inopportune times), are caused by a herpes simplex virus. Although cold sores are a nuisance, they are not serious and usually do not leave scars. They are typically treated with over-the-counter medicine, but if you have a particularly severe cold sore or if you are *immunocompromised* (that is, your immune system is not working properly, as can occur, for example, with some serious diseases such as leukemia, after transplant surgery, and if you're receiving certain forms of cancer chemotherapy), then the herpes simplex virus can lead to more widespread problems. In these circumstances, **antiviral agents** such as **acyclovir, famciclovir,** or **valacyclovir** may be used to help keep things under control.

Conjunctivitis

The *conjunctiva* is the transparent membrane covering the "whites of the eye" and lining the inside part of the eyelid. If the conjunctiva becomes inflamed (a condition called *conjunctivitis*), the eye will look red (hence the other name for this condition: pink eye) and a discharge may form.

Conjunctivitis is classified as being infectious (in which case it's typically caused by a bacteria or virus) or non-infectious (typically caused by allergies). Bacterial conjunctivitis is treated with **antibiotic** eye drops or ointments, typically ones containing **erythromycin, sulfacetamide, polymyxin-bacitracin,** or a **fluoroquinolone.** (**Aminoglycoside** antibiotic therapy is also used — however, it can lead to eye inflammation after several days of treatment.) Neither viral nor allergic conjunctivitis requires prescription drugs for treatment.

Contraception

We admit including a section called "Contraception" in a chapter entitled "Ailments and Their Treatment" is taking liberties (contraception is assuredly *not* an ailment), but seeing as contraceptives are some of the most commonly prescribed medications in Canada we felt it important to include this information. (And, heck, it just seemed to fit best here.)

Contraception refers to the activities people undertake to avoid conception (that is, pregnancy). In this section we look at hormonal therapy available to women to prevent pregnancy. (No male hormonal therapies are available as yet.)

The two general types of hormonal contraceptive therapy are

- ✔ **Preventive therapy:** *Oral contraceptives* (The Pill) and *transdermal contraceptive patches* (that is, a topical medicine you wear on your skin — in this case, in the form of a patch) work by preventing ovulation. A longer-acting, injectable preparation (Depo-Provera) works similarly and is administered in the form of a shot you receive from your physician once every three months. Depo-Provera is a good option if you're in need of a highly effective contraceptive but are unlikely to remember to take an oral or topical medication on a consistent basis. (Other available hormone-containing preventive therapies are progesterone-containing IUDs and *transvaginal contraceptive rings.*)

- ✔ **Emergency (post-coital) contraceptives.** This type of contraceptive is used in emergency situations (for example, if you had unprotected intercourse, your barrier method of contraception failed, or you forgot to take your oral contraceptive). **Levonorgestrel,** known as *Plan B,* is an oral, "behind-the-counter" medication available for this purpose. (See Chapter 2 for a discussion on the classification of drugs.)

None of the drug therapies for contraception protect against sexually transmitted diseases (STDs). To protect yourself against STDs, use a condom and other safe sex practices.

Cough

Everybody coughs from time to time. Many things are known to trigger bouts of coughing, such as exposure to allergens (such as dust mites or ragweed) in people with allergies, exposure to noxious substances such as fumes and smoke, and, surest of all, exposure to the intense and intimidating stare of a symphony conductor as he demands (and fails to obtain) complete and total silence from his audience.

Coughing can be helpful, such as when you cough to clear your airways of mucus. Coughing may also be a clue to the presence of an underlying disease (such as asthma), and treating this underlying condition helps ease the cough that accompanies it. Not infrequently, however, coughing is simply a nuisance. If you experience coughing that's particularly bothersome and does not respond to over-the-counter medicines, you and your doctor may elect to treat it with prescription drugs.

The most widely used prescription drug to treat (that is, to suppress) a cough is **codeine.** Although codeine works well, its use should be confined to brief periods of time because, being a *narcotic ("opioid") analgesic,* it carries a risk of addiction.

Depression

Everyone feels sad from time to time. Sadness is a normal, temporary feeling, typically related to a clearly identifiable cause. *Depression,* on the other hand, is a severe, overwhelming, and unrelenting feeling of despair often leading to sleeplessness, fatigue, poor appetite, aches and pains, and a feeling of hopelessness and helplessness. Regrettably, many people with depression never seek help.

The precise cause of depression is not known; however, often there is a genetic component (that is, the affected person may have a close relative who has experienced mental health problems). Additionally, personal experiences, such as a death in the family or financial difficulties, may play a role. It's also known that people with depression have abnormalities of certain chemical messengers (*neurotransmitters*) within the brain, especially *norepinephrine* and *serotonin.*

Prescription drugs are often required to treat depression, both as initial therapy and then as ongoing therapy to help prevent depression from coming back.

- Most often, the first type of drug used is a *serotonin-norepinephrine reuptake inhibitor (SNRI),* or *selective serotonin reuptake inhibitor (SSRI).*

- If an SNRI or SSRI doesn't help you, other potentially helpful drugs include *tricyclic antidepressants, monoamine oxidase (MAO) inhibitors,* and **bupropion.**

Diabetes

Diabetes is an ailment in which insulin (a hormone made by the pancreas) either is not present in sufficient quantities or does not work properly (a condition called *insulin resistance*) — or both. In *type 1* diabetes (the type typically acquired in childhood or youth) the main problem is a lack of insulin, and in *type 2* diabetes the main problem is insulin resistance. If you have diabetes you have a tendency toward high levels of glucose ("sugar") in your blood. As a result, you're prone to a characteristic symptom that led physicians in 1600s England — when they surely knew how to call a spade a spade — to refer to diabetes as "the pissing evil"!

Treating diabetes has *many* aspects, including appropriate lifestyle measures and maintaining control of your blood pressure, blood glucose levels, and blood cholesterol levels. In this section, we look at prescription drugs to control blood glucose; elsewhere in this chapter we discuss drugs to control blood pressure and cholesterol.

Insulin therapy

Everyone with type 1 diabetes — and many people with type 2 diabetes — requires **insulin** therapy to keep their blood glucose levels controlled. Because it maximizes the ability to fine-tune insulin doses whilst also maximizing flexibility (regarding meal timing, exercise, and so on), a particularly effective approach is to use a combination of

- ✔ "Rapid-acting" insulin (**aspart** or **lispro**) given immediately before meals.
- ✔ Longer-acting insulin (**detemir, glargine,** or **NPH**) given at bedtime.

Regular insulin can be given instead of aspart or lispro (and has the advantage of being less expensive), but is more of a hassle to use because it needs to be given about one-half hour before meals and also it's more likely to lead to low blood glucose (an *insulin reaction*).

Premixed insulin (a mixture of two different insulins) given twice a day is another option for people with type 2 (seldom for people with type 1 diabetes) but, as we look at in Chapter 6, provides less flexibility than taking individual insulins separately.

 If you have type 2 diabetes treated with oral hypoglycemic agents (which we discuss immediately below) and your fasting (that is, before breakfast) blood glucose levels are too high but your values the remainder of the day are excellent, *adding* detemir, glargine or NPH insulin once per day (at bedtime) will often correct the problem.

Insulin reactions can be so bad you become unconscious. In this situation, having someone administer an injection of **glucagon** to you can quickly raise your blood glucose level back to a safe range. We discuss glucagon and other precautions to follow when taking insulin in Chapter 6.

To find out more about insulin therapy (and all other matters regarding diabetes) we (sort of) humbly refer you to *Diabetes for Canadians for Dummies*; a book Ian co-wrote with Alan Rubin.

Oral hypoglycemic agents

Oral hypoglycemic agent (OHA) drugs help to control blood glucose levels in people with type 2 diabetes.

Oral hypoglycemic agents are also referred to as *oral antidiabetic agents* and *oral antihyperglycemic agents.* These terms all refer to the same group of medicines.

Important points about OHA therapy include:

- ✔ In most cases, the preferred OHA for initial therapy is **metformin.**

- ✔ When that is insufficient, a *thiazolidinedione* (**pioglitazone** or **rosiglitazone**) is often added.

- ✔ *Sulfonylurea* drugs such as **glyburide** (by far the most commonly used sulfonylurea) are as effective as metformin and thiazolidinediones at reducing blood glucose levels, but unlike these other drugs they can lead to hypoglycemia and glyburide does not provide as effective long-term glucose control. Also, glyburide often causes weight gain, whereas metformin does not. For these reasons glyburide is less preferred than metformin and thiazolidinediones.

- ✔ If you're taking glyburide and experiencing hypoglycemia, switching to **repaglinide, gliclazide,** or **glimepiride** may be a good idea as these drugs are less likely to cause low blood glucose.

- ✔ Because of problematic flatulence (hmm, is there any other kind?) and limited potency, **acarbose** is not often used.

Some provincial drug benefit programs pay for a thiazolinedione only if you have first been on certain other oral hypoglycemic agents (typically glyburide and/or metformin). We think this is inappropriate, but, alas, we don't make the rules — sure wish we did, though!

Diarrhea

Most people experience diarrhea, or loose stools, from time to time and it seldom requires prescription drug therapy. If, however, your diarrhea is so severe it's interfering with your ability to carry on with your normal activities, you may benefit from a prescription medicine.

 If you have diarrhea lasting beyond a few days, see your doctor so the underlying cause for the problem can be found. Treating the symptom (the diarrhea) while ignoring the cause (infection, inflammation, a tumour) is not wise.

Antibiotic therapy (usually with a *fluoroquinolone*) is often helpful if you have "traveller's diarrhea" (also known as "Montezuma's Revenge" — clearly, someone royally ticked off Montezuma!).

Cholestyramine is occasionally helpful in certain cases of diarrhea caused by inflammatory bowel disease and irritable bowel syndrome (both of which we discuss elsewhere in this chapter).

Codeine can work well but has a significant risk of side-effects, so over-the-counter, codeine-like drugs (such as **diphenoxylate** or **loperamide**), which have fewer side-effects, are preferred. Nonetheless, it's best not to take these on a regular basis unless under the ongoing supervision of your physician.

Dizziness

We can lump most of the various causes of dizziness into two broad groups:

- ✔ **Momentary drop in blood pressure:** This type makes you feel lightheaded or faint. It typically has a quickly reversible cause, such as being in pain, straining too hard while having a bowel movement, witnessing the sight of blood, standing up quickly from sitting or lying, or opening the door to your teenage son's bedroom. No treatment is required in these cases (although you can *try* asking your son to clean up his room). Sometimes, however, serious causes may be responsible, such as a disorder of the heart rhythm; if so, this requires further evaluation by your doctor. If the cause of your faintness is not immediately evident to you and is not clearly harmless, we recommend you seek prompt medical attention.

> ✔ **A problem with the balance mechanism in the inner ear:**
> This type makes you feel as if you or your environment is
> moving or even spinning; it's typically referred to as *vertigo*.
> (We won't quibble over whether James Stewart really experi-
> enced vertigo in the film *Vertigo*.)

TIP

Some drugs (such as ***alpha blockers***) used to treat hypertension
can make your blood pressure fall unduly when you first stand up
from sitting or standing, which may make you feel lightheaded or
faint. In Chapter 6 we discuss precautions you can follow while
you're taking blood pressure medication.

If you have vertigo caused by *acute labrynthitis* (an inner ear problem likely caused by a virus), treatment is primarily with bed rest,
drinking sufficient fluids to maintain your hydration, and, if necessary, taking over-the-counter medicines such as **dimenhydrinate**
(Gravol) for nausea. There is some evidence taking an oral
corticosteroid (usually for three weeks) may also be helpful.

If your vertigo is because of *Meniere's disease* (a condition where
a fluid imbalance exists in the inner ear, and typically associated
with hearing loss and *tinnitus* — "ringing" — in the affected ear),
betahistine and ***diuretics*** are the two types of medicine most
proven to be of benefit.

Ear Infections

Humans may have only two ears, but each ear actually has three
parts; an outer, a middle, and an inner component.

> ✔ The outer part of the ear helps to focus sound and serves as a
> convenient place to hang shiny bits of metal and glass.
>
> ✔ The middle ear is where sound waves are converted into
> mechanical forces through the action of a miniature hardware
> store featuring a hammer, anvil, and stirrup (we kid you not).
>
> ✔ The inner ear is where the mechanical forces are transferred
> into electrical impulses, which travel down a nerve (the
> *auditory nerve*) to the brain, where you then interpret these
> signals as messages saying things such as "I love you father,
> now can I have the car keys?"

Outer ear infections (*otitis externa*) are almost always caused by
bacteria and are more likely to occur if you have psoriasis or
eczema or if you spend a fair bit of time swimming in fresh water
(hence the other name for this condition, "swimmer's ear").

The infection is usually confined to the ear canal itself and causes discomfort and itching, sometimes accompanied by a discharge. Treatment is with **antibiotic** ear drops, of which many equally good ones exist. Sometimes **corticosteroid** ear drops are also prescribed, as these will reduce inflammation and swelling within the ear canal.

Middle ear infections (*otitis media*) typically affect youngsters — indeed, up to 90 percent of children have had at least one episode by the time they reach their third birthday. The affected child often has ear pain and temporary hearing loss. Other symptoms may include fever, irritability, and headache. The preferred antibiotic is oral **amoxicillin.**

We discuss inner ear infections in the "Dizziness" section of this chapter.

Eczema

In this section we discuss the most common form of eczema, *atopic eczema* (also called *atopic dermatitis*), a skin condition that generally begins in childhood and makes the affected area of skin itchy, red, and swollen. People with environmental allergies are more likely to develop atopic eczema.

When prescription drug therapy is required, use of a topical **corticosteroid** cream helps. Oral corticosteroid therapy is sometimes used for severe cases; however, because of the potential for significant side-effects, its use is generally confined to very brief periods. Also sometimes used to treat severe cases are **immunosuppressive drugs** (such as topical **tacrolimus** or **pimecrolimus,** and oral medicines including **cyclosporine, methotrexate, azathioprine,** or **mycophenolate**); however, like oral corticosteroids, the risk of significant side-effects limits their use. Oral **antihistamines** (such as **diphenhydramine** or **hydroxyzine**) can help relieve itching.

Edema

Although a variety of types of edema exist, the term typically refers to fluid retention and swelling in the feet (most noticeably, the ankles) and sometimes the fingers. This is called *peripheral edema* (as opposed to fluid buildup in the lungs, which is called *pulmonary edema*). If you have peripheral edema, your doctor needs to determine the cause — causes can range from as serious as congestive heart failure or kidney or liver disease, to as minor as being in a hot, humid environment or spending a long time in a plane.

If you have bothersome edema, *diuretics* are prescribed. Diuretics help the body rid itself of excess fluid by increasing the amount of urine you make. The specific diuretic prescribed depends, in part, on the cause of your edema. Edema caused by heart failure or kidney disease is typically treated with a *loop diuretic,* such as **furosemide,** whereas edema caused by liver disease is usually treated with a *potassium-sparing diuretic* such as **spironolactone.** If you have mild edema and are otherwise healthy, your doctor may recommend a less potent drug: a *thiazide diuretic.* Sometimes a combination of two different types of diuretics is used.

Regardless of which type of diuretic you're prescribed, your doctor needs to send you for periodic blood tests to make sure the medication has not caused an imbalance of your sodium and potassium levels and that your kidney function is also stable.

Endocarditis Prophylaxis

Endocarditis prophylaxis refers to the prevention of bacterial infections within the heart.

Within your heart are valves that allow blood to flow forward (which is good) but not backward (which would be bad — who wants to drive the wrong way down a one-way street, after all!). If a valve becomes infected, this is called *endocarditis* (also known as *subacute bacterial endocarditis,* or *SBE*). SBE is most likely to occur if you have a scarred or abnormal heart valve or if you have a surgically implanted, artificial valve.

If you have a heart valve problem (and hence are at increased risk of SBE), taking antibiotics before certain procedures — most notably dental work — *may* (it's not scientifically proven) reduce your risk of acquiring endocarditis. The preferred treatment is to take oral **amoxicillin** one hour before the dental work is performed. If you're allergic to amoxicillin, good alternatives include oral **clindamycin** or **azithromycin.**

If your physician advises that you require endocarditis prophylaxis before dental work, be sure to contact your dentist prior to your appointment so appropriate arrangements can be made for you to receive the antibiotics.

Endometriosis

In some women, the lining of the uterus, known as the *endometrium,* can grow abnormally, resulting in endometrial tissue growing outside the uterus (typically in the pelvis or abdomen). This can lead to pelvic and abdominal pain.

Treatment is aimed at controlling this abnormal growth of endometrial tissue by using medicines to reduce the production of female hormones. Lower levels of female hormones reduce the stimulus to endometrial tissue to grow. Prescription drugs found to be helpful are *oral contraceptives,* **Depo-Provera,** *gonadotropin-releasing hormone (GnRH) agonists,* and **danazol.** *Analgesics* or *nonsteroidal anti-inflammatory drugs (NSAIDs)* can be helpful for pain control. When these treatments are insufficient, surgical options can be considered.

Epilepsy

Our brains work using a combination of chemicals (*neurotransmitters*) and electrical impulses. When the electrical pathways in the brain malfunction — think of it as similar to a short-circuit in your home's wiring — an attack of epilepsy (also known as a *seizure* or *convulsion*) may occur. *Grand mal* epilepsy, one of the most common types of seizure disorder, causes sudden attacks of loss of consciousness accompanied by shaking movements of the arms and legs, and incontinence caused by loss of bowel and bladder control.

Sometimes epilepsy occurs because of an area of damage to the brain, for example from a stroke or a brain tumour. More often than not, however, doctors do not find a specific cause. Medications used to treat epilepsy are called *anticonvulsants.*

If you have had only one seizure, prescription drug therapy is not always required. If treatment *is* necessary, a low dose of a single anticonvulsant is used and the dose is then increased until seizures do not recur — the "start low and go slow" approach. If the chosen drug fails to prevent seizures (or if your body is not tolerating the drug), another drug should be chosen. If that, too, fails, then combination therapy with two different drugs should be used. The preferred drugs to treat epilepsy (depending on the form of epilepsy you have) are **carbamazepine, phenytoin, valproic acid** (also called **valproate**), and **topiramate.** If these drugs have not helped, then **lamotrigine, phenobarbital, primidone,** or **levetiracetam** are used.

Erectile Dysfunction

Erectile dysfunction is the condition in which a man is unable to achieve and maintain an erection that is sufficiently firm to allow for sexual intercourse. If this affects you only rarely, therapy is unlikely to be necessary. On the other hand, if erectile dysfunction is a persisting or recurring problem, you do have the option of various available treatments.

Rather than automatically reaching for the prescription pad, a prudent physician will first try to determine the cause for a man's erectile dysfunction (ED). ED may be caused by many things, including

- Peyronie's disease (a condition where the penis becomes abnormally curved because of scar tissue)

- Hormonal disorders (such as an excess of prolactin or a deficiency of testosterone)

- Atherosclerosis ("hardening of the arteries") and/or nerve damage as occurs, for example, in many men with diabetes

- Drug side-effects — ED is a not uncommon side-effect from medications, especially blood pressure pills

- Psychological factors

When oral prescription medication is required to treat ED, the drugs used are from the **phosphodiesterase type 5 (PDE5) inhibitor** family. Members of this family are **sildenafil, tadalafil,** and **vardenafil.** Although they are, in general, equally effective, sometimes an individual responds better to one than the other — so if one doesn't help you, it's worth trying another. One possible advantage of tadalafil is that it remains in the body longer than the other two.

If these oral drugs don't help you, a very effective alternative is to inject into the side of the penis, using a small needle, a medication called **alprostadil** (Caverject), either alone or as **Trimix** (a mixture of alprostadil, **papaverine,** and **phentolamine**). A urologist (a specialist in this area) typically instructs you on how to properly perform the injection. (You might understandably think this sounds like a rather unpleasant form of therapy; however, most men find it not nearly so bad as they expect and, indeed, usually find the results well worth the effort.) Alprostadil can also be given as a tiny pellet you insert into the urethra (the opening at the end of the penis).

Trimix is not pre-made by a manufacturer and so needs to be created from scratch (*compounded*) by a pharmacist. Although most pharmacists routinely compound some basic substances, the preparation of Trimix is typically done only by pharmacists who specialize in compounding. If your regular pharmacist is unable to make Trimix for you, he can refer you to a pharmacist who does. (Your urologist will also likely know which pharmacists in your vicinity perform this task.)

For those men who are not being helped by medication, other treatment options exist including use of a vacuum device (liked by some men, not by others) or surgical implantation of a penile prosthesis (a therapy many men find highly satisfactory).

Fibromyalgia

Fibromyalgia syndrome (FMS) is characterized by widespread muscle and joint pain and is often associated with excess fatigue and the inability to get a good night's sleep. Its cause is unknown, and despite the nature of the musculoskeletal symptoms medical studies have not found inflammation in the muscles or joints.

Treatment includes combinations of aerobic exercise, good neck and back care, trying to have a good night's sleep, and, when needed, judicious use of *analgesics, skeletal muscle relaxants, tricyclic antidepressants, selective serotonin reuptake inhibitors (SSRIs)* and *selective-norepinephrine reuptake inhibitors (SNRIs)*. Used on their own, *nonsteroidal anti-inflammatory drugs (NSAIDs)* are not generally helpful.

Flatulence

Flatulence is the fancy name for, well, farting. We prefer flatulence (so to speak). Our kids prefer farting. We're the parents, so we win (at least on this occasion). Flatulence is a normal part of life; indeed, one of our all-time favourite pieces of trivia (one, so far as we are aware, that has yet to make it into Trivial Pursuit) is that the average person farts (oops; *passes flatus*) 14 times per day. Well, to be precise, 13.6 times per day, but we thought if we rounded it off you wouldn't, ahem, raise a stink.

Sometimes, adjusting the diet helps reduce the amount of gas you pass. The only time prescription drug therapy is likely to be necessary would be if your doctor determines you have an unusual condition called small bowel bacterial overgrowth, in which case she may prescribe two weeks of antibiotic therapy with **metronidazole** or **tetracycline.**

Gastroenteritis

Gastroenteritis is an infection of the *gastrointestinal tract* (in particular, the stomach and intestine) resulting in diarrhea and, sometimes, nausea and vomiting. It's usually caused by a virus or a bacteria (salmonella, shigella, campylobacter, *E. coli,* or Clostridium difficile); less often, it's caused by organisms called protozoa. "Traveller's diarrhea" is gastroenteritis (usually caused by drinking contaminated water) acquired while, well, travelling.

As most cases of gastroenteritis quickly go away on their own, the only therapy usually required is "supportive" in nature (for example, drinking lots of fluids to replace what you're losing). However, antibiotics should be considered if you have a particularly bad case of diarrhea, especially if you also have a fever or blood with your stool or if you have a problem with your immune system. A stool specimen tells your doctor the specific germ responsible and enables him to target the treatment directly at that organism. The preferred ***antibiotic*** is usually a ***fluoroquinolone;*** alternatives include **azithromycin** and **erythromycin.**

Gastro-esophageal Reflux Disease (GERD)

GERD (*gastro-esophageal reflux disease*) is a condition where stomach acid escapes into the esophagus and, typically, causes a burning feeling behind the breastbone. It's treated by lifestyle measures including keeping the head of your bed elevated and avoiding those things (such as fatty foods, colas, and excess alcohol) that aggravate the condition and, when necessary, by taking medicines that reduce stomach acidity.

Although over-the-counter products such as antacids or ***histamine-2 (H2) receptor antagonists*** (for example, Pepcid) usually suffice, sometimes more potent acid-suppressing prescription drugs called ***proton pump inhibitors*** **(PPIs)** are required. With the availability of these powerful drugs, surgery — which used to be done not infrequently — is now typically performed only if an individual prefers this over the prospect (and significant cost) of taking PPI medication on an indefinite basis.

Glaucoma

The eye is largely a hollow organ save for being filled with fluid that goes by the wonderful names *aqueous humour* and *vitreous humour*. Aqueous humour fills the front part of the eye, and vitreous humour fills the back part of the eye. In glaucoma, it's the aqueous humour fluid doctors are concerned with. Like a sink with the tap turned on and the drain open, the eye is constantly making new fluid and constantly removing old fluid. If you have glaucoma, your eye cannot drain the fluid quickly enough, which leads to a buildup of excess fluid within the eye — this excess fluid causes the pressure within the eye to increase.

If glaucoma is left untreated it can lead to blindness. Your eye doctor should routinely test you for this condition during your regular eye check-ups.

Although laser therapy or eye surgery may be performed, the mainstay of therapy for glaucoma involves eye drops. Some eye drops reduce pressure in the eye by slowing down the amount of new fluid being made within the eye; other eye drops work by helping fluid to drain from the eye. Initial therapy is usually with **beta blocker** or **prostaglandin analog** eye drops. Other choices are **carbonic anhydrase inhibitor, adrenergic agonist** (typically **brimonidine**), or **cholinergic agonist** eye drops. Commonly, a combination of different types of eye drops is required (in which case drops from different families are selected). Because of the risk of side-effects, **apraclonidine** eye drops and oral carbonic anhydrase inhibitor medicine are not typically used except in emergencies.

Gonorrhea

Gonorrhea is a sexually transmitted disease (STD) caused by *gonococcus* bacteria. It's acquired during vaginal, rectal, or oral sex. The likelihood of becoming infected with gonorrhea is considerably reduced by use of a condom during sexual activity. Gonorrhea can also be spread from mother to newborn during childbirth, leading to *conjunctivitis* in the child.

Infected men have discomfort when they urinate and a discharge from the urethra (the opening at the end of the penis). Women's symptoms can vary from being nonexistent to discomfort when urinating, fever, and vaginal discharge. In women, the infection can spread to the fallopian tubes, causing scarring that may result in infertility. (Rarely, gonorrhea affects the joints.)

Gonorrhea is curable with ***antibiotic*** therapy. The preferred treatment for vaginal/urethral infections is with a ***cephalosporin*** or a ***fluoroquinolone.*** **Azithromycin** is an effective alternative, but is more expensive and is more likely to cause side-effects.

Because chlamydia and gonorrhea infections often co-exist, if your doctor diagnoses you as having gonorrhea she will recommend treating you for both conditions at the same time.

Gout

Gout is a form of arthritis caused by tiny *uric acid crystals* that create inflammation in one or more joints. Uric acid is created during the body's normal metabolism as it goes about breaking down old or unneeded proteins. Some people, however, make too much uric acid or are unable to excrete sufficient quantities of it; this leads to high levels in the blood that, in turn, can lead to the formation of uric acid crystals in the joints. The crystals may be tiny, but the pain they cause is anything but. Gout typically affects the big toe, but can show up in other joints.

The goals of therapy are to

- ✔ **Decrease pain and inflammation.** This is accomplished by using ***nonsteroidal anti-inflammatory drugs (NSAIDs).*** Of the NSAIDs, **indomethacin** is particularly effective. If NSAIDs don't work or can't be used because of concerns about side-effects, your doctor may prescribe an oral ***corticosteroid*** (or may inject a corticosteroid directly into the affected joint). Because of its tendency to cause side-effects in the high doses needed to treat an acute attack of gout, **colchicine** is not used often. ***Analgesics*** can be added if the pain control provided by an NSAID is insufficient.

- ✔ **Prevent a recurrence**. By reducing the level of uric acid in your blood, you're less likely to have a future attack of gout. This is achieved using either **allopurinol** (a ***xanthine oxidase inhibitor*** that decreases the production of uric acid) or a ***uricosuric agent*** such as **sufinpyrazone** or **probenecid** (these increase the excretion of uric acid from the body).

Don't start taking drugs to prevent a recurrence *during* an acute attack of gout, because doing so can actually make the attack worse. Start taking preventive drugs only after your acute attack has resolved. Along with the preventive drugs, your doctor should also prescribe an NSAID or low-dose colchicine for you to take for a few months to reduce the risk of a recurrence.

Headaches

Tension headaches are typically felt as a pressure over the temples and are commonly brought on by stress. Most people experience tension headaches from time to time. They are typically treated with over-the-counter analgesics. Rarely, ***narcotic ("opioid") analgesics*** are used. (See the warning later in this section.)

Migraine headaches typically are felt as a severe throbbing pain affecting one side of the head and are usually associated with nausea and vomiting. Most people having a migraine headache feel pretty darn rotten. Often, people see flashing lights or geometric patterns before the headache begins. The presence of these warning symptoms enables the prompt use of medicines to help prevent the attack from worsening, as we look at next.

The treatment of migraine headaches has been revolutionized with the discovery of ***serotonin (5-HT) receptor agonist*** therapy. Indeed, Heather, a migraine sufferer, thanks her lucky stars scientists were clever enough to come up with this treatment (and that her neurologist friend, Ralph, figured out what was wrong with her; doctors should *never* try to diagnose themselves!). These prescription medicines are given at the first hint of a migraine developing and typically abort the attack at that early stage. Another medication used for this purpose is ***ergotamine,*** but it's not as effective or as safe as serotonin receptor agonist therapy so it's not prescribed very often.

If your migraines are infrequent, no other treatment is required (apart from pain relief). On the other hand, if migraines are a recurring problem for you, and if you're unable to prevent attacks without prescription drugs, you would benefit from taking prescription medicine to prevent a migraine attack from occurring. The best drug for prevention is a ***beta blocker,*** such as **propranolol.** Other choices include ***calcium channel blockers, tricyclic antidepressants,*** **topiramate,** and **divalproex.** Because of the risk of serious side-effects, **methysergide** is seldom used.

If you have a migraine headache, the pain can be eased with use of over-the-counter ***analgesics,*** such as **acetaminophen;** *nonsteroidal anti-inflammatory drugs (NSAIDs)*, such as **ASA, naproxen,** or **indomethacin;** or *narcotic ("opioid") analgesics* such as **codeine** or **oxycodone.**

Use the least amount of analgesic for the least period of time that gives you sufficient relief from the pain. Overuse of analgesics can actually cause headaches (both tension and migraine) to occur *more* often and also can reduce the effectiveness of preventive medicines.

Heart Attack

A heart attack (*myocardial infarction,* or MI) is permanent damage to a portion of the heart muscle that occurs when a (coronary) artery becomes blocked, leading to insufficient blood flow (and, hence, reduced oxygen delivery) to the affected area of the heart. The blockage comprises a cholesterol *plaque* (or buildup) that slowly develops over years and a blood clot that forms suddenly in the area of the plaque and precipitates the acute attack.

Typically, a heart attack causes a severe, crushing, or heavy discomfort in the chest associated with shortness of breath, sweating, and nausea. The acute management of a heart attack is performed in-hospital and is beyond the scope of this book. In this section we review subsequent, out-of-hospital prescription drug therapy.

Unless some reason (such as a drug allergy or intolerance) prevents you from taking the following medicines, you should be treated with:

- ✔ **ASA.** This is not a prescription drug, but it's so important we're mentioning it here anyhow. ASA is a mild "blood thinner" and helps prevent further blood clots from forming in your coronary arteries. If you're unable to take ASA, **clopidogrel** is an effective alternative.

- ✔ **A *beta blocker*.** Beta blockers reduce the amount of work the heart performs, and reduce your risk of having another heart attack.

- ✔ **An *angiotensin converting enzyme (ACE) inhibitor*.** ACE inhibitors help to widen the arteries and hence make it easier for the heart to pump blood through the circulation. This helps to protect the heart against further damage. If you're unable to take an ACE inhibitor, an *angiotensin receptor blocker (ARB)* is an effective alternative.

- ✔ **A *statin*.** Statins work principally by lowering the bad LDL cholesterol. (We talk more about this under "Lipid Disorders" in this chapter.). This makes your arteries less prone to developing an additional buildup of cholesterol (and, thus, less likely to develop further blockages). In most cases, if you've had a heart attack taking a statin is a good idea even if your blood cholesterol levels are very good to start with.

- ✔ ***Nitroglycerin*.** Always carry with you a quick-acting form of nitroglycerin to take in the event you develop chest discomfort. We discuss this further in the "Angina" section of this chapter.

Heart Failure

The heart is, basically, a glorified pump. A magnificent, incredible, wondrous pump (when's the last time you bought a pump that worked non-stop for 80-plus years?), but a pump nonetheless. And in much the same way that if you have a malfunctioning sump pump in your basement water will eventually accumulate in your house, if you have a malfunctioning heart pump excess fluid will eventually accumulate in your body.

Fluid accumulation in your lungs (*pulmonary edema*) makes you feel short of breath, and fluid accumulation in your legs (*peripheral edema* — or, simply, *edema*) makes your ankles swell. If this collection of fluid in the body is caused by poor heart function, it's known as *congestive heart failure* — or, simply, *heart failure*. Most commonly, heart failure is caused by damage to the heart muscle from one or more heart attacks, but it also can be because of other forms of heart disease including damage from viruses, damage to one or more heart valves, or, occasionally, severe lung disease.

Prescription drugs used to treat heart failure are

- ✔ *Diuretics.* Diuretics help flush out the extra fluid that has accumulated in your body. The preferred diuretic is usually **furosemide.** If you have a badly damaged heart, **spironolactone** may also be used.

  Because in some people spironolactone can cause dangerously high levels of potassium in the blood, your doctor will need to periodically send you for blood tests to monitor your potassium level and kidney function.

- ✔ **An *angiotensin converting enzyme (ACE) inhibitor.*** ACE inhibitors help to widen the arteries and hence make it easier for the heart to pump blood through the circulation. If you're unable to take an ACE inhibitor, an ***angiotensin receptor blocker (ARB)*** is an effective alternative.

- ✔ *Beta blockers.* These drugs are life-saving in the treatment of heart failure. The most important caveat here, however, is that when a beta blocker is used to treat heart failure, it should be started in very low dose and then increased only if you're not getting significant side-effects from it. (Also, not all beta blockers are effective in this role — in particular, *short-acting* **metoprolol,** though useful to treat angina and other conditions, is not used in the treatment of heart failure.)

✔ **Digoxin.** Digoxin, a drug that has been around for generations, has only a secondary role in the treatment of heart failure. It's generally used only if you have not responded to the therapies mentioned earlier in this list or if you also have a heart rhythm problem called *atrial fibrillation* (which we discuss under "Arrhythmias" in this chapter).

✔ **Hydralazine in combination with a long-acting *nitroglycerin*.** This combination is generally used only if you have not responded to the therapies mentioned earlier in this list.

Hemorrhoids

Hemorrhoids are swollen veins in the area of the anus. They typically become apparent either when they bleed, in which case you'll notice red blood on the toilet paper when you wipe yourself after having a bowel movement, or you will see blood streaking your stool, or when a blood clot forms within them, in which case a fairly small, inflamed, itchy, tender lump may protrude from the anus. Of course, "fairly small" is relative. If you're the one with the problem, your hemorrhoid may technically be the size of a grape, but may make you feel like you've become overly intimate with a watermelon.

The treatment of hemorrhoids consists of consuming sufficient fluids and fibre (to avoid constipation) and using over-the-counter, topical medicine. Sometimes, topical **hydrocortisone** (a type of *corticosteroid*) is prescribed to help relieve discomfort and itching. Topical hydrocortisone should *not* be used to treat hemorrhoids for more than a week or so, because more prolonged use can damage the healthy surrounding tissues. If the problem is severe, treatment might involve a "banding procedure," where a surgeon puts a rubber band around the hemorrhoid, which makes it shrink and painlessly drop off, or, on occasion, surgery.

Hepatitis, Viral

Hepatitis means liver inflammation. Although a number of viruses can cause this, the majority of cases are caused by infection with *hepatitis A virus, hepatitis B virus,* or *hepatitis C virus.* The name of the virus and the infection it causes are used interchangeably — so, for example, someone who has developed hepatitis from hepatitis B virus is said to "have hepatitis B."

✔ Hepatitis A is acquired by ingesting contaminated food or water. Hepatitis A is not as serious as hepatitis B or C and typically goes away on its own without leaving any scarring on the liver.

✔ Hepatitis B is acquired by exposure to infected body fluids. Although most people with hepatitis B have a full recovery, in some individuals the virus can remain in the body indefinitely, leading to *chronic hepatitis,* which can cause scarring of the liver, liver failure, or liver cancer. People with chronic hepatitis B sometimes benefit from treatment with **interferon** or **lamivudine** or **adefovir.**

✔ In the past, hepatitis C was typically transmitted through contaminated blood transfusions; nowadays, it's most commonly transmitted between users of illicit drugs who share contaminated needles. It too can lead to chronic hepatitis. People with chronic hepatitis C sometimes benefit from combined treatment with interferon and **ribavirin.**

When viral hepatitis first develops it's called *acute hepatitis.* Doctors don't have specific therapy to speed recovery from acute hepatitis A or B, so treatment is simply "supportive" (ensuring proper hydration, rest, and so on). It's unknown whether treating acute hepatitis C with prescription drugs is helpful; some doctors recommend using **interferon.**

Because the liver is involved with how the body handles *(metabolizes)* many drugs (both prescription and non-prescription), if you have hepatitis it's imperative that you let your doctor know what drugs you're taking as they may need to be discontinued (or, at least, have the dosages adjusted) until you've recovered.

Effective vaccines are now available to prevent hepatitis A and hepatitis B. It's wise to get the hepatitis A vaccine if you're at increased risk of contracting this condition (such as, for example, if you're travelling to parts of the world where this disease is common). Hepatitis B vaccination is recommended for all children in Canada and is also given to adults (such as health care workers) who are at increased risk of exposure to hepatitis B.

Herpes, Genital

Genital herpes is an infection caused by the herpes simplex virus (HSV). Genital herpes typically causes sores to develop on the genitals or buttocks. The virus is spread by sexually intimate contact; however, the risk of becoming infected is reduced (though not eliminated) by using condoms and by avoiding sexual contact when the sores are present.

Antiviral agents such as **acyclovir, famciclovir,** and **valacyclovir** can treat symptoms and can reduce the likelihood of sores recurring, but these medicines do not cure the disease. If you're affected by genital herpes, taking valacyclovir *and* using a condom help protect your partner from contracting your condition.

 Treatment with antiviral drugs works best if started within 24 hours of the appearance of sores. Therefore, it's a good idea to keep a supply of medicine on hand. That way, if sores appear you can start therapy right away rather than going through the hassle of trying to get a prescription on very short notice.

Hirsutism

Hirsutism refers to the presence, in women, of unwanted hair; it's typically on the face and lower abdomen, though the limbs can also be affected. Although all women have both male and female hormones, if you have hirsutism you may have an imbalance of the two, with a relative excess of male hormones.

One particularly common cause is *polycystic ovary syndrome* (PCOS), which we discuss elsewhere in this chapter. Uncommonly, hirsutism is caused by more serious diseases of the ovaries or adrenal glands. On occasion, it occurs as a side-effect from a drug (such as anabolic steroids used — inappropriately — by some bodybuilders and competitive athletes). Sometimes, no cause is found.

Hirsutism is typically treated using physical measures such as plucking, waxing, shaving, or bleaching. A topical prescription medication, **eflornithine,** inhibits hair growth and may be helpful. If these measures are insufficient, oral prescription drugs may be used. These work either by reducing the amount of male hormone your body makes, or by blocking the action on your body of the male hormone that is present. The best drug to first try is generally an *oral contraceptive* (**Diane-35** is particularly effective). If, after six months or so, oral contraceptives haven't helped you, your doctor often will add **spironolactone.** Drugs used less often include **flutamide, finasteride,** and *gonadotropin-releasing hormone (GnRH) analogs.* Because concerns exist that some of these drugs could harm a fetus, if you're sexually active your doctor will likely recommend you use an oral contraceptive along with any of the other therapies just mentioned.

HIV/AIDS

HIV is the abbreviation for the *human immunodeficiency virus.* AIDS is the abbreviation for *acquired immunodeficiency syndrome.* HIV is the virus that leads to the disease AIDS, and because of this connection the two terms are typically linked together as "HIV/AIDS."

HIV infection occurs through activities such as not using a condom during sexually intimate contact with an infected partner, sharing "dirty" needles, or receiving a transfusion of contaminated blood. With currently used precautions, the risk of receiving HIV-contaminated blood products in Canada is very remote.

HIV leads to AIDS by infecting and damaging the cells in our body that help to ward off infections and cancers (that is, it damages the immune system — hence the term *immunodeficiency*). People with HIV/AIDS are especially at risk for pneumonia caused by an organism called *Pneumocystis jiroveci* and for developing a type of cancer called Kaposi's sarcoma.

Treatment is geared toward minimizing the amount of the virus in the body (which helps reduce the likelihood of it causing harm) and, if HIV/AIDS has led to a complication — such as pneumonia or cancer — treating this complication. Current therapies have transformed what until not long ago was a uniformly fatal disease into one that can generally be effectively treated and controlled (though not cured). Many people with HIV/AIDS continue to lead full and active lives. The therapy, however, is very complicated and requires the affected individual to invest a great deal of time and energy into keeping track of (and properly taking) their medicines.

HIV is a type of virus called a *retrovirus* and therefore the medicines used to combat it (which are "anti," or against, the retrovirus) are known as **antiretroviral drugs.** To effectively fight HIV/AIDS you typically must take a minimum of three different antiretroviral drugs, and these are usually taken a number of different times per day. This treatment plan is called HAART (highly active antiretroviral therapy). HAART typically includes two drugs from the **nucleoside reverse transcriptase inhibitor (NRTI)** family in combination with one drug from either the **non-nucleoside reverse transcriptase inhibitor (NNRTI)** family or one or two drugs from the **protease inhibitor (PI)** family. We discuss antiretroviral drugs in more detail in Chapter 6.

Hyperprolactinemia (Enlarged Prostate)

Prolactin is a hormone made by the pituitary gland. High levels of prolactin occur normally in pregnant and breastfeeding women. (Prolactin assists these women with milk production. Its role in men is unclear.) High levels of prolactin (*hyperprolactinemia*) can also occur as a result of health problems including pituitary tumours, hypothyroidism, and drug side-effects. Often, however, doctors do not find a cause.

High prolactin levels can cause women to lose their periods, become infertile, and develop milky breast discharge even if they are not (and have not recently been) pregnant. In men, hyperprolactinemia can lead to loss of sexual drive (that is, decreased libido), breast swelling, and erectile dysfunction.

When hyperprolactinemia occurs because of a disease, the treatment is, ideally, aimed toward the underlying disease (for example, treating a hypothyroid person with thyroid supplements). If, however, no cause is found or if a pituitary tumour is responsible, prescription medication is typically used. Indeed, such medicines work so well surgery to treat pituitary tumours — which used to be commonly performed — is now rarely necessary.

The two prescription drugs available are **bromocriptine** and **cabergoline** (these are members of the ***dopamine agonist*** family of drugs). They are equally effective; however, bromocriptine frequently causes severe nausea and cabergoline costs an arm and a leg. Hmm, some choice, eh? If cost isn't a factor for you, we suggest you go with cabergoline. If cost *is* a consideration, we recommend you go with bromocriptine and, if you're unable to tolerate it, you can then look at switching to cabergoline.

Hypertension

Hypertension is also known as high blood pressure, but we like to economize so we'll stick with the one-word moniker. Blood pressure is measured as *something* over *something* (for example, "120 over 80," written as 120/80). The first number represents the *systolic* value and the second number the *diastolic* value.

- ✔ The systolic value is the amount of pressure in the large arteries as the heart contracts to propel blood through the circulation.

- ✔ The diastolic value is the amount of pressure in the large arteries when the heart is at rest.

In Canada, hypertension is defined as a blood pressure above 140/90 when checked by a doctor in the office, or above 135/85 when checked yourself at home. Because blood pressure varies hour-to-hour and day-to-day, before you're diagnosed as having hypertension your pressure almost always will have been found to be elevated on multiple occasions (not just once).

Most people with hypertension have the so-called "essential" variety. *Essential* in this context is a medical term meaning "of unknown cause." (This is quite different from the way the word is generally used in everyday language, where it means "of the utmost importance.") Only in about five percent of cases of hypertension do doctors ever find a cause.

If not satisfactorily treated, hypertension can lead to a number of complications including strokes, heart attacks, and kidney failure. If you've been diagnosed with hypertension, your target blood pressure is less than 140/90. (Note that these are your targets only if you do not have other diseases such as diabetes or kidney disease, either of which would warrant a lower target of less than 130/80.)

Non-drug therapies include participating in regular exercise, weight loss (if you're overweight), and restricting the amount of salt and alcohol in your diet. Most people, however, also require medication (anti-hypertensive drugs) to control their pressure. Indeed, two, three, or even four types may be necessary.

The 2006 Canadian Hypertension Education Program (CHEP) recommendations are that if you have an elevated diastolic blood pressure (with or without an elevated systolic blood pressure):

- ✔ The first drug used should be either a ***thiazide diuretic,*** a ***beta blocker*** (provided you're under age 60), an ***angiotensin converting enzyme (ACE) inhibitor,*** a long-acting ***calcium channel blocker,*** or an ***angiotensin receptor blocker (ARB).***

- ✔ If a second drug is needed because one alone failed to satisfactorily control your blood pressure, it's best to choose another one from the same list in the first bullet.

For people who have an elevation of only their systolic blood pressure, the CHEP recommendation is treatment with a thiazide diuretic, a long-acting calcium channel blocker (of the dihydropyridine type), or an ARB. If that is insufficient, CHEP recommends adding another drug from this group.

 ACE inhibitors are often less effective in people of African ancestry, so they are typically not recommended as initial therapy for members of this group (unless some other reason to take an ACE inhibitor exists, such as kidney disease).

We discuss anti-hypertensive drugs in detail in Chapter 6. You can find out more about CHEP at www.hypertension.ca/chep.

Hyperthyroidism

The thyroid gland is a small (25 grams or so) organ located just in front of the windpipe (the *trachea*). One of its main jobs is to help maintain normal metabolism. The thyroid does this by manufacturing (and then releasing into the bloodstream) the aptly named substance *thyroid hormone.* Having too much thyroid hormone in your system is called *hyperthyroidism,* and it has the same effect on your body that driving down the Trans-Canada Highway at 200 km/hour would have on your car. It's sure gonna wear things out pretty darn quickly! (Or get you pulled over for speeding, but that's another matter.)

Typical symptoms of hyperthyroidism include fatigue, excess sweating, feeling overly hot, frequent bowel movements, palpitations, tremor, and weight loss. The most common cause of hyperthyroidism is a condition called *Graves' disease.*

Two main forms of therapy are used for hyperthyroidism caused by Graves' disease:

- **Radioactive iodine.** This is typically required only once, is taken orally on an outpatient basis, starts to work within two to three weeks, and almost always cures the problem. Its main downside is that it usually leads to hypothyroidism (which we discuss in the next section).

- *Anti-thyroid agents.* Drugs within this family (which we discuss in Chapter 6) work quickly and effectively, but typically need to be taken for a minimum of 12 to 18 months before an attempt should be made to stop them. When they are discontinued, hyperthyroidism not infrequently will flare.

Because of its simplicity, effectiveness, and safety, most people with hyperthyroidism caused by Graves' disease elect to have radioactive iodine therapy rather than anti-thyroid medication.

If you have hyperthyroidism your doctor may also recommend you take a **beta blocker** such as **propranolol;** this is used purely to help control your symptoms until the other therapies mentioned in the preceding list have had time to bring your thyroid levels down to normal, at which point you can stop taking the beta blocker.

Hypothyroidism

If your thyroid gland (which we describe in the preceding section) is producing insufficient quantities of thyroid hormone, you're said to have *hypothyroidism*. Hypothyroidism can cause a number of symptoms including fatigue, weight gain, constipation, muscle aching, dry skin, and dry coarse hair.

The treatment of hypothyroidism is very simple: you simply take, in pill form, the thyroid hormone your gland has become unable to manufacture. Two types of thyroid hormone pills exist, **levothyroxine** (more typically called L-thyroxine) and **liothyronine.** Liothyronine is seldom used. To determine whether you're on the right dose of L-thyroxine, your doctor uses a blood test to measure the level of a hormone called TSH (sometimes additional hormones called FT4 and FT3 are measured, too) and adjusts your dose, if necessary, based on the result.

A common misconception is that if you have hypothyroidism then you will continue to have symptoms despite being on (appropriate) therapy. This is simply not the case. If you're on the proper dose of L-thyroxine and you continue to have symptoms like those noted at the beginning of this section, then your thyroid condition is not responsible and your doctor needs to look for some other cause.

Incontinence, Urinary

Urinary incontinence refers to the inability to control the bladder resulting in the unplanned release of urine. Urinary incontinence may occur during activities such as coughing or sneezing (this is called *stress incontinence*) or when you're hit with a sudden need to empty your bladder (*urge incontinence*). Urge incontinence is also referred to as an *overactive bladder.*

Treatment of bladder incontinence generally includes a combination of techniques including *bladder training* (wherein you learn methods to help regulate bladder emptying), exercises to strengthen the pelvic muscles, medication, and, in some cases, surgery.

Prescription drug therapy has only a small role to play in the treatment of stress incontinence. Some evidence exists that if you're post-menopausal your symptoms may improve with *menopausal hormone therapy* (also known as *hormone replacement therapy*), given either orally or vaginally.

To help urge incontinence, *anticholinergics* such as **oxybutynin** or **tolterodine** can be helpful. Troublesome side-effects (such as dry mouth) can be reduced by using the long-acting forms of these medicines (Ditropan XL and Detrol LA, respectively).

The full benefit of oxybutynin may not be seen for a few weeks, so it's often best not to give up on the drug prematurely (that is, you and your doctor may need to give it a few weeks before deciding it's not effective for you).

Infertility

Infertility is (somewhat arbitrarily) defined as the inability to conceive despite 12 months of trying. The treatment of infertility is targeted toward the underlying cause (of which there are many). In this section we look at some of the most common causes that doctors can treat with non-injectable drugs.

Many women are infertile because they do not ovulate (or they ovulate, but not consistently). Problems with ovulation can occur if you're overweight (particularly if you have *polycystic ovary syndrome,* which we discuss elsewhere in this chapter), in which case losing weight may restore your fertility. Drugs that can help induce ovulation include **clomiphene** and **letrozole,** and, being used increasingly often, **metformin** (a drug heretofore used only to treat diabetes but now known to help with ovulation if you have polycystic ovary syndrome).

Both men and women may be infertile because of a high prolactin level; in these circumstances, taking a ***dopamine agonist*** medicine such as **bromocriptine** to lower the prolactin level to normal may help restore fertility (for more information, see the "Prolactin, High" section in this chapter).

Men who have low testosterone levels may have improved fertility if given **testosterone** therapy.

Inflammatory Bowel Disease

Inflammatory bowel disease (IBD) is a condition of unknown cause wherein a portion of the gastrointestinal tract (most commonly the bowel) becomes inflamed. This can lead to symptoms such as fever, weight loss, abdominal pain, and (often bloody) diarrhea. IBD includes two different conditions:

- *Crohn's disease* can affect any part of the gastrointestinal tract.
- *Ulcerative colitis* affects just the large bowel.

The treatment of IBD is aimed at reducing the inflammation present.

Crohn's disease affecting the end portion of the small bowel (the *terminal ileum*) is treated with oral **5-ASA.** If you do not respond to this, you will require additional drugs; these may include **antibiotics** and **corticosteroids.** If you have persisting diarrhea, your doctor may recommend anti-diarrhea therapy with **loperamide** or **cholestyramine.** If your Crohn's disease is affecting your large bowel, the preferred prescription drugs are oral 5-ASA or oral **sulfasalazine.** If you do not respond to these, antibiotics and oral corticosteroids may be added.

If you have ulcerative colitis affecting only your rectum (*ulcerative proctitis*) or the last few feet of bowel, the preferred treatment is **5-aminosalicylic acid** (also known as **5-ASA** or **mesalamine**) suppositories or enemas. Another option is to use **corticosteroid** foam enemas such as Cortifoam. If you have ulcerative colitis that is affecting a greater portion of your bowel, you will also require oral drugs. Oral 5-ASA or **sulfasalazine** are most commonly used. If you do not respond to these drugs or if you're having particularly bad symptoms, oral **prednisone** (a form of corticosteroid) is used. If you're having a very severe attack you may require hospitalization and intravenous corticosteroid therapy.

Influenza

Influenza is an infection caused by the influenza virus. Typical symptoms of influenza include the sudden onset of fever, headache, malaise, muscle aching, and cough. If the infection has led to pneumonia, then cough, chest pain, and shortness of breath may occur.

Table 5-1 shows the Canadian Medical Association's guidelines (which we have slightly modified) to help distinguish a common cold from influenza.

Table 5-1 Distinguishing the Common Cold from Influenza

Symptom	Common Cold	Influenza
Fever	Rare	Usual, high fever
Headache	Rare	Usual, can be severe
General aches and pains	Sometimes, mild	Usual, often severe
Fatigue and weakness	Sometimes, mild	Usual, severe
Runny, stuffy nose	Common	Common
Sneezing	Common	Sometimes
Sore throat	Common	Common

Because influenza may occur in outbreaks, if you're at higher risk for infection (as is true if you're elderly or if you have kidney disease, cancer, diabetes, or other conditions where your immune system may not be working properly) it's wise for you to get an influenza vaccination (a "flu shot") annually (typically in the late fall).

The term "the flu" tends to be used rather indiscriminately both by lay people and by a surprising number of health care providers. "The flu," however, actually refers to a very specific viral illness (the one caused by the influenza virus). This is important, because treating most other viral illnesses (like the common cold, for instance) with antiviral drugs is of no value.

The treatment of influenza is mostly *supportive* (that is, making sure you drink sufficient fluids and get appropriate rest, treating aches and pains with *analgesics* such as **acetaminophen**, and so on). *Antiviral* therapy with **zanamavir** or **oseltamivir** may speed up recovery from the infection; however, to get the most benefit from these drugs, take them as soon as possible after you have developed influenza.

Do not take **ASA** if you have influenza. Using ASA while you have influenza can lead to a devastating complication called Reye syndrome, in which the brain and liver can be severely damaged. (Children, teenagers, and young adults are at particular risk.)

Insomnia

Insomnia is a condition where people suffer from an *involuntary* lack of sleep. This is to be distinguished from conditions where people *voluntarily* elect to obtain little sleep; one such example is married physicians who are foolhardy enough to take on projects like writing a book on prescription drugs, which means that instead of sleeping they are word-processing at 2 a.m.

If identifiable causes of insomnia can be found — such as use of tobacco, consumption of caffeine or alcohol, depression, anxiety, or stress — treatment should be geared toward these underlying factors. If you require a drug, it's best to take one that remains in the body for only a few hours; the drug will help you sleep but will not cause you to be groggy the next morning. The typically preferred drugs to treat insomnia are **temazepam, triazolam, zaleplon,** and **zopiclone.** (Longer-acting drugs — including over-the-counter products such as **diphenhydramine** — are generally best avoided.)

Irritable Bowel Syndrome

Irritable bowel syndrome (IBS) is a very common condition in which you're prone to varying degrees of constipation or diarrhea or both, accompanied by abdominal cramping and bloating. The *irritable* in irritable bowel syndrome refers to the *bowel* being irritable (as in easily irritated or upset), not your personality! IBS is sometimes called *spastic colon.*

If you have IBS, you may find some relief by cutting down on your intake of raw fruits and vegetables, fatty foods, caffeinated products, and the sweetener sorbitol. If prescription drug therapy is required, several medicines are available to assist you. **Tegaserod** can be helpful if you're a woman and your main symptoms are constipation, cramps, and bloating. (Tegaserod has not been proven to be effective in treating men with IBS.) **Pinaverium** may be of value when the predominant symptom is abdominal pain or cramps. Rarely, *tricyclic antidepressants,* such as **desipramine,** are used to ease discomfort.

Kidney Failure

Kidney failure (also known as *renal failure*) means your kidneys have been damaged and, as a result, can no longer properly carry out their normal functions. The kidneys can be damaged by many things, including hypertension, diabetes, infections, and inflammation (as can happen with lupus, which we also look at in this chapter). Only if the degree of damage is quite severe will you notice symptoms, such as swollen legs, weight loss, and fatigue.

A key part of therapy is to treat the underlying cause of the kidney damage — for example, controlling high blood glucose if you have diabetes and controlling high blood pressure if you have hypertension. Additionally, *angiotensin converting enzyme (ACE) inhibitors* or *angiotensin receptor blockers (ARBs)* are very helpful at preventing many forms of kidney failure from worsening.

Depending on the severity of your kidney failure, you may also require:

- ✔ *Diuretics.* These are used to remove excess fluids from your body. **Furosemide** is the most commonly used diuretic with kidney failure.

- ✔ **Blood pressure medication** (also called *anti-hypertensive therapy*). Most people with kidney failure have high blood pressure (either as a cause of the kidney failure or as a consequence of it). The preferred anti-hypertensive medications are *ACE inhibitors, ARBs, diuretics,* **diltiazem,** **verapamil,** and *beta blockers.*

✔ **Medicines to prevent bone damage.** *Renal osteodystrophy* is a condition in which the bones become weakened due to a change in their structure. Treatment to prevent this typically includes a form of **vitamin D** called **calcitriol.**

✔ **Drugs to prevent phosphate accumulation in the body.** This is typically accomplished by taking **calcium carbonate** or **calcium acetate** supplements.

✔ **Drugs to correct anemia. Iron** supplements are commonly prescribed. In some cases, it's also helpful to take **erythropoietin** or **darbepoetin;** these drugs stimulate the bone marrow to produce red blood cells.

✔ **Sodium bicarbonate.** This helps reduce acid buildup in the blood.

✔ **Drugs for abnormal lipids.** Kidney failure often causes abnormal levels of cholesterol and triglycerides; these problems can be effectively treated with *statins.*

✔ **Dialysis.** Dialysis rids the body of waste products. Dialysis is required only if you have severe kidney failure (called *end stage renal disease*).

Kidney Stones

Kidney stones are very hard (hence, "stones"), typically very small, masses that form within the kidneys. Kidney stones can be made up of various substances, but in most cases calcium is the main ingredient.

Although not all kidney stones cause symptoms, when they do you may experience an agonizing pain in the small of your back that travels down your side toward your genital region. Apart from *analgesics,* prescription drug therapy has a limited role in the treatment of an *existing* stone; rather, medications are used to prevent *new* stones from forming. If you have had a kidney stone, it's important your physician try to determine whether you have a predisposing condition (such as a disorder of your calcium balance) that led to your problem. If you do, then treating this underlying condition helps prevent further stones from forming.

Because your treatment is influenced by the nature of your stone, it's important to try to collect it as it passes. This is usually done by urinating into a filter that will catch the stone as it leaves your body. When you've caught it, you can take it to your doctor for analysis. Be prepared, by the way, for a surprise as your stone passes. Based on the severity of your pain you may be anticipating something the size of Ayres Rock, only to encounter what more commonly resembles a grain of rice.

To prevent more kidney stones from forming it's important that you maintain excellent hydration by drinking lots of water (unless your doctor directs you otherwise). Medications used to prevent kidney stones have specific purposes:

- To prevent *calcium-containing* stones from forming, **hydrochlorothiazide** is often used. This drug reduces the amount of calcium passing from the blood into the urine. Less calcium in the urine, less calcium present to form a stone.

- To prevent the formation of *uric acid–containing* stones, **allopurinol** is very helpful. This drug reduces the amount of uric acid in your urine.

- To prevent *cystine-containing* stones from forming, **penicillamine** and **captopril** can be of value.

Libido, Reduced

Libido is the desire to engage in sexual activity. To say what "reduced" libido is depends on a number of things, including what your level of libido typically is and what you believe it should be. Reduced libido has *many* different causes, including, importantly, your and your partner's general physical and mental health, any drugs you may be taking, whether you have a deficiency of certain hormones including testosterone, and so on. The treatment of reduced libido is geared, wherever possible, toward the underlying cause.

Some post-menopausal women find that their libido improves with use of **estrogen** and/or **progestin. Testosterone** is effective for men with a deficiency of this hormone (its effectiveness for women is less established; however, it's often prescribed for those women who have low testosterone levels).

Lipid Disorders (Abnormal Cholesterol and Triglyceride Levels)

Cholesterol (a type of naturally occurring steroid) and triglycerides (a type of fat) are collectively known as *lipids*. Not all cholesterol is alike. *LDL* cholesterol is a bad cholesterol (think "L for Lousy"), and you want to have a low level of LDL in your blood. *HDL* is a good cholesterol (think "H for Healthy"), and you want to have a high level of HDL in your blood.

When lipids are present in abnormal levels you're said to have *dyslipidemia*. Abnormal levels of cholesterol can increase the risk of atherosclerosis ("hardening of the arteries"), and very high levels of triglycerides can lead to a serious disease of the pancreas called *pancreatitis* (the role of triglycerides in the development of atherosclerosis is less clear).

Because high LDL cholesterol is closely linked to strokes and heart attacks, aggressively lowering LDL is typically the number one priority in treating dyslipidemia.

The treatment of dyslipidemia includes lifestyle measures, such as consuming a low-fat diet, eating sufficient fibre, avoiding excess alcohol, exercising regularly, and so on. However, even with good adherence to these measures dyslipidemia often persists and prescription drugs are required. The main types of drugs used to treat it are

- *Statins:* Statins are the preferred type of drug for most people who have dyslipidemia. They are very effective at lowering LDL cholesterol levels. They are less effective at raising HDL and lowering triglycerides. Of the many statins available, the ones best able to perform all three of these tasks are **atorvastatin** and **rosuvastatin.**

- *Fibrates:* These drugs are quite effective at lowering triglyceride levels, somewhat effective at raising HDL cholesterol levels, and not very effective at lowering LDL cholesterol levels. Fibrates are typically used if your main lipid problem is high triglycerides.

- **Ezetimibe:** This drug is helpful in reducing LDL cholesterol. It's generally used in combination with a statin if a statin by itself has not succeeded in sufficiently lowering your LDL level. Ezetimibe is also used if you had to stop taking a statin because it was causing you side-effects.

✔ **Cholestyramine:** This drug is somewhat helpful in lowering LDL cholesterol levels. Because it's not very potent (and because it can be a hassle to take), it's not used very often.

✔ **Niacin:** This drug's main role is in reducing triglycerides and raising HDL cholesterol. Because niacin commonly causes side-effects it's not used very often. (Newer, better tolerated versions of niacin are now available, and this may lead to their increased usage in the future.)

Lupus

Lupus, or systemic lupus erythematosis (SLE for short), is a chronic, inflammatory process where an individual's immune system malfunctions and, as a result, a variety of body tissues can become injured. Although lupus can affect virtually any organ, the areas of the body most likely to be involved are the skin, joints, lungs, heart, kidneys, and nervous system (the brain and nerves).

The treatment of lupus depends on which tissues are involved and how severely they are affected.

✔ If you have *Raynaud's phenomenon,* a condition in which your fingertips or toes temporarily turn white upon cold exposure, treatment with **calcium channel blockers** is often helpful. If these haven't worked for you, then **angiotensin converting enzyme (ACE) inhibitors** may be tried, or, on occasion, your doctor may prescribe **phosphodiesterase type 5 (PDE5) inhibitors** (the same drugs, by the way, that are used to treat erectile dysfunction).

✔ If your lupus has caused you to have fatigue, joint pain, or a skin rash, your physician will likely recommend you take a **nonsteroidal anti-inflammatory drug (NSAID)** together with **hydroxychloroquine.**

✔ If your lupus is more severe and is damaging your internal organs, other very potent prescription drugs may be added including **prednisone** (usually together with an **immunosuppressive drug** or, occasionally, a **biological response modifier** such as **rituximab**).

If you have lupus, you may be at risk of *photosensitivity.* Although this sounds like it refers to getting teary when you look at a picture of a puppy, in fact it's a condition where excess sun exposure causes a skin rash. You can help minimize your risk of developing a photosensitive skin rash by making liberal use of good sun protection.

Menopause

Menopause is a phase of a woman's life marked by loss of normal estrogen production and the end of reproductive abilities. It's typically also associated with the end of all menstrual cycles. Most of the time menopause occurs as a natural part of aging, but it also occurs when a woman has had surgery to remove her ovaries. Loss of the ovaries results in a dramatic decrease in estrogen production in the body. (If just the uterus — the womb — is removed and the ovaries are left in place and are still producing estrogen, a woman will not have periods but isn't considered menopausal.)

For some women, menopause is an easy transition. For others, it may involve unpleasant symptoms of hot flashes, night sweats, sleep disturbances, and mood changes.

To help minimize some of the symptoms associated with menopause, many women try over-the-counter and complementary/alternative medications. For some women, the use of prescription drugs can ease the transition. *Menopausal hormone therapy* (also known as *hormone replacement therapy*) was, until recently, commonly used; however, concerns about potential side-effects now limits its use to short-term treatment (usually fewer than four years). Several other, sometimes helpful, therapies are available, including **fluoxetine, paroxetine,** and **gabapentin. Venlafaxine** is sometimes used, but there is very limited evidence it's helpful. **Clonidine** is not used very much nowadays because of its limited benefit and frequent side-effects. (See also "Vaginal Dryness" and "Osteoporosis" in this chapter.)

Menstrual Cramps

Menstrual cramps are pains in the lower part of the abdomen experienced by some women during their menstrual periods. The precise cause of menstrual cramps is not known, but may be related to excess contractions of the muscles within the uterus (because of increased amounts of chemical messengers called *prostaglandins*).

Treatment is geared toward easing your pain by taking *nonsteroidal anti-inflammatory drugs (NSAIDs)*; these are particularly helpful because they reduce the levels of prostaglandins. *Analgesic* medication such as **acetaminophen** can provide some pain relief if NSAIDs are not available or can't be used. If these types of medications are not sufficient or not tolerated, *oral contraceptives* or **Depo-Provera** can also be helpful.

Multiple Sclerosis

Multiple sclerosis (MS) is a condition of unknown cause in which the cells coating the body's nerve fibres (called *myelin cells*) become damaged by inflammation. As a result, electrical signals that normally pass quickly along the nerves become slowed; this in turn can make certain areas of your body feel numb or become weak. MS is characterized by variable periods when symptoms are stable and unchanging interspersed with occasional flares of the disease.

Many different drugs can be used to treat MS, but those most commonly prescribed include:

- **Interferon beta.** This is given by injection and helps to reduce the frequency of flares. It may also help slow down progression of the disease.

- **Glatiramer.** This is given by injection and has benefits similar to interferon beta. It's of particular value if you have mild MS and have had it for only a brief period of time.

- *Corticosteroids.* A brief course of corticosteroids is helpful to treat a flare of MS; long-term therapy with these drugs is generally avoided, as their chronic use can lead to many side-effects.

Other drugs can be used to help alleviate symptoms. These include medications such as **baclofen** (to relieve muscle spasms), **bethanechol** (to treat urinary incontinence), *beta blockers* (to reduce tremor), and **amantadine** (to alleviate fatigue).

Muscle Cramps

Muscle cramps are sudden muscle spasms and typically affect the calves (less often the thighs or feet), often awakening the victim with a jolt. Your muscle cramp may quickly go away on its own. If not, you can try to stretch or massage the affected muscle until the cramp goes away. Stretching your leg muscles before you go to sleep can help prevent attacks.

Prescription drug therapy is seldom needed and should be used only if you're having cramps so frequently and of such severity you feel disabled by them. Although generally of limited value, **quinine** may help some people avoid attacks. To avoid side-effects, use only a low dose for as brief a time as possible. When your cramps have not occurred for a few days, it's best to discontinue the quinine.

Nausea and Vomiting

Literally hundreds of causes of nausea and vomiting exist, ranging from the relatively minor (like a viral ear infection) to the catastrophic (like a brain tumour). Most everyone has experienced nausea and vomiting at some point in their lives. Heather well recalls becoming familiar with every washroom on the Yonge Street subway line when, years ago, she was suffering from what should be called *all-day sickness* but somehow came to be called morning sickness. And Ian recalls more than one party back in the '70s when — well, let's not go there.

The mainstay of therapy for nausea and vomiting is to try to correct the underlying cause. When that's not feasible and when nausea and vomiting are persisting and troublesome, drugs are often used. For nausea and vomiting caused by a migraine headache disorder, commonly used drugs include **metoclopramide** and **prochloperazine.** For inner ear causes, *antihistamines* and *anticholinergics* are often used. For nausea and vomiting caused by chemotherapy, **dexamethasone** (a type of *corticosteroid)* and *serotonin antagonists* (such as **ondansetron**) are typically recommended. And for pregnancy-induced nausea and vomiting, **doxylamine/pyridoxine** (Diclectin) is commonly prescribed.

Obesity

For most adults, overweight is generally defined as having a *body mass index* (BMI) of 25 or more; obesity is defined as having a BMI of 30 or more. BMI is a reflection of weight for a given height.

To find out your BMI, we suggest you look at a chart (you can find one at Ian's Web site, www.ianblumer.com/images/bmiengc.pdf) or use an online calculator (you can find one at http://nhlbisupport.com/bmi/bminojs.htm).

No great prescription medicine is available to help you lose weight, but some people benefit from use of **orlistat** or **sibutramine.** Because of the only very modest degree of weight loss these drugs help achieve, and their risks of side-effects and uncertainties about their long-term safety, these drugs are usually recommended only if you're considerably overweight (BMI 30 or more).

Obsessive-Compulsive Disorder

People affected by obsessive-compulsive disorder (OCD) are obsessed with thoughts and ideas compelling them to perform certain tasks over and over. An example is someone who is so overly concerned about cleanliness they spend inordinate time each day repeatedly and unnecessarily cleaning an already clean item, such as a doorknob.

When drug therapy is required, *selective serotonin reuptake inhibitors (SSRIs)* and **clomipramine** can be effective. Because SSRIs tend to have fewer side-effects, they are typically tried first. A response may not be seen right away, so it's best to wait at least ten weeks before concluding the SSRI is not effective.

Osteoporosis

Osteoporosis is a disease where the bones become weak. Less bone is present (lesser *quantity*), and what is present is not as strong as it should be (lesser *quality*). Osteoporosis puts you at risk of a fracture (especially of the vertebrae, wrists, and hips) with little or no trauma. People used to think of bone as being a permanent, unchanging thing — little did we know how dynamic and ever-changing bone really is. Even as an adult you're constantly making new bone (and, at the same time, removing — *reabsorbing* — old bone). This is normally in a nice balance with equal bone formation and removal. With osteoporosis, however, this balance becomes distorted and you lose more bone than you're making.

Osteoporosis is treated with lifestyle measures — ensuring that you're consuming enough calcium and vitamin D, performing weight-bearing exercise, avoiding excess caffeine — and, when necessary, prescription drugs. Most of the drugs used to treat osteoporosis work by reducing the amount of bone your body is reabsorbing:

- ✔ **Bisphosphonates** are the most commonly used of these drugs and can decrease the likelihood of both vertebral and hip fractures.

- ✔ **Calcitonin** is used in selected circumstances and can help decrease vertebral fractures and may help decrease pain associated with them.

✔ For men, though not used often, **testosterone** can be helpful.

✔ In women, the use of **raloxifene** or, in selected cases, **estrogen** is effective.

✔ Currently, **teriparatide** is the only medication available that works primarily by increasing the amount of bone you create. The best use of teriparatide is still being sorted out.

Pain

Medicines used to treat pain are called *analgesics.* Because of its proven safety and effectiveness, **acetaminophen** is the preferred drug to treat everyday, minor aches and pains. *Nonsteroidal anti-inflammatory drugs (NSAIDs)*, such as **ibuprofen,** are also effective for treating pain and may be preferred over acetaminophen if there is a significant degree of inflammation present. (It can be difficult to tell if there is inflammation, so you may need to consult with your doctor to sort this out.) More severe pains typically require more potent medication, unless the underlying cause can be treated directly. The majority of prescription medicines to treat pain are *narcotic ("opioid") analgesics* either given alone or in combination with other drugs. **Tramadol** is a non-narcotic pain medicine that appears to be similar in potency to some narcotic analgesics.

For unclear reasons, some forms of pain — such as pain in the feet caused by nerve damage, as can be seen, for example, in a condition called diabetic peripheral neuropathy — are improved with *tricyclic antidepressants* (even if you're not depressed) or *anticonvulsants* (even if you don't have convulsions; convulsions are also called seizures).

Parkinson's Disease

Parkinson's disease is a condition in which the cells of the brain responsible for helping control movement become damaged and lose their ability to produce a special chemical called dopamine. Without sufficient dopamine, people develop symptoms such as tremor (especially of the hands), muscle stiffness, slow body movement, and difficulty walking. Sometimes, Parkinson's disease develops as a result of repeated head trauma or other brain injury, but most of the time a specific cause is not identified.

Because Parkinson's disease is a progressive disorder, doctors often talk about "early" disease when symptoms are mild and "late disease" when symptoms are more severe and significant disability may be present.

A variety of different types of medicine are available to help you if you have Parkinson's disease. These include

- ✔ **Levodopa** (L-dopa). Levodopa is an oral form of dopamine. It's given in combination with another drug, **carbidopa,** which helps the dopamine get from your blood into your brain where it's needed. Levodopa has long been the "gold-standard" when it comes to Parkinson's disease treatment.

- ✔ *Dopamine agonists.* These may be as effective as L-dopa and may be used instead of L-dopa to treat early disease. Additionally, they can be helpful in avoiding the fluctuations in muscle function that typically develop as Parkinson's disease progresses. They are also used in the later stages of disease in addition to L-dopa.

- ✔ **Entacapone.** This drug prolongs and enhances the action of L-dopa, and therefore is of value if you're taking L-dopa but it's wearing off too quickly after you take your dose.

- ✔ *MAO-B inhibitors*. **Selegiline,** the first member of this group, is a once-lauded drug that has turned out to offer limited benefit; however, a newer drug, **rasagiline,** may be helpful in early and advanced stages of Parkinson's disease.

- ✔ **Amantadine.** This drug is not very potent, but is sometimes helpful in early disease to lessen tremor.

- ✔ *Anticholinergic drugs.* These medicines can help improve tremor.

Pneumonia

Pneumonia is an infection of the air sacs within the lungs (as opposed to *bronchitis,* in which the problem lies within the bronchial tubes). Most commonly, pneumonia is caused by bacteria, though viruses and certain types of fungus can also be responsible.

Your doctor tries to determine which germ has caused your pneumonia by analyzing samples of sputum, blood, and, sometimes, urine. Because results from these tests seldom provide an immediate answer, the initial choice of antibiotic targets the most likely germs. If the tests reveal a *specific* organism is responsible, the antibiotic is then changed to one that specifically targets it. In up to 50 percent of cases a particular germ is never identified.

If you're otherwise healthy and are well enough to not require admission to hospital, the preferred initial antibiotics are **azithromycin, clarithromycin,** or **doxycycline.** If you're very sick from the pneumonia, you may require hospitalization and intravenous antibiotics.

Polycystic Ovary Syndrome (PCOS)

Polycystic ovary syndrome (PCOS) is a condition caused by an imbalance of female hormones. It's characterized by irregular periods (related to inconsistent ovulation), cysts on the ovaries, infertility, and a tendency toward excess hair growth (*hirsutism*).

If you're overweight, losing weight may help your PCOS. If you do not want to get pregnant, your PCOS may be treated with **oral contraceptives.** If you *are* trying to get pregnant several drugs are available to enhance your fertility, which we discuss in the "Infertility" section of this chapter.

Because PCOS is associated with *insulin resistance* (a condition where the insulin in your body does not work well), sometimes drugs reducing insulin resistance are used. Such drugs are **metformin** and **thiazolidinediones.**

Prostatis

The prostate is a small gland, about the size of a walnut (the world of medicine is full of analogies to food!), that surrounds the internal part of a man's urethra. The urethra is the canal that connects the bladder to the penis (and extends to the tip of the penis). The prostate's function is to produce fluid that mixes with sperm and, as such, it's part of the male reproductive system.

An infection of the prostate is called *prostatis.* Prostatis typically affects young and middle-aged men and causes pain that may be felt in a variety of places including the lower part of the abdomen, the testicles, the penis, and, depending on the cost of the antibiotic you will require, the wallet! Other symptoms you may experience depend on whether your prostatitis is *acute* (in which case you will typically have fever, shaking, chills, and feel downright awful) or *chronic* (in which case symptoms are much more subtle and may be limited to discomfort when you pass urine and needing to pass urine frequently).

If you have acute prostatitis you need to start **antibiotics** right away. Your doctor should obtain a urine sample from you for rapid analysis; this will allow an initial determination of which antibiotic to use pending final results from the lab (which takes some time). The preferred drugs to treat both acute and chronic prostatis are **sulfamethoxazole/trimethoprim** or a **fluoroquinolone,** though other types of antibiotics may also work. Taking a **nonsteroidal anti-inflammatory drug (NSAID)** is also helpful in reducing the inflammation within the prostate and easing your pain. **Alpha blockers** may also help ease your symptoms.

If you have chronic prostatis, your antibiotics need to be used for an extended period (typically 6 to 12 weeks). Chronic prostatis has a tendency to recur, in which case you'll need another course of antibiotics.

Prostatism (Enlarged Prostate)

As we explain in the preceding section, the prostate is a small gland that surrounds the internal part of a man's urethra and is part of the male reproductive system.

As you pass through your middle and later years, your prostate can swell (a condition called *prostatism* or *benign prostatic hypertrophy*). Symptoms include difficulty in initiating urination, needing to pass urine more frequently (especially overnight), having a less forceful urinary stream (intricate geometric patterns etched in the snow are definitely a thing of the past here), and, in the most extreme cases, the inability to urinate at all — which is an emergency and requires you visit a hospital right away.

The traditional treatment for prostatism was surgical (to remove prostate tissue); however, nowadays doctors have medicines that can often help improve — though not eliminate — symptoms. The preferred drugs are ***alpha blockers*** — typically **alfuzosin** and **tamsulosin,** unless you have high blood pressure, in which case **doxazosin** or **terazosin** may be a better choice. A second option is to take an ***alpha-reductase inhibitor;*** these drugs are particularly helpful if your prostate is very enlarged, however they take several months to provide much relief so they are typically used in addition to an alpha blocker, which works quickly. After a year or two, the alpha blocker may be stopped and the alpha-reductase inhibitor continued.

Psoriasis

Psoriasis is a chronic skin disease that causes the appearance of red, scaly, sores (called *plaques*). The areas of the body most likely to be affected are the scalp, elbows, knees, and back. Psoriasis can also affect the nails (causing them to have little depressions called *pits*) and, on occasion, can be associated with joint pain and inflammation (a form of arthritis aptly called *psoriatic arthritis*).

If your psoriasis is mild, non-prescription therapy with topical petroleum jelly such as Vaseline or application of a thick cream or tar is often effective, albeit messy.

If prescription drug therapy is required, the preferred medicine is a topical **corticosteroid.** If this is insufficient, alternative topical therapies include **calcipotriol, tazarotene, tacrolimus,** and **pimecrolimus.** For severe psoriasis, oral *immunosuppressive drugs* or *biological response modifiers* may be used; however, their potential to cause serious side-effects limits their use.

Restless Legs Syndrome

Restless legs syndrome (RLS) is a common condition, especially in older people, in which you experience an ache in your legs (especially the calves) that's relieved only if you move them. Nights tend to be worse than days. The discomfort can be bothersome enough to make sitting in a meeting, movie theatre, or airplane quite a problem (for you *and* the person in front of you — "Ah, excuse me sir, I didn't mean to kick the back of your seat but my legs are killing me..."). RLS is often associated with involuntary jerking movements of the legs while you're asleep.

The cause of RLS is usually unknown, but sometimes it's because of other conditions such as iron deficiency, Parkinson's disease, kidney failure, or diabetes.

RLS sometimes improves with avoidance of alcohol and caffeine. **Iron** supplements may also help (particularly if a blood test shows your iron levels are low). Should prescription drug therapy be necessary, the preferred initial treatment is with **pramipexole** or **ropinirole.** If you're unable to tolerate these drugs, another good option is to take **levodopa.** Other sometimes helpful drugs are **clonazepam** and **gabapentin.** Although *narcotic ("opioid") analgesics* can help, their addictive potential limits their use.

Rosacea

Rosacea is a chronic skin disease of unknown cause, typically onsetting in middle-age, leading to redness of the face (especially the nose and cheeks), recurrent flushing, pimples (similar to acne), eye irritation, and, if severe, swelling of the nose (*rhinophyma*). Certain foods such as hot beverages or spicy food can aggravate the condition. As sun exposure also can make it worse, using an effective sunscreen is important. Contrary to popular wisdom, alcohol does not cause rosacea (though it can make it worse).

If prescription drug therapy is required, the preferred medicine is topical **metronidazole.** If this is not sufficient, oral use of **tetracycline, doxycycline, minocycline,** or **erythromycin** can be helpful. If these strategies are not working sufficiently well, oral **isotretinoin** may be used.

Schizophrenia

Schizophrenia is a condition of disordered brain chemistry that results in impaired thinking, with hallucinations (such as hearing voices), delusions (that is, a fixed, false belief), and a general loss of contact with reality (called a *psychosis*).

Prescription drug therapy works best if given without interruption (stopping medication leads to a relapse in the majority of individuals). The preferred medicines are ***second generation ("atypical") antipsychotics,*** because they cause fewer side-effects than ***first generation ("typical") antipsychotics.*** **Clozapine** (a second generation drug) is the only antipsychotic proven to be more effective than the others; however, its risk of causing very serious side-effects limits its use.

Because the various drugs to treat schizophrenia are typically equally effective, there is no "recommended" drug; rather, the choice of therapy often comes down to how well an individual is responding to and tolerating a particular drug.

Shingles

Shingles refers to a skin infection that initially appears as little clear bubbles (called *vesicles*) on the skin, then changes to open weeping areas, and is then followed by crusting of the lesions. These typically are located in a band-like distribution over a portion of one side of the body, or sometimes over part of the face (occasionally also involving an eye).

Shingles occurs when the chicken-pox (*varicella-zoster*) virus that infected you when you were a child and then remained dormant in some of your nerves becomes re-activated (it's almost like a bear awakening from hibernation — but in this case after decades, not months). Although shingles is seldom serious, it can be very painful, both during the active infection and, more problematically, even after the infection is gone (wherein you can be left with a chronic pain condition called *post-herpetic neuralgia*).

If you have shingles, you can spread the varicella-zoster virus to someone who has never had it; this can cause that person to then develop chicken pox.

To help ease the pain of the acute infection, **acetaminophen with codeine** is preferred over *nonsteroidal anti-inflammatory drugs (NSAIDs). Antiviral agents* (preferably with **valacyclovir** or **acyclovir,** but **famciclovir** can also be used) are of most proven benefit if you're over age 50, and should be started within 72 hours of the onset of the infection. Antiviral therapy helps speed up healing, reduces the severity and duration of pain, and makes it less likely you will be left with post-herpetic neuralgia. If you have particularly severe shingles, sometimes *corticosteroids* are also used.

Sinusitis

The sinuses are a collection of hollow, air-filled spaces within several of the bones of the face. Sinusitis refers to an infection of the sinuses. If you have sinusitis, one or more of your sinuses becomes filled with fluid. Sinusitis can be acute (in which case it goes away within a few weeks) or chronic (in which case it may linger for many months).

Symptoms of acute sinusitis include a stuffy nose, thick nasal discharge, painful teeth, loss of the ability to smell, bad breath, and fever. Most cases of acute sinusitis are caused by viruses, and antibiotics are of no value (though *nonsteroidal anti-inflammatory drugs [NSAIDs]* and *antihistamines* may be).

Sometimes, however, sinuses that have become inflamed by a virus then become infected by bacteria as well. It can be very difficult to determine whether what had been a *viral* sinusitis (which should not be treated with antibiotics) has transformed into a *bacterial* sinusitis (which may require antibiotic therapy); for this reason, it's generally recommended to use antibiotics to treat acute sinusitis only if it hasn't cleared up on its own within seven to ten days. In this case, *antibiotics* (most commonly **amoxicillin, sulfamethoxazole/ trimethoprim,** or **doxycline**) are generally recommended.

 On occasion, acute sinusitis can lead to dangerous complications. Seek immediate medical attention if you have sinusitis and you develop blurred or double vision, an impairment in your thinking, or swelling around an eye.

Chronic sinusitis is treated with *decongestants, antibiotics* (such as **amoxicillin-clavulanate** or **cefuroxime**), and nasal *corticosteroids* (such as **mometasone** or **fluticasone**).

Smoking Cessation

You've probably heard the line, "Quitting smoking is easy; I've done it lots of times." Perhaps that applies to you, too. And perhaps you're now reading this section because you're ready to try once again.

Well, we have good news — effective methods are available to help you. In addition to non-drug therapies such as counselling, hypnosis, and acupuncture, and over-the-counter drug therapy such as nicotine replacement patches or gum, also available is the prescription drug **bupropion.** Bupropion is not a panacea, but if you're motivated to quit, it has a good chance of helping you succeed. (Like many drugs, bupropion is effective at treating more than one condition — it's also used to treat depression.)

Stroke

A stroke is a permanent injury to part of the brain occurring, most commonly, when a blood vessel supplying blood (and, hence, oxygen) to the brain becomes blocked by a blood clot. (A "ministroke," or *transient ischemic attack* [TIA], does not usually cause permanent brain damage.)

The symptoms of a stroke vary depending on which part of the brain has been damaged. Common symptoms are a sudden inability to speak and/or weakness of one side of the body, sometimes accompanied by a severe headache and loss of consciousness. Call for an ambulance immediately if you or someone you are with experiences these symptoms.

Most people who have a stroke have atherosclerosis ("hardening of the arteries") affecting, at a minimum, the blood vessels that supply the brain with blood (a condition called *cerebrovascular disease*). You are more likely to experience a stroke if you have high blood pressure (hypertension), abnormal cholesterol levels (dyslipidemia), diabetes, atrial fibrillation (a type of abnormal heart rhythm), or if you smoke. We discuss these conditions elsewhere in this chapter.

The acute treatment of stroke (that is, the in-hospital treatment you will require) is beyond the scope of this book, as is the management of strokes caused by a brain hemorrhage. Here, we look at the prescription drugs available to help you avoid having another stroke (caused by a blood clot). Unless some reason (such as a drug allergy or intolerance) prevents you from taking the following medicines, almost all people who have had a stroke should be treated with:

- ✔ **ASA.** This is not a prescription drug, but it's so important we're mentioning it here anyhow. ASA is a mild "blood thinner" and helps prevent further blood clots from forming: this in turn reduces your risk of having another stroke. If you're unable to take ASA, **clopidogrel** is an effective alternative. (Sometimes, ASA is given together with another anti-platelet drug, **dipyridamole,** in a combination product called Aggrenox, but typically the extra benefit is very small.)

- ✔ An *angiotensin converting enzyme (ACE) inhibitor.* ACE inhibitors perform a number of functions, including helping to keep blood vessels open. Whether or not everyone who has had a stroke should be treated with an ACE inhibitor is controversial, but it's generally recommended.

- ✔ A *statin.* Statins work principally by lowering the bad LDL cholesterol. (We talk more about this under "Lipid Disorders" in this chapter.) This makes your arteries less prone to developing a buildup of cholesterol and thus helps reduce the likelihood your atherosclerosis will worsen and cause another stroke.

- ✔ Additionally, if you have hypertension, you require blood pressure medication to bring your pressure down. (If you're being treated with an ACE inhibitor, this will help.)

- ✔ If you've had a stroke because of atrial fibrillation, then the *anticoagulant* ("blood thinner") **warfarin** is preferred over ASA or clopidogrel.

Syphilis

Over the past few years syphilis has become increasingly common. Syphilis is a sexually transmitted disease caused by a type of bacteria called *Treponema pallidum.* It's particularly common among gay men and people with HIV/AIDS.

Syphilis can cause such a variety of symptoms it's been said that "If a doctor knows syphilis, a doctor knows all of internal medicine." (Mind you, this has also been said of tuberculosis, diabetes, and probably other diseases, too.)

In *early* syphilis (called the *primary* stage), one develops a raised bump, typically on the genitals, which then becomes an open wound (called a *chancre*) and is associated with swollen lymph glands in the groin. A chancre heals fairly quickly but a few weeks to months later may be followed by the secondary stage of syphilis, in which you have a fever, feel pretty rotten, and have a red rash on your abdomen and arms and legs. If syphilis is not treated, many years later it can lead to a third (*tertiary*) stage, in which serious infections of the heart, brain, and spinal cord may develop.

Fortunately, syphilis is generally very effectively treated with ***antibiotics.*** The most proven therapy is with an injection (given by your doctor) of a long-acting form of ***penicillin.*** If you're allergic to penicillin, you may be treated with oral **tetracycline** or **doxycycline.**

Throat Infections

Pretty well everyone gets an occasional sore throat (*pharyngitis*). It's typically caused by a virus, and in most cases little more is needed than some throat lozenges, perhaps some **acetaminophen,** and our old favourite, tincture of time. Antibiotics don't help you if your sore throat is caused by a virus.

A minority of cases of sore throat are caused by bacteria (typically, a *streptococcus* bacteria — the so-called "strep throat"). ***Antibiotics*** are helpful to treat a strep throat in that they help ease the pain and reduce the risk of complications such as abscesses in the throat and rheumatic fever. Clues that your throat infection is caused by the streptococcus germ (and, hence, needs antibiotics) rather than a virus (which should *not* be treated with antibiotics) are that strep throat is more likely to cause sudden onset of throat pain, swollen lymph glands in the neck, and a fever, and less likely to cause a cough.

Your doctor may seek to confirm the diagnosis by doing a *throat swab* — a cotton-tipped swab is placed in your mouth and rubbed against your throat, then sent off to the lab to test for evidence of streptococcus. The preferred antibiotics to treat a strep throat are **penicillin** and **amoxicillin.** If you're allergic to the penicillin family of drugs, a *macrolide* antibiotic (such as **clarithromycin**) is a good alternative.

Toenail Infections

Infections of the nails (typically the toenails; occasionally the fingernails) are caused by a number of different types of fungus. The infected nail will be discoloured (typically white, yellow, or brownish) and thickened.

Many other conditions can mimic toenail infections, so before treatment is given your doctor should exclude these other things.

For many people, treatment of toenail infections is not required. Treatment is more likely to be needed if you're prone to more serious foot infections (such as a skin infection called cellulitis), if the infection is causing you discomfort, or if you find it cosmetically unacceptable.

The preferred prescription medicines are oral **terbinafine** and **itraconazole. Fluconazole** is somewhat less effective but is easier to use, because it needs to be taken only once weekly. Topical **ciclopirox** can be used, but it's far less likely to get rid of the problem. Regardless of which therapy is used, toenail infections often recur.

You will be less likely to develop an infection (or, if you already have it, passing it on to others) by avoiding walking barefoot or sharing pedicure instruments (such as nail clippers).

Tremor, Essential

Essential tremor is a condition of unknown cause involving repetitive movement of a part of the body (most commonly the arms; less often the head). Stressful situations typically make the tremor worse.

A number of prescription drugs are available to help you if you have this condition.

- ✔ For most people, the first drug to try is a **beta blocker** (typically **propranolol** unless you have asthma, in which case **atenolol** is a better choice).

- ✔ If this is not sufficient, then **primidone** is a good alternative. Taprimidone sometimes provides additional benefit.

- ✔ If neither of these measures are assisting you, other helpful drugs include **gabapentin** and **topiramate.**

- ✔ There is some evidence *benzodiazepines* (such as **alprazolam**) may help, but because of the risk of addiction they are generally not recommended.

If your essential tremor is mild except in stressful situations, taking prescription drug therapy day-to-day may not be necessary. Instead, taking a dose of propranolol shortly prior to the stressful situation may be a better option.

Tuberculosis

Tuberculosis (TB) is an infection caused by a form of bacteria called mycobacteria. Although TB can affect many different organs, it most commonly involves the lungs. TB is classified as being *active* (meaning the bacteria are actively infecting you and making you ill) or *latent* (meaning that the germ has infected you but is not currently causing symptoms). You're more likely to develop TB if you live in crowded, unhygienic conditions or if you have an impaired immune system (as is seen with HIV/AIDS).

Symptoms of active TB include fever, weight loss, drenching sweats occurring during the night, malaise, cough, and sputum production.

Active TB is treated with a combination of different antibiotics, typically including **isoniazid, rifampin, pyrazinamide,** and **ethambutol.** Occasionally, a ***fluoroquinolone*** or **streptomycin** is substituted for one of the aforementioned drugs. Because the treatment program is complex, it's essential your physician and/or public health nurse work closely with you to monitor your therapy.

If you have latent TB you were likely infected years before, with the issue now coming to light only because you had a routine chest X-ray or skin test done. Latent TB may or may not require treatment depending on your individual situation. If you have a weakened immune system, will be treated with immunosuppressive medication, or have certain other conditions such as HIV/AIDS, you will be at risk of your latent TB becoming active and treatment is recommended. When treatment is necessary, the preferred drug is usually **isoniazid** (sometimes in conjunction with **rifampin**).

Because therapy with isoniazid can lead to a deficiency of vitamin B6 (*pyridoxine*), if you're being treated with this drug you're generally also given **pyridoxine** supplements.

Ulcers, Peptic

A peptic ulcer (usually simply called an ulcer) is a small hole in the stomach or the first part of the small intestine (the duodenum), which typically causes pain in the upper part of the abdomen, but also can lead to internal bleeding or, if the hole penetrates right through the stomach (a *perforation*), to life-threatening inflammation within the abdomen.

Most ulcers are caused by an infection with bacteria called *H. pylori.* (See the accompanying sidebar to find out more about how this was discovered.)

I can't believe he ate the whole thing!

For many decades, peptic ulcers were typically attributed to stress and, when therapy was required, surgery was often necessary. In the late 1970s very helpful *histamine-2 (H2) receptor antagonists* (such as Pepcid) came along; however, the cause of peptic ulcers remained obscure.

In 1982, Barry Marshall and Robin Warren, two Australian researchers, were examining stomach biopsies under the microscope and noticed the more inflammation in the sample, the more bacteria (called *H. pylori*) were present. They proposed — to the immense skepticism of the medical community — that the bacteria were causing the inflammation. To prove their point, Dr. Marshall *swallowed* a whole bunch of the bacteria (GEESH!) and, lo and behold, he then developed inflammation in his stomach. A biopsy was done of this area of inflammation and, sure enough, it was chock a block full of *H. pylori*.

The cause of (most) peptic ulcers, something that had eluded medical researchers from time immemorial, had been discovered. In 2005, doctors Marshall and Warren received a Nobel Prize in recognition of their seminal work. (We think Dr. Marshall should have also been given a bravery award, but that's a different matter.)

Ulcers are treated by:

- ✔ Taking **antibiotics.** These are used if it's thought your ulcer is because of an *H pylori* infection (as most are). The preferred treatment is to take **clarithromycin** and **amoxicillin.** If you cannot take amoxicillin (because you're allergic to it or to other members of the *penicillin* family), **metronidazole** is substituted for amoxicillin.

- ✔ Taking medicines to reduce the amount of acid within your stomach. Preferred drugs are the *proton pump inhibitors (PPIs)*.

- ✔ Avoiding things that may be contributing to your having an ulcer, including smoking, excess alcohol, and use of certain drugs such as **ASA** and *nonsteroidal anti-inflammatory drugs (NSAIDs)*.

- ✔ Avoiding foods that make your symptoms worse. Symptoms are typically aggravated by things such as coffee, spicy foods, orange juice, and fatty foods. Note that consuming these foods does *not* cause an ulcer, and avoiding them does not heal an ulcer — it simply lessens your symptoms.

The combination of clarithromycin, amoxicillin (or metronidazole), and a proton pump inhibitor is often called *triple therapy*.

Stomach (not duodenal) ulcers can be caused by a stomach cancer. For this reason, if your doctor determines you have a stomach ulcer, she will need to do appropriate testing to exclude this type of cancer.

Urinary Tract Infections

The urinary tract comprises those organs responsible for producing urine and eliminating it from your body — the kidneys, the ureters (the tubes that take urine from the kidneys to the bladder), the bladder, and the urethra (the tube that takes urine from the bladder to the opening from which urine exits the body). The parts of the urinary tract most prone to infection are the bladder and the kidneys. A bladder infection is called *cystitis,* and a kidney infection is called *pyelonephritis.*

Bladder infections

If you have a bladder infection, you typically have a burning feeling as you pass urine. Also, your bladder may become irritated so that you feel an urge to empty your bladder when you have only small quantities of urine. This typically leads to numerous trips to the bathroom (a condition aptly called *urinary frequency*).

The great majority of the time bladder infections are caused by bacteria that have entered into the bladder through the urethra. In part because the urethra is much shorter in women, women are much more likely than men to develop bladder infections. Most bladder infections are promptly cured with antibiotic therapy, the preferred ones being a *fluoroquinolone,* **nitrofurantoin,** or **sulfamethoxazole/trimethoprim.**

Because men are not typically prone to bladder infections, if you're a man and have this condition it's generally a good idea for your doctor to try to determine whether you have an underlying problem with your urinary tract that may have led to your infection.

Kidney infections

Kidney infections are more serious than bladder infections and typically cause more severe symptoms, including fevers, nausea and vomiting, and back pain (typically beside the back bone, in the small of the back).

If you're very sick from a kidney infection, you may need to be hospitalized and given intravenous antibiotics. If you're able to be treated on an outpatient basis, the preferred antibiotics (pending results of a urine sample, which your doctor should ask you to provide *before* you start antibiotic therapy) are oral ***fluoroquinolones*** or **sulfamethoxazole/trimethoprim**. If your doctor suspects that your infection is caused by a germ called *enterococcus,* she'll typically prescribe **amoxicillin** or **nitrofurantoin.**

Vaginal Dryness

Vaginal dryness can occur in women at almost any age, but is most common after menopause. It's usually related to decreased estrogen levels, but occasionally can be caused by illnesses causing the tissues in the vagina to produce less natural lubrication.

When vaginal dryness is a result of reduced estrogen levels, some women note significant and persistent vaginal discomfort. To help minimize these symptoms, low doses of **estrogen** creams, tablets, and rings can be applied directly into the vagina. Alternatively, when vaginal dryness occurs along with other symptoms of menopause, ***menopausal hormone therapy*** (also known as ***hormone replacement therapy***) can be used, especially if other symptoms of menopause exist. (See also "Menopause" in this chapter.) For less persistent symptoms, occasional use of an over-the-counter vaginal lubricant (such as K-Y Brand Jelly) or a vaginal moisturizer such as Replens can be helpful.

Vaginal Infections

The treatment of a vaginal infection depends on the cause. The main types of vaginal infections (listed in order of decreasing frequency) are

- ✔ **Bacterial.** A variety of different types of bacteria can infect the vagina. Symptoms are often absent. If you do have a symptom, it will likely be a malodorous, "fishy-smelling" vaginal discharge. Treatment with oral or vaginal **metronidazole** usually quickly cures the problem. A good but somewhat less effective alternative is to use **clindamycin** (this drug can be administered in several ways, however topical clindamycin cream works best). If you have a bacterial vaginal infection without symptoms, treatment may not be necessary because the infection often goes away on its own.

✔ **Yeast.** Vaginal yeast infections (usually caused by a type of yeast called *Candida albicans*) typically cause symptoms of painful urination, soreness in the vaginal area, and pain during intercourse. Vaginal discharge may be minimal; when present, it has a white, curd-like or cheesy consistency. Treatment is necessary only if you're having symptoms. The most effective therapy is with oral **fluconazole** or **itraconazole.** Alternatively, you can use antifungal vaginal creams (typically available over-the-counter). Some women are prone to recurrent vaginal yeast infections (that is, four or more per year), in which case six months of therapy may be necessary to prevent further infections.

✔ **Trichomonas.** Trichomonas is a single-celled parasite called a *protozoa.* Trichomonas vaginal infections are almost always acquired during sexual intercourse. Some people do not experience symptoms, whereas others may notice a foul-smelling vaginal discharge (typically "thin" as opposed to the thick discharge seen with a vaginal yeast infection), burning and itching within the vagina, and painful intercourse. The best treatment is with oral **metronidazole.**

Vitiligo

Vitiligo is a skin disease in which the cells that produce pigment are damaged, resulting in loss of normal skin colour eventually turning the skin white. The area of skin involved varies from person to person, ranging from only a small portion (for example, just the hands) to virtually the entire body being affected.

Although the cause of vitiligo is uncertain, it's thought likely to be an *autoimmune* disease (that is, a condition where your immune system is malfunctioning and attacking part of your own body).

Non-prescription drug therapies include sunscreens, makeup, and skin stains. Topical *corticosteroids* can be used if the area of skin to be treated is small. *Phototherapy* in which ultraviolet light (often in combination with medications called *psoralens* that enhance the effect of the ultraviolet light) is often helpful. Oral corticosteroids are sometimes used for particularly severe vitiligo. There is some evidence that **tacrolimus** and **pimecrolimus** may also be helpful, but concern about the safety of these drugs limits their use.

Warts, Genital

Genital warts, more properly called *anogenital warts* because the anus may also be affected, is a sexually transmitted infection caused by certain types of human papilloma virus. In men, the penis is most commonly affected — typically under the foreskin, if the penis is uncircumcised. In women, the cervix, the vagina, and the skin around the vagina are commonly affected. In both men and women the area around the anus (and in the rectum) can be affected (especially from anal intercourse). An anogenital wart begins as a small, red bump and then typically becomes larger and rough.

Because your immune system is often able to get rid of anogenital warts, you may not require medication. However, if your own body hasn't successfully gotten rid of the problem on its own, medication is required. Treatment is primarily with various potent topical therapies administered by a doctor in his office; however, subsequent therapy your doctor may prescribe for you to apply at home may include **podofilox** and **imiquimod.** If you have very large warts, your doctor may recommend surgical removal. Regardless of which therapy is used, anogenital warts may recur.

Warts, Skin

Skin warts are caused by exposure to certain types of human papilloma virus. Exposure may be by direct contact with a wart (even touching a healthy part of your own skin with the area where you have a wart) or by indirect exposure (such as walking on a shower floor that has virus on it). Unlike anogenital warts, skin warts are *not* a sexually transmitted disease.

Skin warts often go away spontaneously. If, however, you find your wart cosmetically or physically unpleasant, medication you can use does exist. Topical **salicylic acid,** an over-the-counter medicine, is typically the best therapy to try first. If that is unsuccessful, other therapies can be used. A doctor may freeze the wart, surgically remove the wart, or treat it with prescription drugs. Some prescription medication must be administered by a physician in the office; however, you may apply other topical therapies yourself (these include **imiquimod, 5-fluorouracil,** and **tretinoin**). Regardless of which therapy is used, skin warts may recur.

Part III
Medications A to Z

The 5th Wave · By Rich Tennant

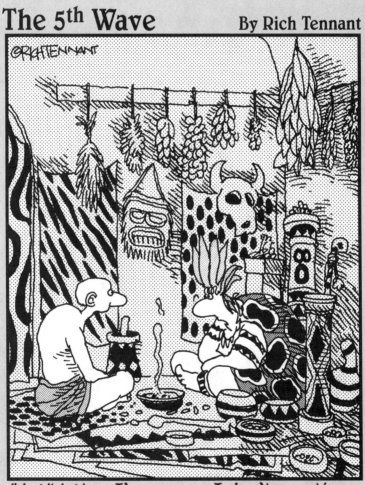

"Antibiotics? I'm sorry — I don't practice alternative medicine."

In this part . . .

You'll find the scoop on well over 200 of the most commonly prescribed medications in Canada. We look at how a medicine works, how it can help you, what side effects it may cause, important precautions to be aware of, when a medicine should not be taken, and how to most effectively take your drug.

Chapter 6

All in the (Drug) Family

In This Chapter

▶ Looking at how your prescription drugs can help you

▶ Knowing what side-effects to watch for

▶ Looking at ways to help you take your medicines safely and effectively

*F*or years now, it's been hard to escape the omnipresent Homer Simpson and his brood. (And, heck, most of us wouldn't want to!) Although the Simpsons are the most disparate of families, we're always struck by the fact that, despite their differences, they're assuredly a family. And so it is with prescription drugs. Prescription drugs have different names and come in all sorts of different colours and shapes and sizes (and costs!), yet with rare exception they share enough in common with some other medicine that, like Homer, Bart, and the rest of the Simpsons, they too are members of a family.

Conventions We Use in This Chapter

In this chapter we group drugs alphabetically by the family to which they belong. (It's worth noting, however, that some drugs engage in what could be considered pharmaceutical polygamy, in that they're members of more than one family. When this is the case, we group the particular drug with the family where it most commonly keeps company, so to speak.) If you're unsure which family your drug belongs to, head to the Drug Index — it will quickly direct you to the page where your drug (and its family) hangs its shingle.

At the beginning of each section in this chapter we list the generic and trade names of the different medicines within a given drug family and, where applicable, by the class of drug within each family (sort of like discussing, say, an imaginary Smith family and then looking separately at the female Smiths and the male Smiths). The names of drugs within a list that are in **bold** are discussed in detail within the section. These drugs typically represent the most commonly used medicine within a family (or class).

As you look at the medicines listed in the tables in this chapter you will find asterisks beside some names. An asterisk indicates that the medicine is actually a combination of two or more different drugs. If your medicine is a combination product you can find the different drugs it contains on the label affixed to the bottle or box your medicine came in. (We show you where this information is located on the example label in Figure 3-2 in Chapter 3.) You can then look up each of those drugs in the Drug Index at the back of this book, which will point you to the right page to find more information.

Although in this chapter we describe the detailed use of prescription drugs, it's always important to bear in mind that each person is unique (ah, you already knew you were special!) and your needs and your doctor's recommendations to meet these needs may differ from "the usual." For this reason, we remind you that the information we provide in this chapter (and throughout the book) is for general information purposes only and should not be taken as a specific recommendation for your own personal care.

Classifying drugs

We think it would be wonderful if there were only one way of classifying drugs. That way, everyone (patients and doctors alike) would immediately know where to locate information on the drug they want to learn more about. Regrettably, life isn't quite so simple. In fact, drugs can be organized in numerous (non–mutually exclusive) ways. Drugs can be classified according to

- ✔ What disease they fight (anticancer drugs, anticonvulsant drugs, etc.).

- ✔ What organ or body system they act on (the so-called "anatomical therapeutic chemical — ATC — classification system" in which A is for alimentary tract, B is for blood, etc.).

- ✔ Their molecular mechanism of action (ACE inhibitors, beta blockers, etc.)

- ✔ Their physical mechanism of action (cholesterol absorption inhibitors, binding resins, etc.).

- ✔ Their chemical structure (aminosalicylates, penicillins, etc.).

- ✔ A combination of things that they are (oral contraceptives), or a combination of things that they are and aren't (nonsteroidal anti-inflammatory agents).

- ✔ How they are taken (inhaled medicines, topical drugs).

- ✔ Alphabetical order. Ah, an old and trusted friend.

Use the Drug Index at the back of this book if you can't find what you're looking for.

Prescription Drugs 101: A Primer

This book is all about *understanding* prescription drugs — so, we look at the most important things for you to know about how to safely and effectively use the medicines your doctor has prescribed. We don't discuss *every* aspect of *every* drug. We *could,* but we thought you would not be well served by the hernia you would get from carrying around the medical equivalent to *War and Peace.* When we look at possible side-effects you might experience from a drug, for example, we point out only those side-effects that are most important for you to be aware of (either because they're the most common or because they're potentially the most dangerous). Also, instead of stating for each drug that it is ill-advised to take a drug to which you're allergic, we will state it now. Oh, we guess we just did.

Understanding Prescription Drugs For Canadians For Dummies looks at those medicines you're most likely to be prescribed for outpatient use. Accordingly, we don't discuss those drugs, for example, that are typically given through an intravenous or by injection into a muscle by your doctor.

Prescription drug use during pregnancy and breastfeeding

The vast majority of drugs have not been sufficiently studied in women who are pregnant or breastfeeding to know with absolute certainty whether they can or cannot be safely used. Nonetheless, many drugs are used — out of necessity — in these circumstances without evidence of harm. In this chapter, when you see the phrase "the safety of drug *x* is unknown during pregnancy and breastfeeding," this doesn't necessarily mean the drug is likely unsafe, or unused in these circumstances (indeed, it might be used commonly); it simply means we don't have *proof* of safety. Therefore, in almost all cases, if you're pregnant (or thinking of becoming pregnant) or breastfeeding, it comes down to you and your physician looking at the potential benefits versus the potential risks and deciding where the balance lies. (We discuss issues surrounding prescription drug use in pregnancy and breastfeeding in Chapter 8.)

Prescription drugs and children

This book is geared toward adult consumers of prescription drugs. Although general principles regarding drug therapy apply to all age groups, there are those issues (including drug doses and, at times, side-effects) that are specific to infants through to older children. For this additional information we recommend you speak to your pharmacist or physician.

Prescription drug interactions and side-effects

As we discuss in detail in Chapter 7, many prescription drugs can interact — typically unfavourably — with other prescription drugs, non-prescription drugs (including antacids), foods (especially grapefruit), mineral supplements (including calcium and iron), and herbs and other "natural" products (such as St. John's wort). It's not feasible in this book to list the thousands of possible interactions that can occur, but your doctor and your pharmacist should routinely check for these using one of a variety of resources available for this purpose.

Medical jargon made simple

In this chapter you will come across certain medical terms. To help you, we define some of these terms here.

Agonist: A drug that acts on a receptor in a way similar to a naturally occurring hormone or neurotransmitter.

Analog: A drug that is structurally similar to a naturally occurring hormone, neurotransmitter, or other (typically older) drug.

Antagonist: A drug that blocks the action on a receptor of a naturally occurring hormone or neurotransmitter.

Blocker: See "Antagonist."

Blood counts: The cells present in the blood. See "Red blood cells," "White blood cells," and "Platelets."

Enzyme: A protein that facilitates a chemical reaction in the body.

Inhibitor: A drug that blunts the action of an enzyme.

Neurotransmitter: A chemical messenger that helps pass messages from one cell to another.

Platelets: Tiny cells in the blood involved in the formation of blood clots.

Receptors: Areas on the surface of a cell to which hormones, neurotransmitters, drugs, and other substances attach.

Red blood cells: Cells in the blood that carry oxygen. A deficiency of red blood cells is called *anemia.*

White blood cells: Cells in the blood that protect against infection and are involved in inflammation.

You can also look up possible drug interactions yourself on the Web. Two excellent Web sites to check for drug interactions are www.drugdigest.org and www.epocrates.com.

Drugs — including inhaled medicines — contain non-medicinal ingredients (such as lactose or gluten) to which some people may react. If you have a history of sensitivities or allergies, before you start taking a medicine be sure to ask your pharmacist what non-medicinal ingredients are in the drug you have been prescribed.

When we look at how often a particular drug causes a particular side-effect, it's important to be aware of the rather startling fact that we seldom know precisely how often drug *x* causes side-effect *y*. We may have a general sense (that is, high, medium, or low likelihood), but sufficient data are seldom available to enable us to be more precise.

Prescription drug choices

It's important to know that drugs are often prescribed to treat conditions for which they have not been officially approved by the Government of Canada. This lack of official approval does not mean the drug does not work for the ailment; indeed, the medicine may work very well. (This type of use is called "off label." When a drug is used for a government-approved purpose it's called a "labelled indication.") When we discuss the use of a drug to treat a condition, that doesn't necessarily mean it has been approved for such use; it just means that, in real life, it *is* being used so we think it's important to discuss it.

Lastly, when we discuss the way (or ways) in which a drug works, we simply present the most widely held *theories* — because, truth be told, although doctors are pretty darn good (if we say so ourselves) at knowing *how* to treat something, we often are not nearly so good at knowing *why* that treatment actually works. (Mind you, how many of us concern ourselves with the details as to how our car engine works, so long as it allows us to get from place A to place B?)

If you want to find out more information on the illnesses we discuss in this chapter, flip back a few pages to Chapter 5 where we look at "Ailments and their Treatment."

Alpha-adrenergic Agonists (Centrally Acting)

(Centrally acting) alpha-adrenergic agonists, a very small family of drugs with but two members, work by stimulating alpha adrenergic receptors in the brain. This results in decreased action within a specialized group of nerves called the *sympathetic nervous system.* This, in turn, leads to widening of the arteries *(vasodilation)* in your body, which reduces blood pressure (and, in the case of clonidine, may provide some degree of relief from menopausal symptoms). Table 6-1 lists the centrally acting alpha-adrenergic agonists available in Canada.

Table 6-1	Centrally Acting Alpha-adrenergic Agonists
Generic Name	*Trade Name(s)*
Clonidine	Apo-Clonidine, Catapres, Dixarit, Novo-Clonidine, Nu-Clonidine
Methyldopa	Apo-Methazide*, Apo-Methyldopa, Nu-Medopa

* This medicine is a combination of different drugs. Refer to the drug label to determine what they are.

 ## Methyldopa

Apo-Methazide*, Apo-Methyldopa, Nu-Medopa

Methyldopa is one of the very, very few drugs for which we have overwhelming evidence of safety during pregnancy. (It can also be safely used during breastfeeding.) For this reason, it's often the drug of choice to treat pregnant women who have high blood pressure. Because it can have significant side-effects with long-term use, it's not often used outside of these circumstances.

How methyldopa can help you

Methyldopa can help you by lowering your blood pressure.

How methyldopa might harm you

Possible side-effects from taking methyldopa include:

✔ *Autoimmune hemolytic anemia,* a form of anemia in which red blood cells are prematurely destroyed because of the formation of antibodies in the body. It's unlikely to occur unless you've been on the drug for at least six months.

✔ *Peripheral edema* (ankle swelling).

✔ Fever.

✔ Abnormal liver tests, hepatitis.

✔ Sleepiness. This is seldom seen after the first few days of therapy.

✔ Faintness (especially upon first arising from a bed or from a chair).

People with the following conditions shouldn't take methyldopa:

✔ Significant liver disease such as hepatitis or cirrhosis.

✔ You shouldn't take methyldopa if you've taken a drug from the monoamine oxidase (MAO) inhibitor family within the past 14 days nor should you start taking an MAO inhibitor within 14 days of stopping methyldopa.

Precautions to follow if you're taking methyldopa

Follow these precautions if you're taking methyldopa:

✔ Before you start taking the drug — then, periodically thereafter — your doctor will need to check your liver tests.

✔ If you start to feel generally unwell and develop poor appetite, nausea, vomiting, dark urine, or yellowing of your skin or eyes (that is, jaundice) you may have developed hepatitis and need to seek urgent medical attention. (Some darkening of the urine can be seen if it's exposed to air: this isn't dangerous.)

✔ Pause for a moment after you get up from bed or from a chair to make sure you're not lightheaded before you walk away. If you feel dizzy, sit or lie back down. (After a few days of taking this medicine, if you're not experiencing lightheadedness you no longer need to follow this precaution.)

✔ This drug may make you drowsy, which would make it unsafe for you to perform activities — like driving — that require you to be alert and focused. This is more likely to be an issue during the first few days of therapy.

✔ Because alcohol may worsen drowsiness, avoid it until you're certain the methyldopa isn't affecting your level of alertness.

How to take methyldopa

The usual starting dose is 250 mg taken two to three times daily. The dose is then adjusted, under your doctor's supervision, based on your response. Your doctor may need to prescribe lower than usual doses if you have kidney failure. Methyldopa may be taken with or without food.

Sometimes, blood pressure initially improves and then, after a few months, the effect of methyldopa wanes. If this happens, your doctor may need to adjust your dose, change you to a different drug, or prescribe an additional anti-hypertensive medicine.

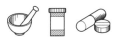

Alpha Blockers

Alpha blockers (sometimes referred to as alpha adrenergic blockers or alpha adrenergic antagonists) are drugs that block stimulation of *alpha receptors*. These receptors are found both in small arteries in the body and also in and around the prostate. Blocking these receptors results in the following:

- ✔ These arteries widen *(vasodilate)*, which enables blood to flow through them more easily resulting in lower blood pressure.

- ✔ Muscles relax within the prostate and at the neck of the bladder (where the bladder and the urethra join). This, in turn, makes it easier for a man with prostatism to have urine flow from the bladder into the urethra (and then out of the body).

Alpha blockers available in Canada are listed in Table 6-2. In this section we look in detail at the most commonly used alpha blocker to treat hypertension (doxazosin) and prostatism (tamsulosin).

Table 6-2	Alpha Blockers
Generic Name	*Trade Name(s)*
Alfuzosin	Xatral
Doxazosin	Apo-Doxazosin, Cardura, Gen-Doxazosin, Novo-Doxazosin
Prazosin	Apo-Prazo, Novo-Prazin, Nu-Prazo
Tamsulosin	Flomax, Flomax CR
Terazosin	Apo-Terazosin, Hytrin, Novo-Terazosin, Nu-Terazosin, PMS-Terazosin, ratio-Terazosin

Doxazosin

Apo-Doxazosin, Cardura, Gen-Doxazosin, Novo-Doxazosin

Doxazosin is used in the treatment of hypertension, but typically only if other, generally more effective, blood pressure medications are not working adequately. It can also help prostatism.

How doxazosin can help you

Doxazosin can help you in the following ways:

✔ Lowering your blood pressure.

✔ Making it easier to empty your bladder. This drug will not help a woman to pass urine as they aren't the proud owners of a prostate. (Mind you, many a man would gladly part with this often troublesome organ.)

How doxazosin might harm you

Possible side-effects from doxazosin include:

✔ Headache, fatigue, ankle swelling, and breathlessness. These are typically fairly mild.

✔ Faintness. Within a few hours of taking a dose of doxazosin, you may have a sudden drop in blood pressure that, when severe, can make you faint. This is especially likely to happen shortly after you start taking the medicine and is more likely to occur if you're standing.

✔ *Priapism,* a persistent painful erection (typically lasting several hours or more). Have it treated right away; otherwise, it can lead to permanent erectile dysfunction. This occurs rarely.

Doxazosin should not be taken if you have had a stroke or heart attack within the preceding six months.

The safety of doxazosin for pregnant and breastfeeding women is unknown. If you're pregnant or breastfeeding, we recommend you discuss it with your physician before taking this medicine.

Precautions to follow if you're taking doxazosin

Watch out for dizziness, especially if you have taken your dose at bedtime then get up during the night — to go to the bathroom, for example. Before you stand, sit for a moment on the side of the bed. Then, if you're feeling okay, stand beside the bed for a moment. Walk away only when you're sure you're not feeling faint. Take special care if you're also taking PDE5 inhibitor drugs such as sildenafil

(Viagra), as this combination may make you especially prone to lightheadedness.

If you're prescribed doxazosin to treat symptoms of an enlarged prostate, you need to first have your prostate examined to exclude prostate cancer because both diseases can cause similar symptoms.

How to take doxazosin

Doxazosin has a very wide dose range (all the way from 1 mg per day to as much as 16 mg per day). It's usually best to start with a very small dose and then, under your doctor's supervision, to have your dose slowly increased, if necessary, so long as you're tolerating the drug well. Doxazosin may be taken with or without food.

If you haven't taken your medicine for several days or more, when you restart it you will need to once again start with a very small dose and gradually increase it.

℞ Tamsulosin

Flomax, Flomax CR

We think the trade name for tamsulosin surely deserves a prize for the "calling a spade a spade" award. Imagine naming a drug to help one urinate "Flomax." Brilliant! A bit over the top, perhaps, but brilliant nonetheless.

How tamsulosin can help you

This drug may help a man by making it easier for him to empty his bladder. This drug will not help women to pass urine as they aren't card-carrying members of the prostate-owner's society.

How tamsulosin might harm you

Possible side-effects from tamsulosin include:

✔ Headache, fatigue, lightheadedness, or palpitations. These are typically mild.

✔ *Priapism,* a persistent painful erection (typically lasting several hours or more). Have it treated right away; otherwise it can lead to permanent erectile dysfunction. This occurs rarely.

✔ Reduced volume of fluid released during ejaculation. This isn't serious.

✔ Within a few hours of taking a dose of tamsulosin, you may have a sudden drop in blood pressure that, if severe, can make you faint. This is especially likely to happen shortly after you start taking the medicine and is more likely to occur if you're standing.

Some people with sulfa drug allergies also react to tamsulosin. For this reason, *before* you start taking tamsulosin be sure to let your doctor know if you have had problems with sulfa medicines.

Precautions to follow if you're taking tamsulosin

Follow these precautions if you're taking tamsulosin:

✔ Because there is some evidence that current or previous use of tamsulosin can increase the risk of eye complications during cataract surgery, if you're going to be having a cataract operation be sure to let your eye doctor know that you're taking or have taken tamsulosin.

✔ If you develop faintness after taking a dose, immediately sit or lie down. This will help you avoid fainting. Take special care if you're also taking PDE5 inhibitor drugs such as sildenafil (Viagra), as this combination may make you especially prone to lightheadedness.

✔ If you're prescribed doxazosin to treat symptoms of an enlarged prostate, you need to first have your prostate examined to exclude prostate cancer because both diseases can cause similar symptoms.

How to take tamsulosin

Take tamsulosin about one-half hour after eating a meal. It doesn't matter which meal you choose, but be consistent day-to-day. The capsule needs to be swallowed whole (that is, not chewed, crushed, etc.). The usual starting dose is 0.4 mg per day with the dose then adjusted, under your doctor's supervision, based on your response to the medicine.

Avoid consuming grapefruit or grapefruit juice because it can affect the level of tamsulosin in your blood.

If you haven't taken your medicine for several days or more, when you restart it you will need to once again initiate with the lower dose.

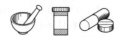

Alpha-Reductase Inhibitors

Alpha-reductase inhibitors (also known as 5 alpha-reductase inhibitors or type II 5 alpha-reductase inhibitors) are useful in the treatment of prostatism and can also help treat male-pattern baldness (that is, a receding hair line and thinning of scalp hair).

With the help of the 5 alpha-reductase enzyme, testosterone (the main male sex hormone) is converted within the body to a more potent hormone called dihydrotestosterone (DHT). DHT causes the prostate to enlarge, which can make urinating difficult (a condition called *prostatism*) and also leads to male-pattern baldness. Alpha-reductase inhibitors block the action of the 5 alpha reductase enzyme and as a result DHT levels fall, the prostate shrinks, and scalp hair follicles function better. Alpha-reductase inhibitors available in Canada are listed in Table 6-3.

Table 6-3	Alpha-Reductase Inhibitors
Generic Name	*Trade Name(s)*
Dutasteride	Avodart
Finasteride	Propecia, Proscar

 ## Finasteride

Propecia, Proscar

Finasteride (given in low doses as Propecia) is used to treat male-pattern hair loss and (given in higher doses as Proscar) is used to treat prostatism.

How finasteride can help you

Finasteride can help you in the following ways:

✔ Making it easier to empty your bladder.

✔ Improving male-pattern baldness. (This benefit is seen only for men and only if there is mild to moderate hair loss.)

It will take a few months of treatment before you notice any improvement in your baldness, and it may take as long as one year before you experience the full benefit. Also, if you stop the medication, the new hair you've grown will be gradually lost.

How finasteride might harm you

Possible side-effects from finasteride include:

- ✔ Sexual problems including erectile dysfunction, decreased libido, impaired ability to ejaculate, and decreased quantity of semen.
- ✔ Breast enlargement (*gynecomastia*) and tenderness.

 Women shouldn't take finasteride. It's especially dangerous for pregnant women because it can cause abnormal genital development in a male fetus.

Precautions to follow if you're taking finasteride

Follow these precautions if you're taking finasteride:

- ✔ To avoid any possible damage to a fetus, a woman who is (or may be) pregnant should avoid physical contact with finasteride; in particular, she should not touch any broken or crushed tablets. A man should wear a condom during intercourse so that the drug that is present within his semen will not get into a woman's system.
- ✔ Because finasteride can lower PSA levels (this is a test for prostate cancer), if a doctor is ordering this test be sure to let him know you're taking the drug.

How to take finasteride

Finasteride is taken once daily with or without food either in a dose of 1 mg (to treat male-pattern baldness) or 5 mg (to treat prostatism).

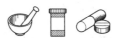

Alzheimer's Disease Medicines

Medical therapy for Alzheimer's disease is aimed at trying to improve, or at least maintain, your ability to function for as long as possible. (We talk more about Alzheimer's disease in Chapter 5.) Although we now have medications to help, they're limited in terms of how much they can achieve. There are two general types of medicine to treat Alzheimer's disease: cholinesterase inhibitors and NMDA receptor antagonists. We look at how they work below. We list the various medications available in Canada to treat Alzheimer's disease in Table 6-4.

Table 6-4	Alzheimer's Disease Medicines	
Class	**Generic Name**	**Trade Name(s)**
Cholinesterase inhibitors	**Donepezil**	Aricept, Aricept RDT
	Galantamine	Reminyl, Reminyl ER
	Rivastigmine	Exelon
NMDA receptor antagonist	**Memantine**	Ebixa

 Donepezil

Aricept, Aricept RDT

Donepezil is the most commonly used cholinesterase inhibitor available in Canada to treat Alzheimer's disease.

 Acetylcholine is a key chemical messenger (*neurotransmitter*) in the brain, helping to pass messages from one cell to another. In Alzheimer's disease, there is a deficiency of acetylcholine in the brain. Donepezil increases the amount of acetylcholine in the brain by blocking the action of an enzyme (*cholinesterase*) that breaks down acetylcholine. This, in turn, helps slow the progression of symptoms of Alzheimer's disease.

How donepezil can help you

Donepezil can help you by slowing the progression of symptoms of mild to moderate Alzheimer's disease (forgetfulness, difficulty in remembering familiar names, places, and activities, and difficulty in carrying out usual day-to-day activities).

How donepezil might harm you

Possible side-effects from taking donepezil include:

- Nausea, vomiting, diarrhea. These are usually mild and go away within about three weeks of starting the medicine. They're less likely to occur if you start with a low dose (see below).

- Insomnia, fatigue, dizziness, headache, seizures.

- Muscle aches.

- Slow heartbeat. This may make you feel faint.

Serious side-effects (such as seizures) seldom occur.

Precautions to follow if you're taking donepezil

Follow these precautions if you're taking donepezil:

- ✔ If you're to undergo surgery, be sure to let the anesthesiologist (anesthetist) — the person who puts you to sleep — know that you're on donepezil, because this drug may affect your response to the anesthetic.

- ✔ If you have asthma or chronic obstructive pulmonary disease (COPD), keep a watch out for worsening of wheezing and, should this happen, promptly let your physician know.

If you're the caregiver for someone with Alzheimer's disease, you will be able to help with these precautions by speaking to the doctor on behalf of the person with the condition.

How to take donepezil

Donepezil is taken once daily, with or without food, and may be taken in the morning or the evening. Donepezil is typically started in a dose of 5 mg once daily with the dose then adjusted, under your doctor's supervision, based on your response.

Memantine

Ebixa

Memantine is a member of the NMDA receptor antagonist drug class. NMDA is short for N-methyl d-aspartate. It's also short for the National Motorcycle Dealers Association, the New Mexico Dental Association and, our favourite, the National Miniature Donkey Association, but we digress.

It's suspected that patients with Alzheimer's disease may have too much *glutamate,* a *neurotransmitter* (chemical messenger) in the brain. Glutamate transmits its message by travelling from one nerve cell (*neuron*) to another where it then attaches to a NMDA receptor, which then causes some of the brain cells to be overstimulated, leading to loss of normal function. Memantine blocks the glutamate from attaching to the nerve cells, and so protects them from this overstimulation.

How memantine can help you

Memantine can help you if you have moderate to severe Alzheimer's disease by slowing the progression of symptoms of dementia. (There's some evidence it may also be helpful in the treatment of other forms of dementia.)

How memantine might harm you

Possible side-effects from taking memantine include:

- ✔ Fatigue, headache, dizziness.
- ✔ Nonspecific aches and pains.
- ✔ High blood pressure.

Most people do not experience any side-effects.

Precautions to follow if you're taking memantine

Follow these precautions if you're taking memantine:

- ✔ Because infections of the urinary tract (kidneys and bladder) can affect the level of memantine in your blood, be sure to let your doctor know if you develop symptoms such as burning pain when you pass your urine, or foul-smelling urine.
- ✔ Avoid ingesting large quantities of sodium bicarbonate (baking soda). Large amounts of sodium bicarbonate can affect memantine levels in your blood.

 If you're the caregiver for someone with Alzheimer's disease, you will be able to help with these precautions by speaking to the doctor on behalf of the person with the condition. In the case of sodium bicarbonate ingestion, we recommend not keeping large supplies of it accessible.

How to take memantine

Memantine is typically started in a dose of 5 mg once daily with the dose then adjusted, under your doctor's supervision, based on your response. The usual full ("maintenance") dose is 10 mg twice daily. Memantine should be swallowed whole, not chewed, crushed, and so on. It can be taken with or without food.

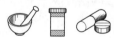

Aminosalicylates

Aminosalicylates have their main role in the treatment of inflammatory bowel disease. One particular member of this family — sulfasalazine — is also used to treat rheumatoid arthritis. We discuss sulfasalazine elsewhere in this chapter (in the section on *immunosuppressive* drugs).

By altering levels of inflammation-causing substances such as prostaglandins, leukotrienes and pro-inflammatory cytokines, 5-ASA reduces inflammation in the bowel. It may also work by acting as a *free radical scavenger*. (Despite the name, these are not dumpster-diving, ex-con, anarchists; rather, free radical scavengers are substances that track down and inactivate disease-causing substances called *free radicals*.) 5-ASA acts on both the small and large bowel, whereas olsalazine, a "delayed-release" medication, acts exclusively on the large bowel. Table 6-5 lists the aminosalicylates available in Canada.

Table 6-5	Aminosalicylates
Generic Name	*Trade Name(s)*
5-Aminosalicylic Acid (5-ASA, Mesalamine)	Asacol, Asacol 800, Mesasal, Novo-5 ASA, Pentasa, Salofalk
Olsalazine	Dipentum
Sulfasalazine	Salazopyrin, Salazopyrin En-tabs

 5-Aminosalicylic Acid (5-ASA)

Asacol, Asacol 800, Mesasal, Novo-5 ASA, Pentasa, Salofalk

5-ASA, though not able to cure inflammatory bowel disease, can help control the condition.

How 5-ASA can help you

5-ASA can help you if you have inflammatory bowel disease in the following ways:

- ✔ Bringing a flare under control.
- ✔ Helping prevent a future flare.
- ✔ Reducing your risk of bowel cancer.

How 5-ASA might harm you

Possible side-effects from 5-ASA include:

- ✔ Headache, malaise (that is, feeling generally unwell), abdominal cramps, and flatus are the most common side-effects — and though they may be a nuisance, they aren't serious.

✔ Skin rash and hair loss occur in only a small percentage of people using this drug.

✔ If you're taking a sulfonylurea drug (such as glyburide) for diabetes, taking 5-ASA may make it more likely that you will develop *hypoglycemia* (low blood glucose).

✔ Serious, but fortunately rare, side-effects include worsening of ulcerative colitis symptoms, a low platelet count, and inflammation of certain organs (lungs, heart, pancreas).

People with the following conditions shouldn't take 5-ASA:

✔ ASA allergy. ASA is present in many medications; one of its trade names is Aspirin.

✔ Stomach or duodenal ulcer.

✔ Urinary tract obstruction (that is, a blockage of the flow of urine from the kidneys or bladder).

✔ Kidney failure.

The safety of 5-ASA in pregnancy and breastfeeding is uncertain, but is generally thought to be safe. If you're pregnant or breastfeeding, we recommend you discuss it with your physician before taking this medicine.

Precautions to follow if you're taking 5-ASA

Follow these precautions if you're taking 5-ASA:

✔ Have your kidney function checked before you start taking this medicine, then periodically after.

✔ If you have diabetes treated with a sulfonylurea drug, monitor your blood glucose readings more often for the first few weeks after you start 5-ASA medication.

✔ If you develop chest or abdominal pain, or unexplained or excessive bleeding, seek urgent medical attention.

How to take 5-ASA

5-ASA is taken, depending on the particular form of the drug, orally or rectally. The dose depends on by which route the drug is being administered and whether you're treating a flare of colitis or are taking it to maintain a remission. (We talk about different treatments for inflammatory bowel disease in Chapter 5.)

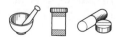

Angiotensin Converting Enzyme (ACE) Inhibitors

ACE inhibitors, around for about a generation now, have contributed to the well being of millions of people; indeed, with each passing year we find additional ways in which to benefit from these medicines.

Angiotensin converting enzyme helps convert a substance called angiotensin I into a powerful substance called angiotensin II. ACE inhibitors block the action of angiotensin converting enzyme, and so less angiotensin II is made. Lower levels of angiotensin II help widen (*dilate*) blood vessels, and as a result blood pressure falls and less stress is placed on various organs in the body.

ACE inhibitors available in Canada are listed in Table 6-6. ACE inhibitors vary *very* little from drug to drug, so we discuss them together. (It's generally thought that all ACE inhibitors are likely equally effective; however, as they have not all been tested in equally large or important drug studies we don't know this for certain.)

Table 6-6	Angiotensin Converting Enzyme Inhibitors
Generic Name	*Trade Name(s)*
Benazepril	Lotensin
Captopril	Apo-Capto, Capoten, Gen-Captopril, Novo-Captopril, Nu-Capto, PMS-Captopril
Cilazapril	Inhibace, Inhibace Plus*, Novo-Cilazapril, PMS-Cilazapril
Enalapril	Vaseretic*, Vasotec
Fosinopril	Apo-Fosinopril, Gen-Fosinopril, Monopril, Novo-Fosinopril
Lisinopril	Prinivil, Prinzide*, Zestoretic*, Zestril
Perindopril	Coversyl, Coversyl Plus*, Preterax*
Quinapril	Accupril, Accuretic*
Ramipril	Altace, Apo-Ramipril
Trandolapril	Mavik, Tarka*

* These medicines are combinations of different drugs. Refer to the drug label to determine what they are.

How an ACE inhibitor can help you

ACE inhibitors can help you in the following ways:

- Lowering your blood pressure.
- Improving (or preventing) congestive heart failure if you have had a heart attack or other forms of damage to the heart muscle.
- Reducing your risk of a heart attack or stroke if you have *atherosclerosis* (hardening of the arteries).
- Helping to prevent (some forms of) existing kidney damage from worsening. (There is also some evidence that ACE inhibitors may prevent some types of kidney damage from developing in the first place.)

How an ACE inhibitor might harm you

Possible side-effects from taking ACE inhibitors include:

- Coughing. This is the most common side-effect, occurring in about 30 percent of people. It's a nagging, dry cough and typically makes you feel like you have a "tickle in the throat."
- Low blood pressure. If severe enough this can make you feel lightheaded or even cause you to faint.
- *Angioedema.* This is a serious form of allergic reaction in which your lips, tongue, and face swell, and you may become wheezy and short of breath.
- Kidney failure. Although ACE inhibitors typically help *prevent* kidney failure, on occasion the opposite effect occurs.
- High potassium levels in the blood.
- Altered taste sensation. When this occurs, it's typically shortly after beginning ACE inhibitor therapy and tends to go away even if the medicine is continued.
- Lower blood glucose levels if you have diabetes. (This isn't necessarily a bad thing; indeed, for most people with diabetes this is beneficial.)
- Abnormal liver tests.
- Decreased numbers of white blood cells. This rarely occurs. If you have a deficiency of white blood cells it puts you at increased risk of infections.

ACE inhibitors should not be taken if you're pregnant because they can harm the developing fetus and even lead to its death.

The safety of ACE inhibitors in breastfeeding is unknown. We recommend before taking this medicine in this circumstance you discuss this with your physician.

Precautions to follow if you're taking an ACE inhibitor

Follow these precautions if you're taking an ACE inhibitor:

- ✔ If you're a sexually active woman of child-bearing age, be sure to use effective contraception. If you find out you're pregnant, immediately notify your physician; in almost all cases you will need to immediately stop taking the drug.

- ✔ Contact your doctor if you develop a fever, bad sore throat, yellow or greenish phlegm, or other symptoms suggesting you have an infection.

- ✔ If your lips, tongue, or face start to swell, and/or you become wheezy or short of breath, immediately stop the medicine and seek urgent medical attention.

- ✔ Don't take "salt substitutes" without first speaking to your doctor. (Salt substitutes are typically rich in potassium and, in the setting of ACE inhibitor use, can sometimes lead to dangerously high potassium levels.)

- ✔ If you have diabetes treated with medicines (such as glyburide or insulin) that lower blood glucose, be extra vigilant for hypoglycemia (low blood glucose) until you determine how the drug affects your blood glucose levels.

- ✔ In most cases, have a blood test done to measure your *creatinine* and potassium levels before you start taking an ACE inhibitor, and then again a few weeks after using the drug. Creatinine is a substance in the blood that is an indicator of kidney health. (If, after starting an ACE inhibitor, your creatinine goes up by more than 30 percent, you may need to stop taking the drug.)

How to take an ACE inhibitor

ACE inhibitors are typically started in low dose and the dose is then adjusted, under your doctor's supervision, based on your response. The dose of the medicine and the frequency you have to take it depends on the particular ACE inhibitor you have been prescribed. Most ACE inhibitors can be taken with or without food; captopril is the exception and should be taken at least one hour before or not sooner than two hours after eating.

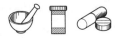

Angiotensin Receptor Blockers (ARBs)

In the few years that angiotensin receptor blockers (also known as AT receptor blockers or angiotensin receptor antagonists) have been around, they've quickly become very popular choices in the treatment of several important conditions including hypertension. One of the reasons for their popularity is that they share many of the very helpful benefits of the highly effective family of drugs known as ACE inhibitors but without the irksome tendency of ACE inhibitors to cause coughing.

Angiotensin II is a substance in the blood that attaches to and stimulates angiotensin II receptors. As a result, blood vessels narrow (*vasoconstrict*), which causes blood pressure to rise. ARBs work by blocking angiotensin II from attaching to the angiotensin II receptors, thus angiotensin II is unable to exert its usual effect.

ARBs available in Canada are listed in Table 6-7. ARBs vary *very* little from drug to drug, so we discuss them together. (It's generally thought that all ARBs are likely equally effective; however, as they have not all been tested in equally large or important drug studies we don't know this for certain.)

Table 6-7	Angiotensin Receptor Blockers
Generic Name	*Trade Name(s)*
Candesartan	Atacand, Atacand Plus*
Eprosartan	Teveten, Teveten Plus*
Irbesartan	Avalide*, Avapro
Losartan	Cozaar, Hyzaar*, Hyzaar DS*
Telmisartan	Micardis, Micardis Plus*
Valsartan	Diovan, Diovan-HCT*

* These medicines are combinations of different drugs. Refer to the drug label to determine what they are.

How an ARB can help you

ARBs can help you in the following ways:

✔ Lowering your blood pressure.

✔ Improving (or preventing) congestive heart failure if you have had a heart attack or other forms of damage to the heart muscle.

✔ Helping to prevent (some forms of) existing kidney damage from worsening. (There is also some evidence that ARBs may prevent some types of kidney damage from developing in the first place.)

How an ARB might harm you

Possible side-effects from ARBs include:

✔ Low blood pressure. If severe enough this can make you feel lightheaded or even cause you to faint.

✔ High potassium levels in the blood.

✔ Kidney failure. Although ARBs typically help *prevent* kidney failure, on occasion the opposite effect occurs.

ARBs can harm a developing fetus and even lead to its death. This risk is likely confined to the second and third trimesters of pregnancy, but it's safest to not take ARBs at *any* stage of pregnancy.

The safety of ARBs in breastfeeding is unknown. We recommend before taking this medicine in this circumstance you discuss this with your physician.

Precautions to follow if you're taking an ARB

Follow these precautions if you're taking an ARB:

✔ If you're a sexually active woman of child-bearing age, be sure to use effective contraception. If you find out you're pregnant, immediately notify your physician; in almost all cases, you will need to immediately stop taking the drug.

✔ In most cases, have a blood test done to measure your *creatinine* and potassium levels before you start taking an ARB, and then again a few weeks after using the drug. Creatinine is a substance in the blood that is an indicator of kidney health.

✔ Don't take "salt substitutes" without first speaking to your doctor. (Salt substitutes are typically rich in potassium and, in the setting of ARB use, can sometimes lead to dangerously high potassium levels.)

How to take an ARB

ARBs are typically started in low dose (which depends on the particular ARB you have been prescribed) and the dose is then adjusted, under your doctor's supervision, based on your response. ARBs are taken once daily, with or without food.

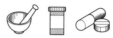

Anti-anxiety Medications

Anti-anxiety medications (sometimes referred to as *anxiolytics*) are medications that are used, as you might guess from the term, to lessen anxiety. The most commonly used anti-anxiety medications have traditionally been benzodiazepines. They can be helpful, but they can also be addictive and thus need to be used with caution.

Zopiclone isn't, strictly speaking, an anti-anxiety medication; however, as both this drug and benzodiazepines share much in common — including being commonly used therapies to treat insomnia — we discuss zopiclone in this section as well.

As we look at in Chapter 5, several other families of drugs, though not classified as "anti-anxiety medications," may be used for this purpose. We discuss these other drugs elsewhere in this chapter.

Benzodiazepines (and trade names for zopiclone) available in Canada are listed in Table 6-8. Benzodiazepines share much in common. In this section we discuss, in detail, lorazepam, a particularly commonly used member of this family.

Table 6-8	Benzodiazepines and Zopiclone	
Class	*Generic Name*	*Trade Name(s)*
Benzodiazepines	Alprazolam	Apo-Alpraz, Apo-Alpraz TS, Gen-Alprazolam, Novo-Alprazol, Nu-Alpraz, Xanax, Xanax TS
	Bromazepam	Apo-Bromazepam, Gen-Bromazepam, Lectopam, Novo-Bromazepam, Nu-Bromazepam
	Chlordiazepoxide	Apo-Chlorax*, Apo-Chlordiazepoxide, Librax
	Clobazam	Apo-Clobazam, Novo-Clobazam, ratio-Clobazam

Class	Generic Name	Trade Name(s)
	Clonazepam±	Apo-Clonazepam, CO Clonazepam, Gen-Clonazepam, Novo-Clonazepam, Nu-Clonazepam, PMS-Clonazepam, ratio-Clonazepam, Rivotril, Sandoz Clonazepam
	Clorazepate	Apo-Clorazepate, Novo-Clopate
	Diazepam	Apo-Diazepam, Diastat, Novo-Dipam, Valium Roche Oral
	Flurazepam	Apo-Flurazepam
	Lorazepam	Apo-Lorazepam, Ativan, Novo-Lorazem, Nu-Loraz, PMS-Lorazepam
	Nitrazepam	Apo-Nitrazepam, Mogadon, Nitrazadon, Sandoz Nitrazepam
	Oxazepam	Apo-Oxazepam
	Temazepam	Apo-Temazepam, CO Temazepam, Gen-Temazepam, Novo-Temazepam, Nu-Temazepam, PMS-Temazepam, ratio-Temazepam, Restoril
	Triazolam	Apo-Triazo, Gen-Triazolam, Halcion
Cyclopyrrolone derivative	**Zopiclone**	Apo-Zopiclone, CO Zopiclone, RAN-Zopiclone, Gen-Zopiclone, Imovane, Novo-Zopiclone, Nu-Zopiclone, PMS-Zopiclone, ratio-Zopiclone, Rhovane, Sandoz Zopiclone

* This medicine is a combination of different drugs. Refer to the drug label to determine what they are.

± We discuss clonazepam in the Anticonvulsants section of this chapter.

 ## Lorazepam

Apo-Lorazepam, Ativan, Novo-Lorazem, Nu-Loraz, PMS-Lorazepam

Lorazepam is an effective short-term treatment for anxiety disorders and insomnia. In contrast to some other benzodiazepines, lorazepam lasts in the body for only a few hours, so it's less likely to cause persisting drowsiness.

Certain specialized areas within the brain are responsible for keeping us alert and, at times, anxious. Activity within these areas of the brain is reduced by the action of a *neurotransmitter* (chemical messenger) called GABA. Lorazepam makes the action of GABA more potent. As a result, feelings of anxiety are eased and your level of alertness may diminish.

How lorazepam can help you

Lorazepam can help you in the following ways:

- ✔ Relieving anxiety.
- ✔ Reducing insomnia (that is, making it easier for you to get to sleep).
- ✔ Easing alcohol withdrawal.
- ✔ Preventing panic attacks.
- ✔ Stopping an attack of epilepsy (given by trained medical personnel, by intravenous injection).

How lorazepam might harm you

Possible side-effects from lorazepam include:

- ✔ Drowsiness. (Lorazepam can be taken as a sleeping pill, so drowsiness isn't a bad thing as long as it's confined to the time when you're trying to fall asleep.)
- ✔ Impaired ability to concentrate, forgetfulness, apathy.
- ✔ Dizziness.
- ✔ Nausea, constipation.
- ✔ *Respiratory failure* (this is severe lung malfunction such that you're not able to maintain normal levels of oxygen and carbon dioxide in your body). This is likely to happen only if you have severe lung disease or if you're taking doses higher than recommended.
- ✔ A paradoxical reaction, becoming agitated and hostile.

- ✔ Addiction (psychological and/or physical) to the drug. To avoid this, lorazepam is typically prescribed only for short-term use lasting no more than two weeks.

People with the following conditions shouldn't take lorazepam:

- ✔ Anxiety not due to a medical disorder.
- ✔ Myasthenia gravis. (This is a rare neurological disease in which the muscles are weak.)

- Certain forms of glaucoma.

- Pregnancy.

- Severe sleep apnea or chronic obstructive pulmonary disease (COPD) with respiratory failure.

- Taking other medications that might also make you sedated.

- Being prone to drug abuse. (Because of lorazepam's addictive potential it's either avoided or, at the very least, used with great caution in people who are susceptible to addictions.)

The safety of lorazepam in breastfeeding is unknown. We recommend before taking this medicine in this circumstance you discuss this with your physician.

Precautions to follow if you're taking lorazepam

Follow these precautions if you're taking lorazepam:

- This drug may make you drowsy, which would make it unsafe for you to perform activities — like driving — that require you to be alert and focused.

- Avoid alcohol, because it may worsen drowsiness.

- If you're elderly or if you have severe kidney, liver, or lung disease, you and your loved ones/caregivers should keep an especially close eye out for excess sedation or confusion after taking lorazepam. Seek prompt medical attention if these develop.

- Unless you've taken it for less than two weeks, lorazepam should be withdrawn *gradually* and under your doctor's close supervision. Suddenly stopping lorazepam can lead to withdrawal symptoms including excess anxiety, agitation, and nightmares.

How to take lorazepam

Lorazepam should be taken in the lowest dose that controls your symptoms and should be taken for as short a time as possible. The usual starting dose to treat anxiety is 1 mg to 2 mg per day divided in two to three doses, and to treat insomnia, 2 mg to 4 mg at bedtime. A lower starting dose is recommended if you're elderly. You can take lorazepam with or without food. If taking it without food upsets your stomach, try taking it with food.

There is also a sublingual form of lorazepam. A dose is placed under the tongue and dissolves in about 20 seconds. After taking a dose, try not to swallow for at least two minutes to allow the medicine to be absorbed into your system.

Zopiclone

Apo-Zopiclone, CO-Zopiclone, Gen-Zopiclone, Imovane, Novo-Zopiclone, Nu-Zopiclone, PMS-Zopiclone, RAN-Zopiclone, ratio-Zopiclone, Rhovane, Sandoz Zopiclone

Zopiclone is a very commonly used sleeping pill — more than 1.5 million prescriptions were dispensed in Canada in 2005. Clearly, many people in this country are having a hard time getting a good night's sleep.

Certain specialized areas within the brain are responsible for keeping us alert and, at times, anxious. Activity within these areas of the brain is reduced by the action of a *neurotransmitter* (chemical messenger) called GABA. Zopiclone makes the action of GABA more potent. This affects your sleep (as we discuss immediately below).

How zopiclone can help you

Zopiclone can help you by making it easier for you to fall asleep and to stay asleep (that is, less awakening overnight and being less likely to awaken prematurely in the morning).

How zopiclone might harm you

Possible side-effects from taking zopiclone include:

- Bitter taste in the mouth.
- Excess sedation. This is especially a concern in the elderly, where it could lead to falls.
- A paradoxical reaction, becoming agitated and hostile.

- Addiction (psychological and/or physical) to the drug. To avoid this, zopiclone is typically prescribed for short-term use lasting no more than two weeks.

People with the following conditions shouldn't take zopiclone:

- Sleeplessness that does not interfere with your ability to function the following day.
- Sleep apnea, or chronic obstructive pulmonary disease (COPD) with *respiratory failure* (that is, such poor lung function you're not able to maintain normal levels of oxygen and carbon dioxide in your body). (We talk more about COPD in Chapter 5.)
- Pregnancy or breastfeeding.

✔ If you will need to be alert a few hours later. For example, taking a dose of zopiclone to help you sleep during a flight would be unwise if, a few hours later, you need to be at a business meeting, driving a car, or operating machinery.

Precautions to follow if you're taking zopiclone

Follow these precautions if you're taking zopiclone:

✔ If you have taken zopiclone for more than three weeks, be sure to see your doctor to have your condition reviewed and, in particular, to see if the medication can be withdrawn.

✔ Unless you've taken it for less than a few weeks, stop taking zopiclone *gradually* and under your doctor's close supervision. Suddenly stopping zopiclone can lead to withdrawal symptoms including excess anxiety, agitation, and nightmares.

✔ This drug may make you drowsy, which would make it unsafe for you to perform activities — like driving — that require you to be alert and focused.

✔ Avoid alcohol because it may worsen drowsiness.

How to take zopiclone

The usual dose is 5 to 7.5 mg taken at bedtime. If you have liver disease or significant lung disease, your doctor may need to prescribe lower doses. You can take zopiclone with or without food.

Avoid consuming grapefruit or grapefruit juice because it can affect the level of zopiclone in your blood.

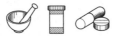

Anti-arrhythmics

Arrhythmia means "without rhythm." Our kids consider Ian's taste in music to make him an expert on this subject. Ian considers our kids ("you call that *music*?") to be the experts. Heather, being equally knowledgeable about music, marriage, and motherhood, takes the fifth (or at least she would if we resided in the U.S.).

Anti-arrhythmics are drugs that work to restore and/or maintain a normal heart rhythm. There are many different types of anti-arrhythmic medication, each having its own special properties. (Most anti-arrhythmic drugs are not in common use, and so are beyond the scope of this book.) The two most widely used oral anti-arrhythmic drugs (apart from beta blockers and calcium channel blockers, which we discuss elsewhere in this chapter) available in Canada are listed in Table 6-9.

Table 6-9	Anti-arrhythmics
Generic Name	Trade Name(s)
Amiodarone	Apo-Amiodarone, Cordarone, Gen-Amiodarone, Novo-Amiodarone, PMS-Amiodarone, ratio-Amiodarone, Sandoz Amiodarone
Digoxin	Lanoxin

 Amiodarone

Apo-Amiodarone, Cordarone, Gen-Amiodarone, Novo-Amiodarone, PMS-Amiodarone, ratio-Amiodarone, Sandoz Amiodarone

Amiodarone is a highly effective drug to control a variety of heart rhythm problems. It can, however, cause serious side-effects, so it needs to be used selectively and under close supervision.

 Certain cells within the heart conduct electricity (much like the wiring in your house). These cells have tiny pathways or openings (called *channels*) that allow sodium and potassium to pass in and out of the cells. Amiodarone works in part by blocking these channels and in part by blunting the action on the heart of hormones such as epinephrine (adrenaline). These combined actions help an out-of-rhythm heart return to and maintain a normal heart rhythm.

How amiodarone can help you

Amiodarone can help you in the following ways:

- Correcting an abnormal heart rhythm (such as atrial fibrillation).
- Preventing life-threatening heart rhythm disturbances such as ventricular tachycardia and ventricular fibrillation.
- Widening the arteries thereby making it easier for the heart to pump blood through the body.

How amiodarone might harm you

Possible side-effects from amiodarone include:

- ✔ Lung inflammation, sometimes leading to permanent damage (*pulmonary fibrosis*).

- ✔ Thyroid malfunction. Both *hyperthyroidism* (that is, thyroid over-functioning) and *hypothyroidism* (thyroid under-functioning) can occur.

- ✔ Heart failure or rhythm abnormalities. (Although amiodarone usually improves the heart rhythm, it has the potential to make things worse, not better.)

- ✔ Impaired vision. Both the cornea and the *optic nerve* (the nerve that connects the eye to the brain) can be damaged.

- ✔ *Photosensitive skin rash.* (That is, a rash that occurs upon sun exposure.)

- ✔ Abnormal liver tests. This is usually mild. Serious liver damage seldom occurs.

People with the following conditions shouldn't take amiodarone:

- ✔ A very slow heartbeat.
- ✔ Hepatitis.
- ✔ A form of lung disease called *interstitial fibrosis*.
- ✔ Breastfeeding.

Amiodarone can lead to damage to the developing fetus and therefore should almost always be avoided by pregnant women.

Precautions to follow if you're taking amiodarone

Follow these precautions if you're taking amiodarone:

- ✔ Use sunscreen and protective clothing to help you avoid getting a photosensitive skin rash (see above).

- ✔ See an eye specialist regularly. Make sure to tell him or her you're taking amiodarone.

- ✔ Notify your doctor promptly if you develop shortness of breath, a persisting cough, abnormal vision (blurring or halos), or faintness.

- ✔ Have your thyroid and liver status assessed with blood tests done before starting amiodarone, then periodically thereafter.

How to take amiodarone

For serious heart rhythm disturbances, the prescribed dose is typically 800 to 1600 mg per day for the first few weeks, then the dose is progressively reduced, under your doctor's supervision, to the lowest possible dose that keeps the heart rhythm controlled (usually 200 to 400 mg per day). For less serious problems, a lower starting dose is generally used. Amiodarone can be taken with or without food.

Avoid consuming grapefruit or grapefruit juice because it can affect the level of amiodarone in your blood.

℞ Digoxin

Lanoxin

Nowadays digoxin is manufactured in huge pharmaceutical plants, but for many years before that digoxin had been manufactured in a plant of quite a different sort: the foxglove plant. This plant was first used medicinally well over 200 years ago.

The two main actions of digoxin are

- ✔ Slowing the passage of electrical signals in a special part of the heart's electrical system called the *atrioventricular node* (the *AV node*).

- ✔ Increasing the force of the heartbeat.

How digoxin can help you

Digoxin can help you in the following ways:

- ✔ Controlling your heart rate if you have a type of heart rhythm disorder called *atrial fibrillation*.

- ✔ Improving congestive heart failure. This action of digoxin is fairly weak and hence it's not prescribed very often for this purpose.

We discuss atrial fibrillation and congestive heart failure in Chapter 5.

How digoxin might harm you

Possible side-effects from digoxin include:

✔ An abnormal heart rhythm. The heartbeat may be too fast, too slow, or irregular. You may notice this as a palpitation or as faintness.

✔ Poor appetite, nausea, vomiting, diarrhea.

✔ Abnormal colour vision (things may appear yellow-tinged), blurred vision.

✔ In males, breast enlargement (*gynecomastia*).

People with the following conditions shouldn't take digoxin:

✔ Low potassium or magnesium levels in the blood.

✔ Very slow heartbeat.

The other conditions that would make it unsafe for you to use digoxin are all quite *un*common heart diseases that your doctor will usually be able to detect by examining you and performing routine heart tests, such as an electrocardiogram (EKG) and heart ultrasound (echocardiogram).

 The safety of digoxin in pregnancy is unknown. It's likely safe to take if you're breastfeeding. If you're pregnant or breastfeeding, we recommend you discuss it with your physician before taking this medicine.

Precautions to follow if you're taking digoxin

Follow these precautions if you're taking digoxin:

✔ Don't stop taking digoxin without first speaking to your doctor. Stopping the drug inappropriately may cause the condition being treated to worsen.

✔ Periodically have blood tests done to measure your potassium level and kidney function. (Your doctor may also need to measure the level of digoxin in your blood.)

How to take digoxin

The dose of digoxin you're prescribed should be based in part on your (ideal) body weight and your kidney function. Digoxin is taken once daily at about the same time each day. It may be taken with or without food.

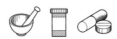

Antibiotics

Antibiotic means "against" (*anti*) "life" (*bios*). Fortunately, the lives that antibiotics are against are not of the human type, but the bacteria that have infected us. (By convention, *antibiotics* refers to anti*bacterial* drugs. We look at antiviral, antifungal, and antituberculosis drugs elsewhere in this chapter.) As there are so many different types of antibiotics, as shown in Table 6-10, we have divided this section into the following classes:

- Aminoglycosides
- Cephalosporins
- Fluoroquinolones
- Lincosamines
- Macrolides
- Nitroimidazoles
- Penicillins
- Sulfas
- Tetracyclines
- Xylophones (Kidding! Just checking to see if you're paying attention!)

These classes differ from one another by virtue of their chemical structure. (Drugs *within* a particular class have a fairly similar structure.) Having different classes of antibiotics available to us is very helpful in two key ways:

- Some antibiotic classes work better than others at attacking particular types of bacteria.
- Because the different classes of antibiotics work in complementary ways, some infections can be treated most effectively by simultaneously using two different antibiotics: one from one class and one from another. (This is done most commonly to treat serious infections in hospitalized patients.)

In this section we discuss in detail a particularly commonly used member of each of the antibiotic classes. (Table 6-10 doesn't include those antibiotics that are given exclusively by injection and hence are given *to* you, not taken *by* you.)

A particular antibiotic will help you only if the bacteria that are being treated (or prevented) are susceptible to this antibiotic. Different germs respond better to some antibiotics than others. When prescribing an antibiotic, your doctor determines what bacteria are most likely responsible for the infection and chooses an antibiotic based on this.

Table 6-10		Antibiotics
Class	**Generic Name**	**Trade Name(s)**
Aminoglycosides±	Framycetin	Proctol*, Proctosedyl*, ratio-Proctosone, SAB-Proctomyxin HC, Sandoz Opticort*, Sandoz Proctomyxin*, Sofra-Tulle, Sofracort*, Soframycin Nasal Spray, Soframycin Skin Ointment, Soframycin Sterile Eye Drops, Soframycin Sterile Eye Ointment
	Gentamicin	Garamycin Ophthalmic Drops, Garamycin Ophthalmic Ointment, Garamycin Otic Drops, Garamycin Topical Preparations, Garamycin Ophthalmic/Optic Solution, Garasone Ophthalmic Ointment, ratio-Gentamicin, Sandoz Pentasone, Valisone-G
	Neomycin	Cicatrin, Cortisporin Eye/Ear Suspension Sterile, Cortisporin Ointment, Cortisporin Otic Solution Sterile, Maxitrol*, Neo-Medrol Acne Lotion*, Neosporin Cream, Neosporin Eye and Ear Solution, Neosporin Irrigating Solution, Neosporin Ointment, Optimyxin Plus Solution, ratio-Triacomb*, Sandoz Cortimyxin Ophthalmic Ointment*, Sandoz Cortimyxin Otic Solution*, Viaderm-K.C.
	Paromomycin	Humatin
	Tobramycin	Tobradex*, Tobrex, TOBI Tobramycin Inhalation Solution

(continued)

Table 6-10 (continued)

Class	Generic Name	Trade Name(s)
Cephalosporins	Cefaclor	Apo-Cefaclor, Novo-Cefaclor, Nu-Cefaclor
	Cefprozil	Cefzil
	Cefuroxime	Apo-Cefuroxime, Ceftin, ratio-Cefuroxime
	Cephalexin	Apo-Cephalex, Novo-Lexin, Nu-Cephalex
Fluoroquinolones	**Ciprofloxacin**	Apo-Ciproflox, Ciloxan, Cipro Oral Suspension, Cipro Tablets, Cipro XL, Ciprodex*, Cipro HC*, CO Ciprofloxacin, Gen-Ciprofloxacin, Novo-Ciprofloxacin, PMS-Ciprofloxacin, RAN-Ciprofloxacin, ratio-Ciprofloxacin, Sandoz Ciprofloxacin, Taro-Ciprofloxacin
	Levofloxacin	Levaquin, Novo-Levofloxacin
	Moxifloxacin	Avelox, Vigamox
	Norfloxacin	Apo-Norflox, CO Norfloxacin, Novo-Norfloxacin
	Ofloxacin	Apo-Oflox, Floxin, Novo-Ofloxacin, Ocuflox
Lincosamine	**Clindamycin**	Apo-Clindamycin, BenzaClin*, Clinda-T, Clindasol, Clindets, Clindoxyl*, Dalacin C, Dalacin C Flavored Granules, Dalacin T Topical Solution, Dalacin Vaginal Cream, Gen-Clindamycin, Novo-Clindamycin, ratio-Clindamycin, Taro-Clindamycin
Macrolides	**Azithromycin**	CO Azithromycin, Novo-Azithromycin, PMS-Azithromycin, ratio-Azithromycin, Sandoz Azithromycin, Zithromax, Z-PAK
	Clarithromycin	Biaxin, Biaxin BID, Biaxin XL, Hp-PAC*, Losec 1-2-3 A*, Losec 1-2-3 M*, Nexium 1-2-3 A*

Class	Generic Name	Trade Name(s)
	Erythromycin	Apo-Erythro Base, Apo-Erythro E-C, Apo-Erythro-ES, Apo-Erythro-S, Benzamycin*, EES 200, EES 400, EES 600, Erybid, Eryc, Erysol*, Novo-Rythro Estolate, Novo-Rythro Ethylsuccinate, Nu-Erythromycin-S, PCE, Pediazole*, Stievamycin Preparations*
	Spiramycin	Rovamycine
Nitroimidazole	**Metronidazole**	Apo-Metronidazole Capsules, Apo-Metronidazole Tablets, Flagyl, Flagystatin*, Florazole ER, Losec 1-2-3 M*, MetroCream, MetroGel, MetroLotion, NidaGel, Noritate, Rosasol
Penicillins	**Amoxicillin**	Apo-Amoxi, Apo-Amoxi Clav*, Clavulin*, Gen-Amoxicillin, Hp-PAC*, Losec 1-2-3 A*, Nexium 1-2-3 A*, Novamoxin, Novo-Clavamoxin 875*, Nu-Amoxi, ratio-Aclavulanate*
	Ampicillin	Novo-Ampicillin, Nu-Ampi
	Cloxacillin	Apo-Cloxi, Novo-Cloxin, Nu-Cloxi
	Penicillin V	Apo-Pen VK, Novo-Pen-VK, Nu-Pen-VK
	Pivampicillin	Pondocillin
Sulfas	Sulfacetamide	Blephamide*, Sulfacet-R*
	Sulfamethoxazole/trimethoprim	Apo-Sulfatrim*, Apo-Sulfatrim DS*, Apo-Sulfatrim Pediatric Tablets*, Apo-Sulfatrim Oral Suspension*, Novo-Trimel*, Novo-Trimel DS*, Novo-Trimel Oral Suspension*, Nu-Cotrimox*, Nu-Cotrimox DS*, Nu-Cotrimox Oral Suspension*
	Sulfisoxazole	Pediazole*
	Sulfur	Medrol Acne Lotion*, Neo-Medrol Acne Lotion*, Sulfacet-R*

(continued)

Table 6-10 *(continued)*

Class	Generic Name	Trade Name(s)
Tetracyclines	Doxycycline	Apo-Doxy, Apo-Doxy-Tabs, Doxycin, Novo-Doxylin, Nu-Doxycycline, Vibra-Tabs
	Minocycline	Apo-Minocycline, Enca, Gen-Minocycline, Minocin, Novo-Minocycline, ratio-Minocycline, Sandoz Minocycline
	Tetracycline	Apo-Tetra, Nu-Tetra

± Many of these aminoglycoside-containing products have several additional medicinal ingredients, one of which is typically a corticosteroid.

* This medicine is a combination of different drugs. Refer to the drug label to determine what they are.

Aminoglycosides

Aminoglycosides may be given by intravenous injection in hospital to treat serious infections. More often, however, they're used in the form of drops, ointments, or creams for self-administration in the home. (These drops and topical preparations often also contain a corticosteroid to reduce inflammation.)

 ## Neomycin

Cicatrin, Cortisporin Eye/Ear Suspension Sterile, Cortisporin Ointment, Cortisporin Otic Solution Sterile, Maxitrol*, Neo-Medrol Acne Lotion*, Neosporin Cream, Neosporin Eye and Ear Solution, Neosporin Irrigating Solution, Neosporin Ointment, Optimyxin Plus Solution, ratio-Triacomb*, Sandoz Cortimyxin Ophthalmic Ointment*, Sandoz Cortimyxin Otic Solution*, Viaderm-K.C.

Neomycin is helpful in preventing and curing a wide variety of bacterial infections.

 All living things have genes; even the lowliest bacteria. One of the most important things that genes do is trigger the creation of proteins within an organism's cells. Neomycin interferes with the ability of bacteria to carry out this function, and as a result the bacteria die (and we survive; sounds fair to us).

How neomycin can help you

Neomycin can help you by treating infections involving the skin, the conjunctiva (*conjunctivitis*) and other superficial parts of the eye, and the outer ear (*swimmer's ear*).

Neomycin also may help prevent infections, for example bladder infections in people with bladder catheters, or skin infections for people who have wounds.

How neomycin might harm you

Possible side-effects from neomycin include the following:

- Skin irritation. Symptoms include itching, redness, swelling, and scaling.
- Eye irritation (if the neomycin is being applied to the eyes). Symptoms include itching, redness, and swelling.
- Hearing loss.
- Kidney damage.

Hearing loss and kidney damage are rare from non-injection use of neomycin and are likely to occur only if the medicine has been used for a long period of time in a high dose applied to an area of skin damage that allows for excess absorption of the medicine into your body.

When you shouldn't use neomycin

These are important "shouldn'ts" about using neomycin *ointment* or *cream*:

- They shouldn't be used if you have hearing loss and your doctor thinks you're at risk of having the medicine absorbed in significant quantities into your body.
- They shouldn't be put in the ear canal or on the outer ear if you have a perforated eardrum.
- They shouldn't be put in the eyes.

Don't use neomycin *ear drops* or *ear solution* if you have a perforated eardrum.

 The safety of neomycin in pregnancy and breastfeeding is unknown. If you're pregnant or breastfeeding, we recommend you discuss it with your physician before taking this medicine.

Precautions to follow if you're taking neomycin

You should notice some improvement in your infection within a few days of starting therapy; if you don't, we recommend you get in touch with your doctor.

Neomycin eye drops may contain a preservative (benzalkonium chloride) that can damage soft contact lenses. For this reason, be sure to remove your contacts before using your eye drops and wait at least 15 minutes before reinserting them.

How to take neomycin

This is how to take the different forms of neomycin:

- ✔ **Cream:** Gently remove any crusts, pus, debris, and so on from the area needing treatment, then apply a small amount of neomycin cream. This should be repeated two to five times daily depending on your doctor's instructions.

- ✔ **Ointment:** Gently remove any crusts, pus, debris, and so on from the area needing treatment, then apply a small amount of neomycin ointment. Spread this so that it makes a thin film. You can then cover this film with a gauze or you can leave it exposed.

- ✔ **Eye or ear drops**: Place one to two drops in the affected eye or ear two to four times daily depending on your doctor's instructions.

We discuss in detail the best way to take medicines in Chapter 4.

Cephalosporins

Many forms of cephalosporin are given by injection in a hospital setting. Of the oral cephalosporins, cephalexin is particularly popular.

 ## Cephalexin

Apo-Cephalex, Novo-Lexin, Nu-Cephalex

Cephalexin is effective in the treatment of many non–life-threatening infections and is generally very well tolerated.

Bacteria have a protective coating called a *cell wall*. Cephalexin causes bacteria to make a defective cell wall; one that is weakened and, like a collapsing house of cards, implodes.

How cephalexin can help you

Cephalexin can help you by treating infections involving the sinuses (*sinusitis*), the bladder (*cystitis*), the prostate (*prostatitis*), bone (*osteomyelitis*), the middle ear (*otitis media*), and skin (*cellulitis*).

How cephalexin might harm you

Possible side-effects from taking cephalexin include:

- ✔ Nausea, vomiting, diarrhea; these are the most common side-effects.
- ✔ Kidney damage and elevated liver tests; these seldom occur.

People with the following conditions shouldn't take cephalexin:

- ✔ Allergy to cephalexin or to other members of the cephalosporin family.
- ✔ Severe allergy to a drug from the penicillin family. (If you had a *minor* allergic reaction, taking cephalexin or another type of cephalosporin is *usually* safe.)

Cephalexin is generally considered safe to take during both pregnancy and breastfeeding. Nonetheless, if you're pregnant or breastfeeding, we recommend you discuss it with your physician before taking this medicine.

Precautions to follow if you're taking cephalexin

If you get severe or persisting diarrhea notify your physician, because this may indicate you have developed a serious bowel infection due to an organism called *C. difficile.*

How to take cephalexin

The usual dose of cephalexin is 500 mg taken every six to eight hours. It may be taken with or without food. Your doctor may need to prescribe lower than usual doses if you have kidney failure.

Fluoroquinolones

We well remember the buzz of excitement in the medical community when fluoroquinolones first came onto the scene. They were recognized as being powerful antibiotics that could target a wide variety of bacteria. Unfortunately, this excitement led to such widespread use of fluoroquinolones that over time a number of bacteria have developed resistance to (that is, are no longer affected by) this class of antibiotic. Nonetheless, fluoroquinolones do retain an important role in therapy. These drugs share many properties in common; their chief difference is that some types of infections respond better to one fluoroquinolone than another.

Ciprofloxacin

Apo-Ciproflox, Ciloxan, Cipro Oral Suspension, Cipro Tablets, Cipro XL, Ciprodex*, Cipro HC*, CO Ciprofloxacin, Gen-Ciprofloxacin, Novo-Ciprofloxacin, PMS-Ciprofloxacin, RAN-Ciprofloxacin, ratio-Ciprofloxacin, Sandoz Ciprofloxacin, Taro-Ciprofloxacin

Ciprofloxacin is a particularly commonly used member of the fluoroquinolone class of antibiotics.

DNA is the substance within cells that controls their function. Ciprofloxacin enters into bacteria and damages their DNA. As a result, the bacteria die.

How ciprofloxacin can help you

Ciprofloxacin can help you by treating infections involving the following:

- Conjunctiva (*conjunctivitis*). This is treated with topical ciprofloxacin.
- Sinuses (*sinusitis*), bronchial tree (*acute exacerbations of COPD*), lungs (*pneumonia*).
- Kidney (*pyelonephritis*), bladder (*cystitis*), prostate (*prostatitis*).
- Bone (*osteomyelitis*), joint (*septic arthritis*).
- Urethra, cervix, rectum (if due to *gonorrhea*).
- Bowel (*gastroenteritis*); if due to some types of food poisoning or traveller's diarrhea.

How ciprofloxacin might harm you

Possible side-effects from taking ciprofloxacin include the following:

- Nausea, vomiting, indigestion, diarrhea, abnormal liver tests are the most common side-effects, but occur in only a small percentage of users.
- Tremor, restlessness, confusion, drowsiness.
- *Myasthenia gravis* (a rare neurological disease in which the muscles are weak) can be made worse.

✔ Inflammation of tendons (*tendonitis*), most commonly affecting the Achilles tendon. This is rare and is most likely to occur if you're elderly and also taking *corticosteroid* medicine.

✔ *Photosensitive skin rash* (that is, a rash that occurs upon sun exposure).

Don't take ciprofloxacin if you're allergic to it *or to other members* of the fluoroquinolone family.

The safety of ciprofloxacin in pregnancy and breastfeeding is unknown. If you're pregnant or breastfeeding, we recommend you discuss it with your physician before taking this medicine.

Precautions to follow if you're taking ciprofloxacin

Follow these precautions if you're taking ciprofloxacin:

✔ Use sunscreen and protective clothing to help you avoid getting a photosensitive skin rash (see above).

✔ If you develop diarrhea or worsening of diarrhea you were already having, notify your physician because this may indicate you have developed a serious bowel infection due to an organism called *C. difficile*.

✔ This drug may make you drowsy, which would make it unsafe for you to perform activities — like driving — that require you to be alert and focused.

✔ Because alcohol may worsen drowsiness, it may be unwise to consume it. We recommend you check with your doctor to find out whether drinking (small amounts of) alcohol would be okay.

How to take ciprofloxacin

When taken orally, the usual dose for most types of infections is 500 mg twice daily. Your doctor may need to prescribe lower than usual doses if you have kidney failure. Take ciprofloxacin on an empty stomach. Ciprofloxacin shouldn't be taken within a few hours (before or after) of taking calcium or iron supplements, because these supplements will interfere with the absorption of ciprofloxacin into your body.

Lincosamines

Mention the word "lincosamine" to a doctor and you'll get a quizzical look. Mention the word "clindamycin" to a doctor and you'll get a nod of recognition. Basically, the word "lincosamine" is of value only insofar as it allows us to see where clindamycin fits into the (drug classification) scheme of things.

R̡ *Clindamycin*

Apo-Clindamycin, BenzaClin*, Clinda-T, Clindasol, Clindets, Clindoxyl*, Dalacin C, Dalacin C Flavored Granules, Dalacin T Topical Solution, Dalacin Vaginal Cream, Gen-Clindamycin, Novo-Clindamycin, ratio-Clindamycin, Taro-Clindamycin

Clindamycin is used in a variety of ways, including topically, vaginally, orally, and, in a hospital setting, by injection.

Clindamycin works by blocking the ability of bacteria to make life-sustaining proteins and nucleic acids (such as DNA).

How clindamycin can help you

Used topically, clindamycin is helpful in the treatment of acne. Clindamycin is also used vaginally to treat certain types of vaginal infection.

Taken orally, clindamycin can help you by treating the following infections:

- ✔ Lung, abdominal, and bone infections caused by susceptible bacteria (such as staphylococcal and streptococcal bacteria).
- ✔ *Pelvic inflammatory disease* (this is a serious type of gynecological infection).
- ✔ Pneumonia caused by *Pneumocystis jiroveci* (this is a common form of pneumonia affecting people with HIV/AIDS).

Clindamycin is also used for endocarditis prophylaxis. (See Chapter 5 for a discussion of this topic.)

How clindamycin might harm you

Possible side-effects from using topical clindamycin include dry, burning, itchy or scaly skin. Headaches may also occur. Gastro-intestinal symptoms as described below rarely occur with topical use.

Possible side-effects from taking oral clindamycin include:

- ✔ Nausea, vomiting, abdominal pain.
- ✔ Diarrhea. This is usually minor, however one particular form of diarrhea (*pseudomembranous colitis*; more commonly known as *C. difficile,* as this is the germ that causes this problem) can be very serious, especially in the elderly and the debilitated.

✔ Skin rash occurs in about 10 percent of people taking oral clindamycin.

✔ Abnormal liver tests.

✔ Rarely, abnormal blood counts, arthritis, or kidney malfunction.

Don't take clindamycin if you're allergic to it or to other members of the lincosamine family.

People with the following conditions shouldn't take clindamycin:

✔ Previous pseudomembranous colitis.

✔ Inflammatory bowel disease. (We discuss this in Chapter 5.)

Precautions to follow if you're taking clindamycin

Follow these precautions if you're taking clindamycin:

✔ If you get diarrhea, seek prompt medical attention. Even if you stopped the antibiotic *weeks before* the diarrhea started, still see your doctor because *C. difficile* (see above) may be responsible.

✔ If you're taking the medicine orally for more than a few weeks, your doctor will send you for periodic blood tests to monitor your liver and kidney function (and possibly your blood counts).

✔ If you're using intra-vaginal clindamycin, it may weaken a condom or diaphragm. Therefore, don't rely on these forms of contraception during intra-vaginal treatment (or for up to five days after treatment has been completed.)

 Clindamycin is generally thought to be safe during pregnancy, but this isn't proven. Its safety during breastfeeding is also unproven. If you're pregnant or breastfeeding, we recommend you discuss it with your physician before taking this medicine.

How to take clindamycin

When used topically (as in the treatment of acne), a thin film of clindamycin is applied twice daily.

When used orally, the dose depends on the severity of the infection being treated. The dose may range from 150 mg to 450 mg taken every six hours. Clindamycin may be taken with or without food, but to avoid irritating the esophagus it should be swallowed with a full glass of water.

If taking clindamycin without food is making you feel nauseated, taking it with food may help.

Macrolides

Erythromycin was, for years, a very popular (and effective) macrolide antibiotic, but because it tends to cause troublesome nausea it's now largely replaced by newer, better-tolerated members of this class.

℞ Azithromycin

Novo-Azithromycin, PMS-Azithromycin, ratio-Azithromycin, Sandoz Azithromycin, Zithromax, Z-PAK

Azithromycin is one of the most commonly used antibiotics in Canada. In fact, if you took every azithromycin pill sold in Canada last year and placed them end-to-end, you would have a lot of people wondering why you don't have something better to do!

Azithromycin works by interfering with the ability of bacteria to make proteins necessary for their survival.

How azithromycin can help you

Azithromycin can help you by treating infections involving the middle ear (*otitis media*), tonsils (*tonsillitis*), throat (*pharyngitis*), bronchial tree (*acute exacerbations of COPD*), lungs (*pneumonia*), skin (*cellulitis*), and urethra and cervix (if due to gonorrhea).

How azithromycin might harm you

Possible side-effects from taking azithromycin include:

- ✔ Nausea, abdominal pain, and diarrhea are the most common side-effects.
- ✔ Abnormal liver tests.
- ✔ Skin rash. Rarely, this may be severe.

Don't take azithromycin if you're allergic to it *or to other members* of the macrolide family.

The safety of azithromycin in pregnancy and breastfeeding is unknown. If you're pregnant or breastfeeding, we recommend you discuss it with your physician before taking this medicine.

Precautions to follow if you're taking azithromycin

Follow these precautions if you're taking azithromycin:

- If you have liver or kidney disease you may be more susceptible to side-effects, so keep an especially close eye out for these.

- If you get severe or persisting diarrhea, notify your physician because this may indicate you have developed a serious bowel infection due to an organism called *C. difficile.*

How to take azithromycin

The dose of azithromycin depends on the type of infection you have; however, one common schedule is to take 500 mg on the first day of treatment, then 250 mg once daily for four more days (that is, a total of 1.5 g). Another common schedule — used to treat infections such as those caused by chlamydia — is to take a single 1g dose. Take azithromycin with or without food.

Nitroimidazoles

We think the most interesting thing about the name applied to this class of drug (that is, "nitroimidazole") is that until we wrote this chapter we'd never heard of the word! (And we suspect you'd have a hard time finding a doctor who ever has.) We have, however, not only heard of metronidazole (the only member of this class available in Canada), but have frequently prescribed it. If ever you're prescribed metronidazole we suggest you don't even bother mentioning its class name; just refer to it by its generic name or whatever trade name you were dispensed.

 ## Metronidazole

Apo-Metronidazole Capsules, Apo-Metronidazole Tablets, Flagyl, Flagystatin*, Florazole ER, Losec 1-2-3 M*, MetroCream, MetroGel, MetroLotion, NidaGel, Noritate, Rosasol

Metronidazole is helpful in the treatment of a variety of different infections, including those caused not only by bacteria, but other types of organisms as well.

 That metronidazole works is well known. *How* it works is largely a mystery. It may be that oral metronidazole works by damaging a germ's DNA and that topical metronidazole works by reducing inflammation. Of course, it may be that the moon is made of green cheese. No, wait, Neil Armstrong proved that wrong...

How metronidazole can help you

Metronidazole can help you by treating the following infections:

- ✔ *C. difficile gastroenteritis* (also known as *pseumomebranous colits*). This is a sometimes very serious bowel infection that may develop as a side-effect from having taken other antibiotics.

- ✔ *Bacterial vaginosis.* This is a condition in which the vagina is inflamed and a variety of different organisms may be present.

- ✔ *Periodontitis, gingivitis.* These are forms of mouth/dental infections.

- ✔ *Ameba* and *giardia* (*beaver fever*) infections of the bowel, *trichomonas* infections of the vagina, and other infections caused by small parasites called *protozoa.*

- ✔ Stomach or duodenal ulcers (if due to *H. pylori*). This requires the use of other medicines as well.

- ✔ Rosacea.

- ✔ Certain other serious bacterial infections including brain abscesses and infections within the abdomen.

How metronidazole might harm you

Possible side-effects from taking metronidazole include:

- ✔ Nausea, vomiting, diarrhea.

- ✔ Seizures, unsteady gait, numbness and tingling in the fingers and toes.

- ✔ Your urine may turn a dark or reddish-brown colour. This isn't dangerous.

Because of safety concerns, it's generally recommended that metronidazole *not* be taken during pregnancy and breastfeeding. If you're pregnant or breastfeeding, we recommend you discuss it with your physician before taking this medicine.

Precautions to follow if you're taking metronidazole

Follow these precautions if you're taking metronidazole:

- ✔ Seek urgent medical attention if you develop any of the neurological side-effects noted above (seizures, unsteady gait, numbness and tingling of the fingers and toes).

- ✔ Don't consume alcohol. (Consuming alcohol may result in flushing, headache, nausea, and vomiting.)

How to take metronidazole

The dose of metronidazole depends on the nature of the infection being treated and the particular form of this antibiotic you're taking. Your doctor may need to prescribe lower than usual doses if you have kidney failure or liver disease.

Penicillins

Penicillins refers to a class of antibiotic, whereas *penicillin* refers to the founding member of the class. Nowadays there are many different members within this group, including the immensely popular antibiotic amoxicillin.

 ## Amoxicillin

Apo-Amoxi, Apo-Amoxi Clav*, Clavulin*, Gen-Amoxicillin, Hp-PAC*, Losec 1-2-3 A*, Nexium 1-2-3 A*, Novamoxin, Novo-Clavamoxin 875*, Nu-Amoxi, ratio-Aclavulanate*

Amoxicillin is the most frequently prescribed antibiotic in Canada: a whopping 5.7 million prescriptions for amoxicillin were filled in 2005!

How amoxicillin works

 Of all the ways that drugs work, we think amoxicillin's technique is one of the neatest. Bacteria have a protective coating called a *cell wall*. Amoxicillin causes bacteria to make a weakened protective coating, so, in the same way a demolition crew often brings down buildings in densely developed urban areas, its infrastructure is destroyed and it collapses in on itself. Way cool.

How amoxicillin can help you

Amoxicillin can help you by treating infections involving the middle ear (*otitis media*), sinuses (*sinusitis*), throat (*pharyngitis*), bronchial tree (*acute exacerbations of COPD*), lungs (*pneumonia*), bone (*osteomyelitis*), kidneys (*pyelonephritis*), bladder (*cystitis*). It's also used to treat ulcers in the stomach or duodenum caused by *H. pylori* (we talk about these ulcers in Chapter 5).

And that's not all! Amoxicillin is also used to treat chlamydia infections, Lyme disease, typhoid fever, and to prevent heart valve infections (this use is termed *SBE prophylaxis,* which we explain in Chapter 5). No wonder amoxicillin is so popular.

How amoxicillin might harm you

Possible side-effects from taking amoxicillin include:

- ✔ Nausea, vomiting, diarrhea.

- ✔ Skin rash. This is especially common if you take amoxicillin at the same time as having infectious mononucleosis.

- ✔ Yeast infections of the mouth or throat (*thrush*) or, in women, of the vagina.

People with the following conditions shouldn't take amoxicillin:

- ✔ Infectious mononucleosis.

- ✔ Allergy to amoxicillin or to other members of the penicillin family.

- ✔ Severe allergy to a drug from the cephalosporin family. (If you had a *minor* allergic reaction, taking amoxicillin or another type of penicillin is *usually* safe.)

Amoxicillin is generally considered safe to take during both pregnancy and breastfeeding. Nonetheless, if you're pregnant or breastfeeding, we recommend you discuss it with your physician before taking this medicine.

Precautions to follow if you're taking amoxicillin

Follow these precautions if you're taking amoxicillin:

- ✔ If you get a white coating in your mouth or throat, or, for women, if you develop a vaginal discharge, this may indicate you have a yeast infection. If this happens, seek (non-urgent) medical attention.

- ✔ If you get severe or persisting diarrhea notify your physician, as this may indicate you have developed a serious bowel infection due to an organism called *C. difficile*.

How to take amoxicillin

The dose of amoxicillin will vary widely depending on what type of infection is being treated. For most infections, the prescribed dose is either 250 mg to 500 mg taken every eight hours, or 875 mg taken every 12 hours. Your doctor may need to prescribe lower than usual doses if you have kidney failure. Amoxicillin may be taken with or without food. If taken with food, we know this great Greek restaurant in downtown Penticton...

Sulfas

Sulfas are medications with a sulfur component (or *base*). Because many different medicines have this property, "sulfas" are more properly referred to as "sulfa antibiotics." In this section we discuss in detail a particularly commonly used sulfa antibiotic: sulfamethoxazole (which is used in combination with another antibiotic: trimethoprim).

Sulfamethoxazole/Trimethoprim

Apo-Sulfatrim*, Apo-Sulfatrim DS*, Apo-Sulfatrim Pediatric Tablets*, Apo-Sulfatrim Oral Suspension*, Novo-Trimel*, Novo-Trimel DS*, Novo-Trimel Oral Suspension*, Nu-Cotrimox*, Nu-Cotrimox DS*, Nu-Cotrimox Oral Suspension*

Sulfamethoxazole/trimethoprim is also referred to as trimethoprim/ sulfamethoxazole. Either way you look at it, the name is a mouthful!

The actions of sulfamethoxazole and trimethoprim are complementary (hence their combined use). Working together, they block different steps in a chemical pathway that bacteria use to manufacture folic acid. With insufficient folic acid, bacteria cannot survive. (Our own folic acid is seldom affected.)

How sulfamethoxazole/trimethoprim can help you

Sulfamethoxazole/trimethoprim can help you by treating infections involving the sinuses (*sinusitis*), bronchial tree (*acute exacerbations of COPD*), kidneys (*pyelonephritis*), bladder (*cystitis*), prostate (*prostatitis*), bowel (*gastroenteritis*, including *traveller's diarrhea*), and lungs (*pneumonia*). It's particularly effective in the treatment of pneumonia due to *Pneumocystis jiroveci*.

Sulfamethoxazole/trimethoprim is also used to prevent Pneumocystis jiroveci pneumonia in people at risk of developing it, such as those with HIV/AIDS.

How sulfamethoxazole/trimethoprim might harm you

Possible side-effects from taking sulfamethoxazole/trimethoprim include:

- Nausea, vomiting.
- Skin rash. Rarely, this may be severe.
- Bone marrow injury.
- Liver injury.
- Kidney stones. This seldom occurs.

People with the following conditions shouldn't take sulfamethoxazole/trimethoprim:

✔ Allergy to trimethoprim or sulfamethoxazole or to other members of the sulfa antibiotic family.

✔ Anemia due to low folic acid.

✔ Severe liver or kidney disease.

✔ Porphyria (this is a rare, genetic disease).

The safety of sulfamethoxazole/trimethoprim in pregnancy will depend, at least in part, on how far along your pregnancy is. Its safety during breastfeeding will depend, in part, on the health of the baby. We recommend before taking this medicine in these circumstances you discuss this with your physician.

Precautions to follow if you're taking sulfamethoxazole/trimethoprim

Follow these precautions if you're taking sulfamethoxazole/trimethoprim:

✔ If you develop a skin rash, sore throat, fever (or, if you already had a fever, a worsening of it) or other symptom suggesting you may have developed a new infection, seek prompt medical attention. People who are elderly or have AIDS are at particularly high risk of complications and therefore need to be especially vigilant.

✔ If you're elderly or malnourished, your doctor should monitor your blood counts.

✔ Maintain good hydration. This will reduce your likelihood of getting kidney stones.

How to take sulfamethoxazole/trimethoprim

Your dose and duration of therapy depends on the infection being treated; however, the most common amounts of these medicines are 800 mg of sulfamethoxazole and 160 mg of trimethoprim taken twice daily. You can take it with or without food (however, it's less likely to bother your stomach if taken with food).

Tetracyclines

Tetracycline is the original and most commonly used member of the class of antibiotics called tetracylines.

Tetracylcine

Apo-Tetra, Nu-Tetra

Tetracycline was patented the same year that the first McDonald's opened. And, like McDonald's, billions have been served. It was once one of the most popular antibiotics, but as time has passed it has largely been replaced by newer drugs. Nonetheless, it still has a role to play in specific circumstances.

Tetracycline works by interfering with the ability of bacteria to make proteins necessary for their survival. It may also work by damaging the protective membrane that surrounds bacteria.

How tetracycline can help you

Tetracycline can help you by treating the following infections:

- Acne, rosacea.

- Periodontitis. (This is a form of dental infection.)

- Mycoplasma pneumonia.

- Lyme disease.

- Stomach or duodenal ulcers (if due to *H. pylori*). This requires the use of other medicines as well.

- Acute exacerbations of COPD.

- Sexually transmitted diseases due to gonorrhea or syphilis.

- Those caused by organisms called rickettsiae. These germs can cause uncommon diseases such as Rocky Mountain spotted fever and Q fever.

How tetracycline might harm you

Possible side-effects from taking tetracycline include:

- *Photosensitive skin rash* (that is, a rash that occurs upon sun exposure).

- Irritation to the esophagus (*esophagitis*), nausea, vomiting, diarrhea.

- *Tinnitus* (ringing in the ears), hearing loss.

- Blurred vision.

- Liver damage. This is most likely to occur if you're taking high doses for long periods of time, especially if you have kidney malfunction.

People with the following conditions shouldn't take tetracycline:

- ✔ Allergy to tetracycline or to other members of the tetracycline family.

- ✔ Severe liver or kidney disease.

Because tetracycline can damage the teeth of a fetus and infant, it's almost always avoided during pregnancy and breastfeeding. If you're pregnant or breastfeeding, we recommend you discuss it with your physician before taking this medicine.

Precautions to follow if you're taking tetracycline

Follow these precautions if you're taking tetracycline:

- ✔ Use sunscreen and protective clothing to help avoid getting a photosensitive skin rash.

- ✔ If on long-term treatment, have your blood counts, liver, and kidney function tested from time to time.

How to take tetracycline

To avoid tetracycline irritating your esophagus, take it during the daytime (not at bedtime), standing or sitting, on an empty stomach and with a large glass of water. The dose of tetracycline you require depends on the specific disease being treated, however a common dose is 250 mg to 500 mg taken four times per day. Your doctor may need to prescribe lower than usual doses if you have kidney failure.

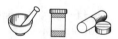

Anticancer Drugs for Breast and Prostate Cancer

Breast and prostate cancer are two of the most common malignancies for which anticancer drugs are taken outside of a hospital setting. Some of the most important drugs used in their treatment work, as we discuss in more detail below, by blocking the action of certain hormones that influence the growth of these cancers. In Table 6-11 we list those drugs. (Tamoxifen is also used to treat breast cancer; however, as it differs in important ways from the other drugs in this section, we discuss it elsewhere in this chapter.)

Table 6-11	Anticancer Drugs for Breast and Prostate Cancer	
Class	**Generic Name**	**Trade Name(s)**
Aromatase inhibitors	**Anastrozole**	Arimidex
	Exemestane	Aromasin
	Letrozole	Femara
Anti-androgens	**Bicalutamide**	Casodex, CO Bicalutamide, Novo-Bicalutamide, PMS-Bicalutamide, ratio-Bicalutamide, Sandoz Bicalutamide
	Flutamide	Apo-Flutamide, Euflex, Novo-Flutamide
	Nilutamide	Anandron
GnRH agonists	Buserelin	Suprefact, Suprefact Depot
	Goserelin	Zoladex 3.6mg, Zoladex LA
	Leuprolide	Eligard, Lupron, Lupron Depot

 Anastrozole

Arimidex

Aromatase inhibitors (also known as anti-estrogens) such as anastrozole are used in the treatment of breast cancer.

 Breast cancers typically get worse if there is estrogen in your body. Even post-menopausal women (that is, women who no longer ovulate or have periods) still have some estrogen present. Aromatase inhibitors work by blocking the action of *aromatase*, an enzyme that helps produce estrogen in tissues other than the ovaries. This leads to reduced levels of estrogen in the body (hence the reason why these drugs are also referred to as *anti-estrogens*), making breast cancer less likely to grow and spread.

How anastrozole can help you

Anastrozole can help you if you're post-menopausal and have breast cancer by reducing the risk that your cancer will grow and spread.

How anastrozole might harm you

Possible side-effects from taking anastrozole include:

- ✔ Hot flushes, vaginal dryness, thinning hair. These are common though not serious side-effects.

- ✔ Loss of appetite, nausea, vomiting, diarrhea.

- ✔ Osteoporosis. Estrogen is important in protecting women from getting osteoporosis. Because anastrozole reduces estrogen levels, you will be at increased risk of osteoporosis.

- ✔ Muscle aches and pains.

People with the following conditions shouldn't take anastrozole:

- ✔ Using tamoxifen.

- ✔ Pre-menopausal women.

- ✔ Serious liver or kidney disease.

Precautions to follow if you're taking anastrozole

Follow these precautions if you're taking anastrozole:

- ✔ Take preventive measures to avoid osteoporosis (or, if you already have osteoporosis, to help prevent it from worsening), such as consuming sufficient calcium and vitamin D, performing weight-bearing exercise, and, in some women, taking *bisphosphonate* medication.

- ✔ Have your *bone density* checked regularly. This is done with a special type of x-ray procedure your doctor can arrange for you.

How to take anastrozole

Anastrozole is taken as a once-daily, 1-mg tablet and is typically used for a total duration of five years. It may be taken with or without food.

If you find the anastrozole is making you nauseated, try taking it *after* you've eaten. You may find you tolerate it better that way.

℞ Bicalutamide

Casodex, CO Bicalutamide, Novo-Bicalutamide, PMS-Bicalutamide, ratio-Bicalutamide, Sandoz Bicalutamide

Anti-androgens such as bicalutamide are used in the treatment of prostate cancer.

Male hormones, such as testosterone, are known as *androgens*. Prostate cancer typically worsens if there is androgen in your body. Anti-androgens work by blocking the effect of testosterone on the prostate, resulting in less stimulation of the prostate cancer cells to grow.

How bicalutamide can help you

Bicalutamide can help you if you have prostate cancer by reducing the risk your cancer will grow and spread.

How bicalutamide might harm you

Possible side-effects from taking bicalutamide include:

- ✔ Hot flushes, breast swelling, and tenderness. These are the most common side-effects, and although not dangerous they can be unpleasant.
- ✔ Nausea, diarrhea, constipation.
- ✔ Reduced sex drive (*libido*).
- ✔ *Peripheral edema* (ankle swelling), congestive heart failure.
- ✔ Abnormal liver tests. These typically return to normal after the medicine has been stopped; however, rarely, people taking this drug develop hepatitis.

Women should not take bicalutamide.

Follow these precautions if you're taking bicalutamide:

- ✔ Have your liver enzyme levels checked periodically on a blood test. If they're significantly abnormal you may need to stop taking the medicine.
- ✔ See your doctor if you develop shortness of breath or swollen ankles.

How to take bicalutamide

Bicalutamide is typically taken once per day in a dose of 50 mg. You may take it with or without food. Bicalutamide is generally prescribed together with other anticancer drugs such as goserelin or leuprolide.

 ## Goserelin

Zoladex 3.6mg, Zoladex LA

GnRH (gonadotropin-releasing hormone) agonists such as goserelin are used in the treatment of prostate cancer, breast cancer, and certain gynecological problems.

Prostate cancers typically get worse if there is testosterone in your body, and breast cancers typically get worse if there is estrogen in your body. The pituitary gland (a tiny structure located in the brain) releases hormones (LH, FSH) that stimulate a man's testicles to produce testosterone and a woman's ovaries to produce estrogen. GnRH agonists work by blocking the pituitary's production of LH and FSH. As a result, in a man there is less testosterone and this helps to control prostate cancer; in a woman, there is less estrogen and this helps to control breast cancer and certain estrogen-requiring gynecological conditions.

How goserelin can help you

Goserelin can help you in the following ways:

- ✔ If you have prostate cancer, it may reduce the risk your cancer will grow and spread.

- ✔ If you're a woman who is either pre-menopausal or around the time of menopause (*peri-menopausal*) and you have breast cancer, it may reduce the risk your cancer will grow and spread.

- ✔ Improving endometriosis. We discuss endometriosis in Chapter 5.

- ✔ Helping to prepare the uterus for a procedure called endometrial ablation.

How goserelin might harm you

Possible side-effects from taking goserelin include:

- ✔ Hot flushes and sweats. These common side-effects are not dangerous, but can be unpleasant.

- ✔ Reduced sex drive (*libido*) and, in men, erectile dysfunction. These occur commonly.

- ✔ Headache, emotional swings, feeling depressed. These are more common in women.

- ✔ Insomnia. This commonly occurs in men.

- ✔ Low blood pressure (which might make you feel faint) or, conversely, raised blood pressure. These both typically go away as treatment is continued.

- ✔ Congestive heart failure; blood clots (such as phlebitis). These serious side-effects are uncommon.

- ✔ Osteoporosis.

People with the following conditions shouldn't take goserelin:

- ✔ Severe liver disease.
- ✔ Pregnancy, breastfeeding.
- ✔ Women who have vaginal bleeding the cause of which isn't yet known.

Precautions to follow if you're taking goserelin

Follow these precautions if you're taking goserelin:

- ✔ Shortly after starting therapy you may experience temporarily increased pain in your bones. This is more likely to happen if you're male. If this happens, speak to your physician because you may require strong analgesics to tide you over until the problem settles. (Taking an anti-androgen for a few weeks prior to starting goserelin will help minimize this side-effect.)

- ✔ Take preventive measures to avoid osteoporosis (or, if you already have osteoporosis, to help prevent it from worsening), such as consuming sufficient calcium and vitamin D, performing weight-bearing exercise, and, in some cases, taking bisphosphonate medication.

- ✔ Have your bone density checked regularly. This is done with a special type of x-ray procedure your doctor can arrange for you.

How to take goserelin

This medication is given as a *subcutaneous injection* (that is, an injection immediately under the surface of the skin) typically administered by the physician in the office. Goserelin is given every 4 to 12 weeks, the frequency of the injections varying based on the disease being treated and the dose of the medicine.

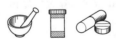

Anticholinergics (for Overactive Bladder)

Anticholinergic drugs are used to treat many different and unrelated illnesses. In this section we look at anticholinergics used specifically to treat overactive bladder.

The cells that line the bladder have receptors that are stimulated by a chemical messenger called acetylcholine. When stimulated, these cells cause the bladder muscle to contract and will typically cause you to feel that your bladder needs to be emptied. This is helpful if, indeed, your bladder is full and you have time to get to a bathroom, but is anything but helpful if your bladder isn't really full, just being overly sensitive (a symptom of overactive bladder). Oral anticholinergics block the bladder's acetylcholine receptors and enable the bladder to hold more urine — this will help give you better control over your bladder function.

Table 6-12 lists prescription anticholinergic medications used to treat overactive bladder. Oxybutynin, the most commonly used drug in this family, is discussed in detail below.

Table 6-12	Anticholinergics for Overactive Bladder
Generic Name	**Trade Name(s)**
Darifenacin	Enablex
Flavoxate	Apo-Flavoxate
Oxybutynin	Apo-Oxybutynin, Ditropan, Ditropan XL, Gen-Oxybutynin, Novo-Oxybutynin, Nu-Oxybutynin, Oxytrol, PMS-Oxybutynin, Uromax
Tolterodine	Detrol, Detrol LA

 Oxybutynin

Apo-Oxybutynin, Ditropan, Ditropan XL, Gen-Oxybutynin, Novo-Oxybutynin, Nu-Oxybutynin, Oxytrol, PMS-Oxybutynin, Uromax

Oxybutynin has been a mainstay of the treatment of overactive bladder for many years.

How oxybutynin can help you

Oxybutynin can help you by reducing your symptoms of overactive bladder. As we discuss in Chapter 5, symptoms of overactive bladder include *urinary incontinence* (that is, losing control of your bladder and wetting yourself), a feeling of needing to urgently empty your bladder, and needing to pass urine overly frequently.

How oxybutynin might harm you

Possible side-effects from taking oxybutynin include:

- ✔ Dry mouth and throat. These are the most common side-effects and, though not serious, can be quite bothersome.
- ✔ Drowsiness.
- ✔ Nausea, constipation.
- ✔ Difficulty emptying your bladder.
- ✔ Worsening of glaucoma.
- ✔ Decreased sweating and/or blurred vision. These seldom occur.

All these side-effects are directly related to the drug's *anticholinergic* effect (that is, blocking acetylcholine receptors) in various organs in the body. In other words, what's good in the bladder is often bad in other organs.

You may find some relief from a dry mouth by taking sips of water or by sucking on hard candy or chewing sugarless gum. Also, having a persistent dry mouth can increase your risk of cavities, so be sure to look after your teeth well and have regular dental care.

People with the following conditions shouldn't take oxybutynin:

- ✔ Glaucoma.
- ✔ Serious bowel diseases (such as having a blockage or ulcerative colitis).
- ✔ Myasthenia gravis. This is a rare neurological disease in which the muscles are weak.
- ✔ Blockage of the urinary tract (such as might occur with prostatism).

The safety of oxybutynin in pregnancy and breastfeeding is unknown. If you're pregnant or breastfeeding, we recommend you discuss it with your physician before taking this medicine.

Precautions to follow if you're taking oxybutynin

Follow these precautions if you're taking oxybutynin:

- ✔ Be sure to maintain adequate hydration, especially in hot weather.
- ✔ If you get blurring of your vision or become unable to pass urine, seek urgent medical attention.

✔ This drug may make you drowsy, which would make it unsafe for you to perform activities — like driving — that require you to be alert and focused.

✔ Because alcohol may worsen drowsiness, it may be unwise to consume it. We recommend you check with your doctor to find out whether drinking (small amounts of) alcohol would be okay.

How to take oxybutynin

The usual starting dose of oxybutynin is 5 mg to 10 mg per day (taken as a single dose or divided into 2 doses depending on the particular brand you're given). The dose is then adjusted, under your doctor's supervision, based on your response. Take regular (short-acting) oxybutynin on an empty stomach with water; take long-acting oxybutynin with or without food.

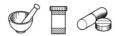

Anticoagulants

Anticoagulants are powerful "blood thinners" used to prevent and treat serious blood clots such as deep vein thrombosis (phlebitis) and pulmonary thromboembolism. We discuss these conditions in Chapter 5.

As we discuss in Chapter 5, anticoagulant therapy may be given orally (with a type of coumarin called warfarin) or by injection (typically with a low molecular weight [LMW] heparin). Because warfarin takes a few days to take effect whereas LMW heparin works immediately, both are initially given. Then, after a week or so, the LMW heparin is withdrawn while the warfarin is continued. (The situation is different if you're pregnant or have cancer, in which case LMW heparin is used instead of warfarin for reasons of safety and efficacy, respectively.)

Table 6-13 lists the coumarins and low molecular weight heparins available in Canada.

Table 6-13	Anticoagulants	
Class	**Generic Name**	**Trade Name(s)**
Coumarins	Nicoumalone*	Sintrom
	Warfarin	Apo-Warfarin, Coumadin, Gen-Warfarin, Novo-Warfarin, Taro-Warfarin

Class	Generic Name	Trade Name(s)
Low molecular weight heparins	**Dalteparin**	Fragmin
	Enoxaparin	Lovenox, Lovenox HP
	Nadroparin	Fraxiparine, Fraxiparine Forte
	Tinzaparin	Innohep

* Nicoumalone is seldom used. (Its main role occurs when you require an oral anticoagulant but are allergic to warfarin.)

 Warfarin

Apo-Warfarin, Coumadin, Gen-Warfarin, Novo-Warfarin, Taro-Warfarin

There are few drugs that deserve more respect than warfarin. Each and every year, warfarin protects countless numbers of people — perhaps including you — from the devastation of a stroke or other serious blood clot. Yet, at the same time, this drug has its all too real dangers, such as catastrophic bleeding. To succeed with warfarin therapy, caution is the buzzword.

 Clotting factors are substances in the blood that are directly involved in the clotting process. Several of these factors are made with the help of vitamin K and are called vitamin K dependent clotting factors. Warfarin blocks the action of vitamin K and, as a result, fewer of these factors are made. With fewer of these clotting factors in the blood, you're less likely to form a blood clot.

 People often call warfarin a "blood thinner." (Indeed, we did the same in the introduction to this section!) Figuratively, this is true insofar as it prevents clotting; however, warfarin does not actually make your blood less thick, less viscous, less molasses-like, or make you "thinner" in any other sense of the word. (Except if you walk to the drugstore to buy it, in which case it will help thin your waist, but we digress...)

How warfarin can help you

Warfarin can help you by preventing blood clots from forming or an existing clot from getting bigger.

It's a commonly held misperception that warfarin dissolves clots that have already formed. It doesn't. If you already have a clot, the body has its own natural processes to deal with it. Warfarin is used to prevent *additional* clots from forming while your body deals with the one you already have.

How warfarin might harm you

Possible side-effects from taking warfarin include:

- ✔ Bleeding. This appropriately feared complication is by no means rare.

- ✔ Severe skin damage. Fortunately, this seldom occurs.

- ✔ *Purple toes syndrome.* Yes, Virginia, there really is a purple toes syndrome. This condition is characterized by, as you might guess, a purplish discolouration of the toes and is caused by cholesterol deposits breaking off from blood vessels and travelling to other parts of the body, including the toes.

People with the following conditions shouldn't take warfarin:

- ✔ Pregnancy. (Warfarin can damage the fetus.)

- ✔ Having a significantly increased risk of bleeding. Examples include having a bleeding disorder or recent bleeding episode (such as a brain hemorrhage), having had some types of recent surgery (such as a brain or eye operation), having had a recent stomach or duodenal ulcer, or having severe (uncontrolled) hypertension.

- ✔ Inability to follow the careful monitoring required to safely take warfarin. People who potentially would be in this group are inadequately supervised individuals with dementia or alcoholism, or people who, for whatever reason, are unable or unwilling to maintain the close medical follow-up that is required.

The safety of warfarin to the child of a breastfeeding woman is unknown. We recommend before taking this medicine in this circumstance you first discuss this with your physician.

Precautions to follow if you're taking warfarin

Follow these precautions if you're taking warfarin:

- ✔ Warfarin therapy must be very closely supervised, with frequent blood tests called an INR (international normalized ratio). The INR level indicates whether you're sufficiently protected from blood clots or if you're at undue risk of bleeding. An INR that is too low indicates your warfarin dose is too low and you're at risk of clotting. An INR that is too high indicates your warfarin dose is too high and you're at risk of bleeding.

- ✔ As is true of most any other prescription drug, warfarin can interact with other prescription drugs *and* non-prescription therapies. In the case of warfarin, however, the outcome from too high or too low a level of the medicine in your system can be far more devastating (see the preceding bullet) than for most other drugs. For this reason, it's essential you review *all* your therapies with your doctor and not take *any* new therapy without first consulting your physician.

✔ Your daily dietary intake of vitamin K should remain consistent. (A change in your intake of vitamin K may alter your INR and, hence, the effectiveness and safety of the medication.) Many foods, including green leafy vegetables and beef liver, are rich in vitamin K. (We discuss this further in Chapter 4.)

✔ Because injections into muscle may cause bruising, such injections should, if possible, be avoided. If such injections are required, it's best to use the arm rather than the leg or buttock.

✔ Check your stools for blood on a daily basis: if you see red blood or if your stools are tarry and black (which can indicate bleeding within the gut), seek urgent medical attention.

✔ Don't consume more than one or two alcohol-containing drinks per day.

If you're taking warfarin and you also need a mild *analgesic* (pain killer), take acetaminophen rather than ASA as acetaminophen will not increase your risk of bleeding.

How to take warfarin

Your dose of warfarin will be tailored to your individual needs. The warfarin dose that achieves the desired blood levels is variable, but *usually* people are started on 5 mg to 10 mg per day for the first two days of treatment, then 2 mg to 10 mg per day thereafter. You may take warfarin with or without food.

Low molecular weight heparins

Because the various low molecular weight (LMW) heparins are so similar, we discuss them together. LMW heparin is an injectable medicine that is usually started in the emergency department (after a diagnosis of a blood clot is made). Further doses are then given by health care professionals or, increasingly often, by the patient who is taught how to do this.

Clotting factors are substances in the blood that are directly involved in the clotting process. LMW heparin interferes with the action of certain clotting factors, and as a result you're less likely to form a blood clot.

How low molecular weight heparins can help you

LMW heparins may help you by preventing blood clots from forming or an existing clot from getting bigger.

How low molecular weight heparins might harm you

Possible side-effects from taking LMW heparins include:

- Bleeding.
- Bruising in the area of the injection(s).
- Low platelet count. This seldom occurs.
- Elevated liver tests. This is typically very mild and insignificant.
- Osteoporosis. This occurs only with long-term therapy (many months or longer).

People with the following conditions shouldn't take LMW heparins:

- Having a significantly increased risk of bleeding. Examples include having a bleeding disorder or recent bleeding episode (such as a brain hemorrhage), having had some types of recent surgery (such as a brain or eye operation), having had a recent stomach or duodenal ulcer, or having severe (uncontrolled) hypertension.
- Allergy to heparin or to pork products (LMW heparin is derived from pigs).

Although LMWH heparin can be safely taken during pregnancy (and breastfeeding), some multidose vials of LMW heparin contain a preservative (benzyl alcohol) that, in high enough doses, may harm a fetus. Although the amount present in LMW heparin vials is likely safe, it's nonetheless recommended that if you're pregnant you use single dose vials (which don't contain this preservative). Your pharmacist can tell you if the particular type of LMW heparin you have been prescribed contains benzyl alcohol.

Precautions to follow if you're taking low molecular weight heparins

Check your stools for blood on a daily basis: if you see red blood or if your stools are tarry and black (which can indicate bleeding within the gut), seek urgent medical attention.

If you're taking a LMW heparin and you also need a mild *analgesic* (pain killer), take acetaminophen rather than ASA because acetaminophen will not increase your risk of bleeding.

How to take low molecular weight heparins

LMW heparins are given as subcutaneous injections (that is, an injection only slightly under the skin surface). Depending on which specific preparation you're using, the medication is injected either once or twice daily. Injections are given into the abdomen or the side of your thigh. Your dose depends on the particular type of LMW heparin you're prescribed and your particular situation (including, for example, your body weight).

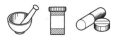

Anticonvulsants

Another name for an attack of epilepsy is a *seizure* or a *convulsion*. (We talk more about this condition in Chapter 5.) Medications to prevent a convulsion are called *anticonvulsants* (you may also see them referred to as *anti-epileptic drugs*). In recent years a large number of new anticonvulsant drugs have become available, however some of the older drugs continue to have an important role to play. Although these drugs are called "anticonvulsants," many of them are used for totally different purposes such as treating painful conditions, especially pain in the feet due to nerve damage (as may happen from, for example, diabetes). Oral anticonvulsants available in Canada are listed in Table 6-14. In this section we discuss those that are most commonly used.

Table 6-14	Anticonvulsants
Generic Name	*Trade Name(s)*
Carbamazepine	Apo-Carbamazepine, Gen-Carbamazepine CR, Novo-Carbamaz, Nu-Carbamazepine, PMS-Carbamazepine, Sandoz Carbamazepine, Taro-Carbamazepine, Tegretol
Clobazam	Apo-Clobazam, Novo-Clobazam, ratio-Clobazam
Clonazepam	Apo-Clonazepam, CO Clonazepam, Gen-Clonazepam, Novo-Clonazepam, Nu-Clonazepam, PMS-Clonazepam, ratio-Clonazepam, Rivotril, Sandoz Clonazepam
Divalproex	Apo-Divalproex, Epival, Novo-Divalproex, Nu-Divalproex
Ethosuximide	Zarontin

(continued)

Table 6-14 *(continued)*

Generic Name	Trade Name(s)
Gabapentin	Apo-Gabapentin, CO Gabapentin, Gen-Gabapentin, Neurontin, Novo-Gabapentin, PMS-Gabapentin, ratio-Gabapentin
Lamotrigine	Apo-Lamotrigine, Gen-Lamotrigine, Lamictal, Novo-Lamotrigine, PMS-Lamotrigine, ratio-Lamotrigine
Levetiracetam	CO Levetiracetam, Keppra
Oxcarbazepine	Trileptal
Phenobarbital	Bellergal Spacetabs*, PMS-Phenobarbital
Phenytoin	Dilantin Capsules, Dilantin Infatabs, Dilantin-30 Suspension, Dilantin-125 Suspension, Taro-Phenytoin
Primidone	Apo-Primidone
Topiramate	Gen-Topiramate, Novo-Topiramate, PMS-Topiramate, ratio-Topiramate, Sandoz Topiramate, Topamax
Valproic Acid	Apo-Valproic Acid, Depakene, Gen-Valproic, Novo-Valproic, Nu-Valproic, PMS-Valproic Acid, PMS-Valproic Acid E.C., ratio-Valproic, Sandoz Valproic, Sandoz Valproic EC
Vigabatrin	Sabril

* This medicine is a combination of different drugs. Refer to the drug label to determine what they are.

 ## Carbamazepine

Apo-Carbamazepine, Gen-Carbamazepine CR, Novo-Carbamaz, Nu-Carbamazepine, PMS-Carbamazepine, Sandoz Carbamazepine, Taro-Carbamazepine, Tegretol

Carbamazepine, an older anticonvulsant, remains one of the most effective drugs available to treat certain forms of epilepsy.

 Nerves contain tiny pathways or openings (called *channels*) that allow sodium to pass into the cells. By blocking these channels, carbamazepine slows down the amount of electrical activity going on within nerve cells; this in turn lowers the likelihood of a seizure.

How carbamazepine can help you

Carbamazepine can help you in the following ways:

- ✔ Reducing your risk of having certain types of seizures.

- ✔ Reducing pain from certain forms of nerve injury, such as trigeminal neuralgia (tic *douloureux*) and diabetic peripheral neuropathy.

- ✔ Improving bipolar disorder.

How carbamazepine might harm you

Possible side-effects from carbamazepine include:

- ✔ Dizziness, drowsiness, blurred vision, headache.

- ✔ Dry mouth, nausea, vomiting.

- ✔ Low blood counts.

- ✔ Abnormal liver tests. Actual hepatitis, however, seldom occurs.

- ✔ Skin rash.

Minor side-effects occur quite often, but serious side-effects seldom develop.

Side-effects from carbamazepine are most likely to occur in the first few weeks to months of treatment or if you're on a high dose or are elderly.

People with the following conditions shouldn't take carbamazepine:

- ✔ Liver disease.

- ✔ Bone marrow disease or serious blood disorders.

- ✔ You shouldn't take carbamazepine if you have taken a drug from the monoamine oxidase (MAO) inhibitor family within the past 14 days, nor should you start taking an MAO inhibitor within 14 days of stopping carbamazepine.

- ✔ A disorder of the heart's electrical system called *heart block*.

- ✔ A history of allergy to this drug or to tricyclic antidepressants. (If you've reacted to tricyclic antidepressants you will be at increased risk of reacting to carbamazepine.) We discuss tricyclic antidepressants elsewhere in this chapter.

There is evidence that carbamazepine can lead to damage to a developing fetus, therefore it's generally recommended that, whenever possible, it not be taken during pregnancy. Nonetheless, if you're pregnant and taking carbamazepine don't discontinue this medicine without first speaking to your doctor. It's *probably* safe to be taken during breastfeeding. Again, we recommend you discuss this with your physician.

Precautions to follow if you're taking carbamazepine

Follow these precautions if you're taking carbamazepine:

- ✔ Don't stop the drug without first speaking to your doctor. (Suddenly stopping carbamazepine may cause you to have a seizure.)

- ✔ Your doctor should send you for a blood test to check your liver function, blood counts, and kidney function before and then periodically after starting the drug.

- ✔ Let your physician know if you develop a fever, bad sore throat, yellow or greenish phlegm, or unexpected bruising.

- ✔ See an eye doctor regularly, especially if you have glaucoma. (Eye problems, including a worsening of glaucoma, occasionally occur in people taking carbamazepine.)

How to take carbamazepine

Carbamazepine is generally started in a low dose (100 mg to 200 mg once or twice daily) and then increased, under your doctor's supervision, based on your response.

Avoid consuming grapefruit or grapefruit juice because it can affect the level of carbamazepine in your blood.

 ## Clonazepam

Apo-Clonazepam, CO Clonazepam, Gen-Clonazepam, Novo-Clonazepam, Nu-Clonazepam, PMS-Clonazepam, ratio-Clonazepam, Rivotril, Sandoz Clonazepam

Clonazepam is a member of the benzodiazepine family of drugs. We look at other members of this family elsewhere in this chapter, but we discuss clonazepam here because its main role is as an anticonvulsant.

How clonazepam works

Clonazepam enhances the action of a chemical messenger in the brain called GABA. GABA has a calming influence on nerve signals and clonazepam enhances this effect.

How clonazepam can help you

Clonazepam can help you in the following ways:

✔ Reducing your risk of having certain types of seizures.

✔ Lessening sudden muscle spasms (*myoclonic jerks*).

✔ Improving restless legs syndrome, panic disorder, and schizo-phrenia. These benefits are less proven.

How clonazepam might harm you

Possible side-effects from taking clonazepam include:

✔ Drowsiness.

✔ Unsteadiness when you walk (*ataxia*).

✔ Abnormal behaviour.

People with the following conditions shouldn't take clonazepam:

✔ Liver disease.

✔ Certain types of glaucoma.

✔ Breastfeeding.

There is evidence that clonazepam can lead to damage to a develop-ing fetus and therefore it's generally recommended that, whenever possible, it not be taken during pregnancy. Nonetheless, if you're pregnant and taking clonazepam don't discontinue this medicine without first speaking to your doctor.

Precautions to follow if you're taking clonazepam

Follow these precautions if you're taking clonazepam:

✔ Don't stop the drug without first speaking to your doctor. Suddenly stopping the drug may make you feel unwell and may result in a seizure.

✔ This drug may make you drowsy, which would make it unsafe for you to perform activities — like driving — that require you to be alert and focused.

✔ Because alcohol may worsen drowsiness, it may be unwise to consume it. We recommend you check with your doctor to find out whether drinking (small amounts of) alcohol would be okay.

How to take clonazepam

Clonazepam is started in a low dose (of 0.5 mg three times daily), and the dose is then adjusted, under your doctor's supervision, based on your response. You may take it with or without food.

Avoid consuming grapefruit or grapefruit juice because it can affect the level of clonazepam in your blood.

℞ *Divalproex, Valproic Acid*

Apo-Divalproex, Epival, Novo-Divalproex, Nu-Divalproex

Apo-Valproic Acid, Depakene, Gen-Valproic, Novo-Valproic, Nu-Valproic, PMS-Valproic Acid, PMS-Valproic Acid E.C., ratio-Valproic, Sandoz Valproic, Sandoz Valproic EC

Divalproex and valproic acid are very similar anticonvulsant drugs, so we discuss them together.

Divalproex and valproic acid enhance the action of a chemical messenger in the brain called GABA. GABA has a calming influence on nerve signals, and these drugs enhance this effect. As a result, convulsions and other symptoms (see below) are less likely to occur.

How divalproex and valproic acid can help you

These drugs can help you in the following ways:

✔ Reducing your risk of having certain types of seizures.

✔ Helping prevent migraine headaches.

✔ Controlling episodes of mania if you have bipolar disorder.

How divalproex and valproic acid might harm you

Possible side-effects from these two drugs include:

✔ Nausea, vomiting, indigestion, drowsiness, hair loss. These typically go away as the medicine is continued.

✔ Weight gain.

✔ Inflammation of the pancreas (*pancreatitis*).

✔ Liver damage.

People with liver disease shouldn't take either of these two drugs.

There is evidence that these drugs can lead to damage to a developing fetus, therefore it's generally recommended that, whenever possible, they not be taken during pregnancy. Nonetheless, if you're pregnant and taking one of these drugs don't discontinue the medicine without first speaking to your doctor. These drugs are *probably* safe to use while breastfeeding.

Precautions to follow if you're taking divalproex or valproic acid

Follow these precautions if you're taking divalproex or valproic acid:

- ✔ If you have diabetes and test your urine for ketones, these drugs can give you a false result.

- ✔ Have a blood test to assess your liver function and to ensure your blood clotting system is working properly before starting the medicine, and then periodically thereafter.

- ✔ This drug may make you drowsy, which would make it unsafe for you to perform activities — like driving — that require you to be alert and focused.

- ✔ Because alcohol may worsen drowsiness, it may be unwise to consume it. We recommend you check with your doctor to find out whether drinking (small amounts of) alcohol would be okay.

How to take divalproex and valproic acid

These drugs are started in a low dose and the dose is then adjusted, under your doctor's supervision, based on your response. To treat seizures the dose is based on how much you weigh, with the usual starting dose for divalproex being 15 mg per kg per day and for valproic acid being 10 mg to 15 mg per kg per day. You can take these medicines with or without food.

℞ *Gabapentin*

Apo-Gabapentin, CO Gabapentin, Gen-Gabapentin, Neurontin, Novo-Gabapentin, PMS-Gabapentin, ratio-Gabapentin

Although, comparatively speaking, gabapentin is one of the newer anticonvulsant drugs on the block, it has quickly established itself as an important medication in the treatment of epilepsy and several other neurological ailments as well.

Gabapentin appears to work by affecting how calcium passes through tiny little passageways in the lining of nerves called *voltage-gated ion channels*. (Sounds like a fancy name for an electrified drawbridge in Venice!)

How gabapentin can help you

Gabapentin can help by reducing your risk of having certain types of seizures. It's also taken to lessen pain from peripheral neuropathy and post-herpetic neuralgia. We discuss these conditions in Chapter 5.

Other, less proven, uses include the treatment of bipolar disorder and mood problems.

How gabapentin might harm you

Possible side-effects from gabapentin include:

✔ Drowsiness, unsteady gait, dizziness. These are usually mild and go away as you continue to take the medicine.

✔ *Peripheral edema* (ankle swelling).

✔ Weight gain.

The safety of gabapentin in pregnancy and breastfeeding is unknown. If you're pregnant or breastfeeding, we recommend you discuss it with your physician before taking this medicine.

Precautions to follow if you're taking gabapentin

Follow these precautions if you're taking gabapentin:

✔ Don't stop the drug without first speaking to your doctor. (Suddenly stopping the drug may result in a seizure.)

✔ This drug may make you drowsy, which would make it unsafe for you to perform activities — like driving — that require you to be alert and focused.

✔ Because alcohol may worsen drowsiness, it may be unwise to consume it. We recommend you check with your doctor to find out whether drinking (small amounts of) alcohol would be okay.

How to take gabapentin

Gabapentin is started in a low dose (typically 300 mg three times per day) and the dose is then adjusted, under your doctor's supervision, based on your response. You may take it with or without food.

If you have kidney failure, your doctor may need to prescribe lower than usual doses.

 ## Lamotrigine

Apo-Lamotrigine, Gen-Lamotrigine, Lamictal, Novo-Lamotrigine, PMS-Lamotrigine, ratio-Lamotrigine

Lamotrigine is an anticonvulsant that can help not only in the treatment of epilepsy, but several mood disorders as well.

Lamotrigine affects the passage of sodium through tiny little passageways (*sodium channels*) in the lining of nerve cells. By acting on these channels, there is a reduction in certain naturally occurring, epilepsy-promoting body chemicals (glutamine, aspartate). Less epilepsy-promoting chemicals, less epilepsy. Sounds pretty simple — so clearly it must be more complicated than that! (Just like Albert Einstein said: "Make everything as simple as possible, but not simpler.")

How lamotrigine can help you

Lamotrigine can help you in the following ways:

- ✔ Reducing your risk of having certain types of seizures.

- ✔ Lessening depression in some people with epilepsy.

- ✔ Making it less likely for you to experience episodes of mania or depression if you have bipolar disorder.

How lamotrigine might harm you

Possible side-effects from lamotrigine include:

- ✔ Dizziness, headache, drowsiness, nausea. These are the most common side-effects and sometimes can be eased by reducing the dose under your doctor's guidance.

- ✔ Hepatitis. This seldom occurs.

- ✔ Skin rash. This can range from being very mild to being very serious. See your doctor if you get a rash when taking this medication.

Don't take lamotrigine if you're breastfeeding (it passes into breast milk and thus will get into the baby's system).

 There is evidence that lamotrigine taken during pregnancy increases the risk of cleft palate and cleft lip. We recommend before taking this medicine during pregnancy you discuss this with your physician.

Precautions to follow if you're taking lamotrigine

Follow these precautions if you're taking lamotrigine:

- ✔ Seek prompt medical attention if you get *any* type of skin rash — especially within the first few weeks of starting treatment.

- ✔ Stop taking the drug gradually if you need to come off it, unless side-effects (such as a skin rash) make it necessary to immediately stop the drug.

✔ This drug may make you drowsy, which would make it unsafe for you to perform activities — like driving — that require you to be alert and focused.

✔ Because alcohol may worsen drowsiness, it may be unwise to consume it. We recommend you check with your doctor to find out whether drinking (small amounts of) alcohol would be okay.

One of the trade names for this drug, Lamictal, is similar enough to several other drug names (such as Lamisil and Lomotil) that there is the risk of a medication error. If you have been prescribed lamotrigine, be sure to double-check the label on the prescription bottle to make sure it says lamotrigine before you take your dose.

How to take lamotrigine

Lamotrigine is started in a low dose (usually 25 mg every one to two days) with the dose then adjusted, under your doctor's supervision, based on your response. Your doctor may need to prescribe lower than usual doses if you have kidney or liver disease. You can take lamotrigine with or without food.

℞ *Phenytoin*

Dilantin Capsules, Dilantin Infatabs, Dilantin-30 Suspension, Dilantin-125 Suspension, Taro-Phenytoin

No matter how many new drugs show up to try to push phenytoin off its pedestal, this drug, first used for epilepsy in 1938, continues to be a key player in the treatment of this condition.

Phenytoin reduces the amount of sodium that accumulates within nerve cells. This makes nerve cells in the brain less prone to trigger an epilepsy attack.

How phenytoin can help you

Phenytoin can help you in the following ways:

✔ Reducing your risk of having certain types of seizures.

✔ Lessening pain from certain forms of neuropathy. We discuss neuropathy in Chapter 5.

✔ Preventing some forms of heart rhythm disturbance (*arrhythmia*). It's rarely prescribed for this purpose.

How phenytoin might harm you

Possible side-effects from phenytoin include:

✔ Slurred speech, dizziness, unsteady gait, confusion. These symptoms are usually caused by too high a level of phenytoin in your blood.

✔ A low white blood cell count (which would put you at increased risk of infections) and low platelet count (which would put you at increased risk of bleeding).

✔ Hypothyroidism. We discuss this condition in Chapter 5.

✔ A variety of skin rashes, some serious, may occur. These are more likely to occur within the first few weeks of starting therapy.

✔ Osteoporosis, enlarged gums, or excessive body hair (*hirsutism*). These are more likely to occur if you have taken the medicine for a long time.

There is evidence that phenytoin can lead to damage to a developing fetus and therefore it's generally recommended that, whenever possible, it not be taken during pregnancy. Nonetheless, if you're pregnant and taking phenytoin don't discontinue the medicine without first speaking to your doctor. Phenytoin is generally considered safe to use while breastfeeding.

Precautions to follow if you're taking phenytoin

Follow these precautions if you're taking phenytoin:

✔ Don't stop the drug without first speaking to your doctor. Suddenly stopping the drug may result in a seizure.

✔ Your thyroid hormone blood levels should be checked from time to time.

✔ Seek prompt medical attention if you get *any* type of skin rash — especially within the first few weeks of starting treatment.

✔ Good dental hygiene will help minimize any gum swelling that may occur from the drug.

✔ This drug may make you drowsy, which would make it unsafe for you to perform activities — like driving — that require you to be alert and focused.

✔ Because alcohol may worsen drowsiness, it may be unwise to consume it. We recommend you check with your doctor to find out whether drinking (small amounts of) alcohol would be okay.

✔ Have your bone density and blood levels of vitamin D, calcium, and folic acid measured from time to time.

How to take phenytoin

The usual dose of phenytoin is 300 mg per day (taken either as a single dose or divided up into multiple, smaller doses). Your dose may need to be adjusted from time to time, under your doctor's supervision, based on the level of the drug on a blood test.

You may take phenytoin with or without food but *be consistent.*

 ## *Topiramate*

Gen-Topiramate, Novo-Topiramate, PMS-Topiramate, ratio-Topiramate, Sandoz Topiramate, Topamax

Though an anticonvulsant, topiramate has also been found to be helpful in the prevention of migraine headaches. Gotta love the brand name one company chose for this product: "Topamax." Top...max. My, my, my...

 Topiramate works in several ways, including enhancing the action of a chemical messenger in the brain called GABA. GABA has a calming influence on nerve signals. As a result, convulsions are less likely to occur.

How topiramate can help you

Topiramate can help you in the following ways:

✔ Reducing your risk of having certain types of seizures.

✔ Helping prevent migraine headaches. (Topiramate isn't of value in the treatment of an attack after it has already begun.)

Other, less proven uses, include the treatment of bipolar disorder, post-traumatic stress disorder, binge eating, and cluster headaches.

How topiramate might harm you

Possible side-effects from topiramate include:

✔ Numbness, tiredness, drowsiness, dizziness, and decreased appetite are some of the most common side-effects and are seldom dangerous.

✔ Reduced bone quality (which would put you at increased risk of fractures) and kidney stones may occur after long-term therapy.

✔ Heat stroke and glaucoma are rare but serious side-effects.

The safety of topiramate in pregnancy and breastfeeding is unknown; it's generally recommended this drug not be taken if you're breast-feeding. If you're pregnant or breastfeeding, we recommend you discuss it with your physician before taking this medicine.

Precautions to follow if you're taking topiramate

Follow these precautions if you're taking topiramate:

- ✔ Stay well hydrated. This will reduce your risk of getting kidney stones.

- ✔ This drug may make you drowsy, which would make it unsafe for you to perform activities — like driving — that require you to be alert and focused.

- ✔ Because alcohol may worsen drowsiness, it may be unwise to consume it. We recommend you check with your doctor to find out whether drinking (small amounts of) alcohol would be okay.

- ✔ Seek immediate medical attention if you get sudden blurring of your vision or painful, red eyes. These may be clues you have developed an attack of glaucoma.

- ✔ Your blood bicarbonate level should be measured from time to time. A low level is related to a buildup of acid in your blood, which can put you at increased risk of side-effects.

How to take topiramate

Topiramate is started in a low dose (usually 25 mg to 50 mg per day), with the dose then gradually increased, under your doctor's supervision, based on your response. The full ("maintenance") dose you require will be less if you have kidney disease. You can take topiramate with or without food.

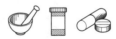

Antidepressants

Antidepressants are, as a group, the most widely used drugs in Canada, with more than 25 million prescriptions filled in 2005. There are several classes of antidepressants, as we list in Table 6-15. Missing from this table are tricyclic antidepressants, which, because of their common use for conditions other than depression, we discuss in their own section in this chapter.

Although the various classes of antidepressants share the common property of helping lessen depression, the way in which they do this differs considerably; therefore, we look at these classes separately below.

Table 6-15	Antidepressants	
Class	Generic Name	Trade Name(s)
MAO inhibitors	Moclobemide	Apo-Moclobemide, Manerix, Novo-Moclobemide, Nu-Moclobemide, PMS-Moclobemide,
	Phenelzine	Nardil
	Tranylcypromine	Parnate
SNRIs	Atomoxetine	Strattera
	Venlafaxine	Effexor XR
SSRIs	**Citalopram**	Apo-Citalopram, Celexa, CO Citalopram, Gen-Citalopram, Novo-Citalopram, PMS-Citalopram, RAN-Citalopram, ratio-Citalopram, Sandoz Citalopram
	Escitalopram	Cirpralex
	Fluoxetine	Apo-Fluoxetine, CO Fluoxetine, FXT, Gen-Fluoxetine, Novo-Fluoxetine, Nu-Fluoxetine, PMS-Fluoxetine, Prozac, ratio-Fluoxetine, Sandoz Fluoxetine
	Fluvoxamine	Apo-Fluvoxamine, CO Fluvoxamine, Luvox, Novo-Fluvoxamine, Nu-Fluvoxamine, PMS-Fluvoxamine, ratio-Fluvoxamine, Sandoz Fluvoxamine
	Paroxetine	Apo-Paroxetine, CO Paroxetine, Gen-Paroxetine, Novo-Paroxetine, Paxil, Paxil CR, PMS-Paroxetine, ratio-Paroxetine, Sandoz Paroxetine
	Sertraline	Apo-Sertraline, Gen-Sertraline, Novo-Sertraline, Nu-Sertraline, PMS-Sertraline, ratio-Sertraline, Sandoz Sertraline, Zoloft

Class	Generic Name	Trade Name(s)
Miscellaneous	**Bupropion**	Novo-Bupropion SR, Sandoz Bupropion SR, Wellbutrin SR, Wellbutrin XL, Zyban
	Mirtazapine	CO-Mirtazapine, Gen-Mirtazapine, Novo-Mirtazapine, Novo-Mirtazapine OD, PMS-Mirtazapine, ratio-Mirtazapine, Remeron, Remeron RD, Sandoz Mirtazapine, Sandoz Mirtazapine FC
	Trazodone	Apo-Trazodone, Apo-Trazodone D, Desyrel, Desyrel Dividose, Gen-Trazodone, Novo-Trazodone, Nu-Trazodone, Nu-Trazodone-D, PMS-Trazodone, ratio-Trazodone

 Venlafaxine

Effexor XR

Venlafaxine is a member of the SNRI (_serotonin-norepinephrine reuptake inhibitor_) group of antidepressants. Clearly there was a sale on polysyllabic words when this class was named.

 Norepinephrine is a chemical messenger (_neurotransmitter_) in the brain, helping to pass messages from one cell to another. Venlafaxine increases the amount of norepinephrine in the brain by inhibiting its uptake by certain nerve cells. Having more norepinephrine in the brain eases certain symptoms, such as those seen with depression. This drug also increases levels of serotonin and dopamine, which may also play a part in its function.

How venlafaxine can help you

Venlafaxine can help you by easing the symptoms of

- ✔ Depression.
- ✔ _Generalized anxiety disorder._ (Anxiety due to normal day-to-day stresses typically does not require drug therapy.)
- ✔ _Social anxiety disorder_ (also known as social phobia).
- ✔ Fibromyalgia.
- ✔ Panic disorder.

How venlafaxine might harm you

Possible side-effects from venlafaxine include:

- ✓ Headache, fatigue, sleepiness, insomnia, anxiety, and dizziness. These occur in up to about 30 percent of people.
- ✓ Dry mouth, decreased appetite, nausea, vomiting, and constipation. These also occur in up to about 30 percent of people.
- ✓ High blood pressure (or, if you already had high blood pressure, worsening of it).
- ✓ Erectile dysfunction.
- ✓ High cholesterol.
- ✓ Bleeding. This seldom occurs.

You shouldn't take venlafaxine if you have taken a drug from the monoamine oxidase (MAO) inhibitor family within the past 14 days, nor should you start taking an MAO inhibitor within 14 days of stopping venlafaxine. Doing so could cause dangerously high blood pressure.

There is evidence that venlafaxine can damage a fetus, especially if taken during the second half of pregnancy. Because of this safety concern, this drug should almost always be avoided during pregnancy. The safety of venlafaxine taken during breastfeeding is unknown and is generally not recommended.

Precautions to follow if you're taking venlafaxine

Follow these precautions if you're taking venlafaxine:

- ✓ Don't stop the drug without first speaking to your doctor. If venlafaxine is to be discontinued, this should be done gradually, not suddenly as sudden discontinuation may lead to agitation, dizziness, or other unpleasant and potentially dangerous symptoms.
- ✓ This drug may make you drowsy, which would make it unsafe for you to perform activities — like driving — that require you to be alert and focused.

- ✓ Because alcohol may worsen drowsiness, it may be unwise to consume it. We recommend you check with your doctor to find out whether drinking (small amounts of) alcohol would be okay.
- ✓ Have your blood pressure checked before starting this medicine, then regularly thereafter. If your blood pressure rises, the drug may have to be stopped or the dose reduced.

✔ There is evidence that taking antidepressants — particularly in the early stages of treatment — can lead to thoughts of suicide. If you have such thoughts, seek urgent medical care.

How to take venlafaxine

Venlafaxine is currently available in Canada only as Effexor XR. The usual starting dose of Effexor XR is 37.5 mg to 75 mg taken once daily, either in the morning or the evening, with the dose then gradually increased, under your doctor's supervision, based on your response.

Swallow the medication whole and take it with food. Your doctor may need to prescribe lower than usual doses if you have kidney failure or liver disease.

Avoid consuming grapefruit or grapefruit juice because it can affect the level of venlafaxine in your blood.

 ℞ *Citalopram*

Apo-Citalopram, Celexa, CO Citalopram, Gen-Citalopram, Novo-Citalopram, PMS-Citalopram, RAN-Citalopram, ratio-Citalopram, Sandoz Citalopram

Citalopram is a very popular member of the SSRI (selective serotonin reuptake inhibitor) class of antidepressants.

Serotonin is a chemical messenger (*neurotransmitter*) in the brain, helping to pass messages from one cell to another. Citalopram increases the amount of serotonin in the brain by inhibiting its uptake by certain nerve cells. With more serotonin in the brain, certain symptoms such as those seen with depression are eased.

How citalopram can help you

Citalopram can help you by easing symptoms of depression. (An unproven role for this drug is the treatment of alcoholism.)

How citalopram might harm you

Possible side-effects from taking citalopram include:

✔ Sleepiness, insomnia, dry mouth, nausea, and excess sweating. These are the most common side-effects.

✔ Bleeding. This seldom occurs.

✔ Erectile dysfunction. This typically resolves if the drug is stopped.

There is evidence that citalopram can damage a fetus, especially if taken during the second half of pregnancy. Because of this safety concern, this drug should almost always be avoided during pregnancy. The safety of citalopram taken during breastfeeding is unknown and is generally not advised. We recommend before taking citalopram during pregnancy or breastfeeding, you discuss this with your doctor.

You shouldn't take citalopram if you have taken a drug from the monoamine oxidase (MAO) inhibitor family within the past 14 days, nor should you start taking an MAO inhibitor within 14 days of stopping citalopram. Doing so could cause dangerously high blood pressure.

Precautions to follow if you're taking citalopram

Follow these precautions if you're taking citalopram:

✔ Don't stop the drug without first speaking to your doctor. If citalopram is to be discontinued, this should be done gradually, not suddenly as sudden discontinuation may lead to agitation, dizziness, or other unpleasant and potentially dangerous symptoms.

✔ This drug may make you drowsy, which would make it unsafe for you to perform activities — like driving — that require you to be alert and focused.

✔ Because alcohol may worsen drowsiness, it may be unwise to consume it. We recommend you check with your doctor to find out whether drinking (small amounts of) alcohol would be okay.

✔ There is evidence that taking antidepressants — particularly in the early stages of treatment — can lead to thoughts of suicide. If you have such thoughts, seek urgent medical care.

How to take citalopram

The usual starting dose of citalopram is 20 mg taken once daily in the morning or evening, with the dose then gradually increased, under your doctor's supervision, based on your response. Your doctor may need to prescribe lower doses if you have liver disease. You may take citalopram with or without food.

Avoid consuming grapefruit or grapefruit juice because it can affect the level of citalopram in your blood.

Bupropion

Novo-Bupropion SR, Sandoz Bupropion SR, Wellbutrin SR, Wellbutrin XL, Zyban

In Canada, bupropion is used to treat depression and to help people quit smoking. Different trade names are used depending on which of these two conditions is being treated, although the medicine is the same. When used to treat depression, buproprion is called Wellbutrin (as in, it will get you *well*). When used to help you quit smoking bupropion is called Zyban (as in, it will help you *ban*ish smoking). When used to treat depression in someone who is trying to quit smoking, the drug is called Optimism. (Just kidding.)

 Exactly how bupropion works isn't known; however, it may be connected to its ability to increase brain levels of two chemical messengers (*neurotransmitters*): norepinephrine and dopamine.

How bupropion can help you

Bupropion can help you in the following ways:

- ✔ Making it easier to quit smoking. (Of course, as most smokers report, *easier* is definitely not the same as *easy*.)
- ✔ Easing symptoms of depression.

How bupropion might harm you

Possible side-effects from bupropion include:

- ✔ Headache, dizziness, insomnia, anxiety. Of these, insomnia is particularly common.
- ✔ Dry mouth, nausea, constipation.
- ✔ Seizures and severe allergic reactions. These are very uncommon but serious side-effects.

Side-effects are more likely to occur if you have liver disease.

People with the following conditions shouldn't take bupropion:

- ✔ A seizure disorder.
- ✔ Anorexia nervosa, bulimia.
- ✔ Alcohol withdrawal syndrome.
- ✔ Recent discontinuation of *benzodiazepine* or other sedative medication.

✔ You shouldn't take bupropion if you have taken thioridazine or a drug from the monoamine oxidase (MAO) inhibitor family within the past 14 days, nor should you start taking an MAO inhibitor or thioridazine within 14 days of stopping bupropion. Doing so could cause dangerously high blood pressure in the case of MAO inhibitors and dangerous heart rhythm problems in the case of thioridazine.

There is evidence that bupropion can damage a fetus, especially if taken during the second half of pregnancy. Because of this safety concern, this drug should almost always be avoided during pregnancy. The safety of bupropion taken during breastfeeding is unknown and is generally not recommended. We recommend before taking bupropion during pregnancy or breastfeeding, you discuss this with your doctor.

Precautions to follow if you're taking bupropion

Follow these precautions if you're taking bupropion:

✔ Even though bupropion is sold as Zyban for smoking cessation and Wellbutrin (and other brands) for depression, they're the same drug and should not both be taken at the same time.

✔ This drug may interfere with your thinking, making it unsafe for you to perform activities — like driving — that require you to be alert and focused.

✔ Because alcohol may worsen thinking problems, it may be unwise to consume it. We recommend you check with your doctor to find out whether drinking (small amounts of) alcohol would be okay.

✔ There is evidence that taking antidepressants can lead to thoughts of suicide — particularly in the early stages of treatment. If you have such thoughts, seek urgent medical care.

How to take bupropion

When taken for depression, the dose of bupropion varies depending on the particular brand you're prescribed.

If you're taking buproprion to help with smoking cessation, you start taking it while you're still smoking. This helps the medicine build up to a good level in your body before you actually stop smoking and will, therefore, improve the odds that you will successfully quit. The starting dose is 150 mg once daily for three days, then 150 mg twice daily thereafter. Swallow Zyban tablets whole. Treatment should generally continue for 7 to 12 weeks. You may use nicotine replacement products at the same time as using Zyban. If, after seven weeks of therapy, you have not come any closer to quitting smoking (for example, you have not cut down the number of cigarettes you smoke per day), the drug isn't likely to be helping you and continuing it isn't usually of value.

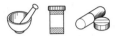

Antifungal Agents

Fungal infections can range from the mild (such as a toenail infection) to the life-threatening (such as a heart valve infection). Fortunately, serious fungal infections are rare. In this section we look at the most commonly used antifungal medicines. Although they all fight off fungal infections, these drugs are used in different ways depending on where your infection is. Table 6-16 lists the antifungal agents available in Canada for outpatient use. (The names in italics are of those antifungal agents that are available over-the-counter.)

Table 6-16	Antifungal Agents
Generic Name	*Trade Name(s)*
Butoconazole	Gynazole_1
Ciclopirox	Loprox, Penlac, Stieprox
Clioquinol	Locacorten Vioform Cream*, Locacorten Vioform Ear Drops*, Vioform Hydrocortisone*
Clotrimazole	*Canesten Topical, Canesten Vaginal, Clotrimaderm*, Lotriderm*
Econazole	Ecostatin
Fluconazole	Apo-Fluconazole, Apo-Fluconazole-150, Diflucan, Diflucan-150, Gen-Fluconazole, Novo-Fluconazole, Taro-Fluconazole
Itraconazole	Sporanox Capsules, Sporanox Oral Solution
Ketoconazole	Apo-Ketoconazole, Ketoderm, Nizoral Cream, Nizoral Shampoo, Novo-Ketoconazole
Miconazole	*Micatin, Micozole, Monistat 7 Vaginal Cream, Monistat 7 Dual-Pak*
Nystatin	*Candistatin, Mycostatin Topical Powder, Nyaderm, ratio-Nystatin*, ratio-Triacomb*
Terbinafine	Apo-Terbinafine, CO Terbinafine, Gen-Terbinafine, Lamisil, Novo-Terbinafine, PMS-Terbinafine, Sandoz Terbinafine

(continued)

Table 6-16 *(continued)*

Generic Name	Trade Name(s)
Terconazole	Taro-Terconazole, Terazol
Voriconazole	Vfend

* This medicine is a combination of different drugs. Refer to the drug label to determine what they are.

 Fluconazole

Apo-Fluconazole, Apo-Fluconazole-150, Diflucan, Diflucan-150, Gen-Fluconazole, Novo-Fluconazole, Taro-Fluconazole

Fluconazole is most commonly used to treat *candida* (yeast) infections. It's a very effective drug and most people tolerate it well.

 Candida organisms are surrounded by a cell membrane. Fluconazole causes these germs to make a defective, weakened cell membrane, rendering the organisms more vulnerable to our immune system, which then attacks and destroys them. We are truly looking at a microscopic battlefield when it comes to germs and the weapons we use to attack them.

How fluconazole can help you

Fluconazole can help you by treating candida infections affecting the mouth, throat, esophagus, lungs, vagina, or bladder, and *cryptococcal meningitis,* a very serious infection of the tissues that surround the brain and spinal cord.

Fluconazole is also used to help *prevent* certain diseases, including cryptococcal meningitis if you have AIDS and have previously had this form of meningitis, and *candida* infections if you're undergoing a bone marrow transplant.

How fluconazole might harm you

Possible side-effects from taking fluconazole include:

- ✔ Nausea, vomiting, diarrhea. These are the most common side-effects.
- ✔ Severe skin rash, which can lead to dangerous blistering of the skin. This rarely occurs.
- ✔ Liver damage.
- ✔ Heart rhythm problems.

Serious side-effects seldom occur.

 The safety of fluconazole in pregnancy and breastfeeding are unknown. If you're pregnant or breastfeeding, we recommend you discuss it with your physician before taking this medicine.

Precautions to follow if you're taking fluconazole

Follow these precautions if you're taking fluconazole:

- ✔ If you get a skin rash, seek prompt medical attention.

- ✔ If you experience episodes of faintness or palpitations, see your doctor (she will need to ensure your heart rhythm is normal).

How to take fluconazole

The dose of fluconazole depends on what particular condition it's treating. Your doctor may need to prescribe lower than usual doses if you have kidney failure. You can take fluconazole with or without food.

℞ *Terbinafine*

Apo-Terbinafine, CO Terbinafine, Gen-Terbinafine, Lamisil, Novo-Terbinafine, PMS-Terbinafine, Sandoz Terbinafine

Terbinafine is used to treat less serious fungal infections, such as jock itch and athlete's foot (hmm, seems to be a theme here), and fungal toenail infections. It's very safe when used topically or when taken for a short period of time orally; however, there are recent safety concerns about longer term (a few months or more) oral therapy (see below).

 Terbinafine interferes with the metabolism of a fungus cell (yes, even the lowly fungus has a metabolism) leading to a buildup of a substance with the awful-sounding name of *squalene*. Well, squalene is clearly awful in other ways, too, because high levels of this within the fungus cell are toxic to it and lead to its death.

How terbinafine can help you

Terbinafine can help you by curing certain types of fungal infections affecting your skin and nails.

 This drug will get rid of your infection only if it's caused by a fungus that is susceptible to the effects of this drug. Not all are. Also, other conditions can mimic fungal infections, so your doctor generally needs to obtain samples of the affected region for analysis before treating you.

How terbinafine might harm you

Side-effects (particularly serious side-effects) seldom occur with topical therapy. Possible side-effects from taking oral terbinafine include:

- ✔ Nausea, abdominal discomfort, diarrhea.
- ✔ Skin rash.
- ✔ Taste abnormalities.
- ✔ Abnormal liver tests. Rarely, hepatitis.
- ✔ Heart failure. (This is uncertain.)

The risk of liver or heart damage appears to be greater if you have been taking the oral drug for several months or more.

People with the following conditions shouldn't take terbinafine:

- ✔ Liver disease.
- ✔ Kidney failure.

The safety of terbinafine in pregnancy and breastfeeding are unknown. If you're pregnant or breastfeeding, we recommend you discuss it with your physician before taking this medicine. (If you're applying topical terbinafine to your breast, don't breastfeed with this breast.)

Precautions to follow if you're taking terbinafine

Follow these precautions if you're taking terbinafine:

- ✔ If you develop malaise (that is, feeling generally unwell), poor appetite, nausea, vomiting, dark urine, or yellowing of your skin or eyes (that is, jaundice), you may have developed hepatitis; seek urgent medical attention.
- ✔ If you develop shortness of breath, this may indicate you have developed heart failure; seek urgent medical attention.
- ✔ If you're using terbinafine spray and it gets in your eyes, rinse them out with water.
- ✔ Your doctor should check your liver enzyme levels (on a blood test) before prescribing oral terbinafine.
- ✔ It may take several months of oral therapy before a toenail infection goes away (and, after you have completed your treatment, it may take many more months before a healthy nail has fully grown back in). Because the risks of serious side-effects from oral terbinafine increase with such prolonged therapy (see above), and because toenail infections are primarily cosmetic, oral terbinafine therapy for this condition is generally not recommended.

One of the trade names for this drug, Lamisil, is similar enough to several other drug names (such as Lamictal and Lomotil) that there is the risk of a medication error. If you have been prescribed terbinafine, be sure to double-check the label on the prescription bottle to make sure it says terbinafine before you take your dose.

How to take terbinafine

Terbinafine comes in oral and topical (cream and spray) forms. The former is taken once daily (with or without food), and the latter is taken once or twice daily. The duration of treatment can be anywhere from one week to three months depending on the particular type of infection that is being treated.

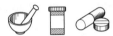

Antihistamines

Antihistamines are primarily used to fight off allergy symptoms caused by histamine (that is, they're *anti* — or against — *histamine*). Most antihistamines are very similar in how they work, however some antihistamines fulfill other roles such as helping control nausea or insomnia. Most antihistamines are available as over-the-counter drugs; in this section, we exclusively look at *prescription* antihistamines. Antihistamines available in Canada by prescription are listed in Table 6-17.

Table 6-17	Prescription Antihistamines
Generic Name	*Trade Name(s)*
Azatadine	Optimine, Trinalin*
Doxylamine/Pyridoxine	Diclectin*
Emedastine	Emadine
Hydroxyzine	Apo-Hydroxyzine, Atarax, Novo-Hydroxyzin
Ketotifen	Apo-Ketotifen, Novo-Ketotifen, Zaditen, Zaditor
Levocabastine	Livostin Eye Drops, Livostin Nasal Spray
Olopatadine	Patanol
Trimeprazine	Panectyl

* This medicine is a combination of different drugs. Refer to the drug label to determine what they are.

Doxylamine/Pyridoxine

Diclectin*

Diclectin, a combination of doxylamine (an antihistamine) and pyridoxine (vitamin B6), is used to treat morning sickness (that is, to lessen the nausea and vomiting many pregnant women experience). It's one of those rare breeds of drugs that has overwhelming evidence of being safe for a woman to take during pregnancy. (Many drugs are *thought* to be safe in pregnancy, but are not necessarily proven to be.)

 The way Dicletin works isn't completely sorted out, however it appears that the two active ingredients (that is, doxylamine and pyridoxine) have a direct influence on the areas of the brain responsible for creating the feeling of nausea.

How doxylamine/pyridoxine can help you

Diclectin can help you if you're pregnant by reducing the amount of nausea and vomiting you may be experiencing.

How doxylamine/pyridoxine might harm you

Possible side-effects from taking Diclectin include:

- ✔ Drowsiness. This is the most common side-effect, but even this occurs in only a minority of users.

- ✔ Dizziness, headache, palpitations, diarrhea, difficulty passing urine.

 The safety of Diclectin when breastfeeding is unknown. We recommend before taking this medicine in this circumstance you discuss this with your physician.

Precautions to follow if you're taking doxylamine/pyridoxine

Follow these precautions if you're taking Diclectin:

- ✔ This drug may make you drowsy, which would make it unsafe for you to perform activities — like driving — that require you to be alert and focused.

- ✔ Avoid alcohol because it may worsen drowsiness. Pregnant women should avoid alcohol in any event.

✔ Don't suddenly discontinue the medicine; rather, you need to gradually wean yourself from it to minimize the likelihood your symptoms will suddenly act up.

How to take doxylamine/pyridoxine

Diclectin should be taken regularly. The usual starting dose is four tablets per day (one tablet in the morning, one tablet in the mid-afternoon, and two tablets at bedtime). Your dose may be subsequently changed, under your doctor's supervision, based on your response. You may take diclectin with or without food, but it sometimes works better when taken on an empty stomach.

Hydroxyzine

Apo-Hydroxyzine, Atarax, Novo-Hydroxyzin

Hydroxyzine is an antihistamine used to treat both allergic and non-allergic conditions.

 Hydroxyzine competes with histamine for histamine receptors in a variety of organs, including the gut, the blood vessels, and the lungs. By attaching to these receptors, hydroxyzine prevents histamine from stimulating these cells to carry out certain functions.

How hydroxyzine can help you

Hydroxyzine can help you by

✔ Easing anxiety.

✔ Improving itchy eyes and runny nose if caused by allergies.

✔ Reducing skin itching if it's caused by allergies.

✔ Lessening nausea and vomiting.

How hydroxyzine might harm you

The majority of people taking hydroxyzine experience no side-effects — if they do occur, they tend to be mild and to go away as you continue the medication. Possible side-effects from taking hydroxyzine include:

✔ Dry mouth.

✔ Drowsiness, headache, blurred vision, hallucinations.

If you're elderly, you're at particular risk of experiencing drowsiness from this drug.

Hydroxyzine is generally considered safe to take during *early* pregnancy; however, its safety in mid and late pregnancy is unknown. It's generally considered to be *unsafe* during breastfeeding. We recommend before taking this medicine during pregnancy or breastfeeding you discuss this with your physician.

Precautions to follow if you're taking hydroxyzine

Follow these precautions if you're taking hydroxyzine:

- ✔ This drug may make you drowsy, which would make it unsafe for you to perform activities — like driving — that require you to be alert and focused.

- ✔ Because alcohol may worsen drowsiness, it may be unwise to consume it. We recommend you check with your doctor to find out whether drinking (small amounts of) alcohol would be okay.

- ✔ If you're prescribed other medicines that can also cause drowsiness, you may need to reduce the doses of these medicines to minimize your risk of getting excessively drowsy from the combination of these drugs.

How to take hydroxyzine

The dose of hydroxyzine varies considerably. Depending on your particular requirements, your dose may range from 25 to 100 mg taken three or four times per day. You can take hydroxyzine with or without food.

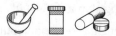

Anti-obesity Drugs

Very few drugs are currently available in Canada for the specific purpose of helping you lose weight. Unfortunately, the value of these drugs is limited for most people either because of only minimal weight loss or side-effects or both. Having said that, the occasional person does meet up with good results. The various anti-obesity drugs share little in common apart from their intended effect (that is, helping you lose weight). In this section we look in detail at the most commonly used anti-obesity drug. Table 6-18 lists the anti-obesity drugs available in Canada.

Table 6-18	Anti-obesity Drugs
Generic Name	*Trade Name(s)*
Diethylpropion	Tenuate, Tenuate Dospan
Orlistat	Xenical
Sibutramine	Meridia

 Orlistat

Xenical

Orlistat has minimal absorption into the body, which means that the likelihood of serious side-effects is very small; however, less serious but decidedly unpleasant side-effects are common and most people taking it don't lose all that much weight. Hmm.

 Orlistat inactivates important digestive enzymes in the stomach and bowel. This prevents fats you've eaten from being broken down into small enough molecules to be absorbed into the body. The fat has got to go somewhere, and because it can't be absorbed *into* the body it heads *out of* the body in the stool. Orlistat causes up to 30 percent of the fat you eat — and hence the calories fat contains — to be lost from the body this way.

How orlistat can help you

Orlistat can help you lose weight. It has also been found to reduce the risk of developing diabetes and, if you already have diabetes, orlistat can help improve your blood glucose control. (These benefits likely result from the weight loss rather than being a direct effect of the drug on glucose metabolism.)

 Because orlistat works by blocking fat absorption from your gut, in order for this drug to help you, you need to be eating sufficient fat. If you eat very little fat, there will be nothing for this drug to do. (On the other hand, if you eat too much it will cause unpleasant side-effects, as we look at next.)

How orlistat might harm you

Possible side-effects from taking orlistat include:

- Abdominal discomfort, flatulence, diarrhea, incontinence of stool, oily droplets escaping from your rectum and soiling your clothes. These common side-effects can be lessened if you sufficiently reduce the fat in your diet.

- Kidney stones. This seldom occurs.

- Deficiency of *fat-soluble vitamins* (vitamins A, D, E, and K). This is seldom of sufficient magnitude to be significant.

People with the following conditions shouldn't take orlistat:

- *Malabsorption,* a condition in which you're not able to properly absorb nutrients into your body from the bowel.

- *Cholestasis,* a condition in which bile is unable to flow from the liver into and through the bile ducts.

- BMI (body mass index) less than 30 (less than 27 if you have other, weight-related health problems, such as high blood pressure or high cholesterol).

To find out your BMI, we suggest you look at a chart (you can find one at Ian's Web site: www.ianblumer.com/images/bmiengc.pdf) or use an online calculator (you can find one at http://nhlbisupport.com/bmi/bminojs.htm).

The safety of orlistat in pregnancy and breastfeeding is unknown. If you're pregnant or breastfeeding, we recommend you discuss it with your physician before taking this medicine.

Precautions to follow if you're taking orlistat

To avoid becoming deficient in fat-soluble vitamins (A, D, E, and K), take a daily multivitamin supplement that contains these. Take the supplement once daily, at least two hours before or after a dose of orlistat.

How to take orlistat

Orlistat is taken with each meal (or up to one hour after eating), but no more than three doses daily. If you miss a meal or consume a meal that does not have fat you can skip your dose.

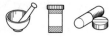

Antiparkinsonian Drugs

Antiparkinsonian drugs are used to treat symptoms of Parkinson's disease. They're also sometimes used in the treatment of similar symptoms when they occur due to other diseases, so-called parkinsonism. We discuss Parkinson's disease in Chapter 5. Whereas the different classes of antiparkinsonian drugs work by very different mechanisms (and have different side-effects, and so on), the drugs within a class share more in common. In this section we look in more detail at the most commonly prescribed drugs to treat parkinsonism. Antiparkinsonian drugs available for use in Canada are listed in Table 6-19.

Table 6-19	Antiparkinsonian Drugs	
Class	*Generic Name*	*Trade Name(s)*
Anticholinergic drugs	Benztropine	Apo-Benztropine, Benztropine Omega
	Ethopropazine	Parsitan
	Trihexyphenidyl	Apo-Trihex
NMDA receptor antagonist	Amantadine	Endantadine, Gen-Amantadine, Symmetrel
COMT inhibitor	Entacapone	Comtan
MAO-B inhibitors	Rasagiline	Azilect
	Selegiline	Apo-Selegiline, Gen-Selegiline, Novo-Selegiline, Nu-Selegiline
Dopamine precursors	Levodopa/ Benserazide	Prolopa
	Levodopa/ Carbidopa	Apo-Levocarb, Apo-Levocarb CR, Novo-Levocarbidopa, Nu-Levocarb, Sinemet, Sinemet CR
Dopamine agonists	Bromocriptine±	Apo-Bromocriptine, Parlodel, PMS-Bromocriptine
	Pergolide	Permax
	Pramipexole	Mirapex
	Ropinirole	ReQuip

± We discuss bromocriptine therapy for prolactin disorders in the "Dopamine Agonist" section of this chapter.

Levodopa/Carbidopa

Apo-Levocarb, Apo-Levocarb CR, Novo-Levocarbidopa, Nu-Levocarb, Sinemet, Sinemet CR

Levodopa has been in the forefront of Parkinson's disease therapy since the 1960s. As we look at next, in order for levodopa to work effectively it's given in combination with another, complementary drug (usually carbidopa or, sometimes, benserazide).

 Symptoms of Parkinson's disease are due to insufficient amounts in the brain of a hormone called *dopamine*. Because dopamine is unable to get from the blood into the brain (that is, it's unable to cross the blood–brain barrier), it's given as levodopa — which *is* able to overcome this barrier. When it's inside the brain, levodopa is converted into dopamine and can then carry out its normal functions, such as helping control the body's movements. (The process is akin to a spy who dons a disguise to pass through security, then when inside disrobes and performs her, well, spy stuff.) To prevent levodopa from changing into dopamine in the blood before it has a chance to get into the brain, carbidopa is added to the levodopa medicine; carbidopa blocks this process.

How levodopa/carbidopa can help you

Levodopa/carbidopa can help you by

- Controlling symptoms of Parkinson's disease (such as tremor and difficulty walking).
- Improving restless legs syndrome.

How levodopa/carbidopa might harm you

Possible side-effects from levodopa/carbidopa include:

- Abnormal, involuntary movements of the body. These are often the most troublesome side-effects.
- Altered thinking including feeling paranoid, confused, or depressed.
- Making a malignant melanoma worse. (See below.)
- Faintness (especially upon first arising from a bed or from a chair).
- Sleepiness. This can occur suddenly and without warning, however this seldom happens.

People with the following conditions shouldn't take levodopa/carbidopa:

✔ Glaucoma

✔ Melanoma (even if it has been treated) or possible melanoma (if you have a suspicious skin lesion, melanoma will need to be excluded before you're started on levodopa/carbidopa).

✔ You shouldn't take levodopa/carbidopa if you have taken a drug from the monoamine oxidase (MAO) inhibitor family within the past 14 days, nor should you start taking an MAO inhibitor within 14 days of stopping levodopa/carbidopa. (This does not apply to all MAO inhibitors.)

 The safety of levodopa/carbidopa in pregnancy and breastfeeding is unknown. If you're pregnant or breastfeeding, we recommend you discuss it with your physician before taking this medicine.

Precautions to follow if you're taking levodopa/carbidopa

Follow these precautions if you're taking levodopa/carbidopa:

 ✔ Sometimes people experience a sudden, temporary worsening of their Parkinson's symptoms (the *on-off phenomenon*). If this happens to you, let your doctor know.

✔ This drug may make you drowsy, which would make it unsafe for you to perform activities — like driving — that require you to be alert and focused.

 ✔ Because alcohol may worsen drowsiness, it may be unwise to consume it. We recommend you check with your doctor to find out whether drinking (small amounts of) alcohol would be okay.

✔ To avoid fainting when you rise from your chair or bed, stand for a moment and start walking only if you're sure you don't feel faint. If you do feel faint, sit (or, if necessary, lie) back down.

 ✔ Don't suddenly discontinue taking this medicine. Doing so can cause a very serious (but fortunately very rare) condition called *neuroleptic malignant syndrome*. Symptoms of this syndrome include fever, rigid muscles, and confusion.

How to take levodopa/carbidopa

Levodopa/carbidopa is typically started in a low dose of 100/25 (that is, 100 mg of levodopa in combination with 25 mg of carbidopa) taken three times daily (as close to every eight hours as possible), with the dose then adjusted every three days — under your doctor's supervision — until you're at the dose that provides you with the best control of your symptoms without causing excessive side-effects.

You can take levodopa/carbidopa with or without food; however, it's less likely to upset the stomach if taken with food. It's recommended that you avoid a high-protein diet as large quantities of protein in the gut can interfere with absorption of the medicine into your body.

 ## Pramipexole

Mirapex

Pramipexole, a relative newcomer on the Parkinson's treatment scene, has, with its sister drug, ropinirole, quickly established an important place in therapy.

 Pramipexole is a dopamine *agonist,* which means that it acts on the body in the same way as if it were dopamine (even though it isn't). Pramipexole travels from the blood into the brain, where it stimulates dopamine receptors; this results in improvement in Parkinson's symptoms such as tremor and difficulty walking.

How pramipexole can help you

Pramipexole can help you by improving symptoms of Parkinson's disease such as tremor and difficulty walking. It can also lessen depression. (The role of pramipexole in the treatment of depression isn't fully sorted out yet.)

How pramipexole might harm you

Possible side-effects from pramipexole include:

- Nausea. This is the most common side-effect.

- Hallucinations, dizziness, sleepiness, confusion. These occur in only a small percentage of people taking this drug.

- Sleepiness. This can occur suddenly and without warning, however this seldom happens.

- Faintness (especially upon first arising from a bed or from a chair).

- Pathological (compulsive) gambling. This has been observed in some people taking this medicine.

 You can lessen nausea by eating small, frequent meals and by sucking hard candies or chewing (sugar-free) gum.

The safety of pramipexole in pregnancy and breastfeeding is unknown. If you're pregnant or breastfeeding, we recommend you discuss it with your physician before taking this medicine.

Precautions to follow if you're taking pramipexole

Follow these precautions if you're taking pramipexole:

✔ This drug may make you drowsy, which would make it unsafe for you to perform activities — like driving — that require you to be alert and focused.

 ✔ Because alcohol may worsen drowsiness, it may be unwise to consume it. We recommend you check with your doctor to find out whether drinking (small amounts of) alcohol would be okay.

✔ To avoid fainting, when you rise from your chair or bed, stand for a moment and start walking only if you're sure you don't feel faint. If you do feel faint, sit (or, if necessary, lie) back down.

 ✔ Don't suddenly discontinue taking this medicine. Doing so can cause a very serious (but fortunately very rare) condition called *neuroleptic malignant syndrome*. Symptoms of this syndrome include fever, rigid muscles, and confusion.

How to take pramipexole

Pramipexole is typically started in dose of 0.125 mg taken three times daily, then increased weekly, under your doctor's supervision, as necessary and as tolerated. Your doctor may need to prescribe lower than usual doses if you have kidney failure. Pramipexole may be taken with or without food (however, it's less likely to upset the stomach if taken with food).

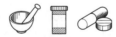

Antiplatelet Agents

Platelets are tiny cells in the blood that help it to clot. Being able to clot is essential; if we couldn't, we would bleed to death. On the other hand, some blood clots — such as those that form in arteries in the heart or brain — can lead to devastating complications such as heart attacks or strokes, respectively. Drugs that counter the action of platelets are called *antiplatelet agents*.

Antiplatelet agents available in Canada are listed in Table 6-20. Antiplatelet drugs share much in common. (Except for cost! ASA, at pennies a day, is immensely cheaper than the other antiplatelet agents.) Below, we look in detail at the two most commonly prescribed antiplatelet agents in Canada: ASA and clopidogrel. ASA, although not a prescription drug per se, is by far the most widely used antiplatelet agent and thus we discuss that drug here. (Incidentally, because health care plans typically require a prescription even for over-the-counter drugs, there were more than 10 *million* prescriptions written in Canada for ASA in 2005!)

Table 6-20	Antiplatelet Agents
Generic Name	*Trade Name(s)*
ASA±	Aggrenox*, Asaphen, Asaphen E.C., Aspirin, Bufferin, Novasen
Clopidogrel	Plavix
Dipyridamole	Aggrenox*, Apo-Dipyridamole, Persantine
Ticlopidine	Apo-Ticlopidine, Gen-Ticlopidine, Novo-Ticlopidine, Nu-Ticlopidine, Sandoz Ticlopidine, Ticlid

± This is only a partial list of trade names for ASA. Also, many ASA-containing products contain one or more other drugs.

* This medicine is a combination of different drugs. Refer to the drug label to determine what they are.

℞ *ASA (Acetylsalicylic Acid)*

Aggrenox*, Asaphen, Asaphen E.C., Aspirin, Bufferin, Novasen

ASA finds its, ahem, roots in willow bark, which has been used to treat various ailments for a few years. Well, more than a few, really. How few? Suffice to say that it was very old news by the time Julius Caesar was in diapers. Or whatever they used as diapers back then.

Because ASA can relieve inflammation (as we discuss below), you will sometimes see it referred to as a *nonsteroidal anti-inflammatory drug (NSAID)* rather than as an antiplatelet agent. Both terms are correct.

ASA can be a life-saving drug and, on rare occasion, a life-threatening drug. That it's available over-the-counter does not in any way lessen its importance, and we strongly recommend you include ASA in your discussions when you review your prescription drugs with your health care providers.

ASA works by blocking the action of an enzyme called cyclo-oxygenase. Blocking this enzyme results in decreased levels of prostaglandins (and, as a result, lessens fever, pain, and inflammation) and thromboxane A2 (and, as a result, makes platelets less likely to form a clot).

How ASA can help you

ASA can help you in the following ways:

- ✔ Lowering fever.

- ✔ Easing pain.

- ✔ Reducing inflammation.

- ✔ Preventing blood clots that cause strokes and heart attacks.

How ASA might harm you

Possible side-effects from taking ASA include:

- ✔ Bleeding.

- ✔ Nausea, vomiting, abdominal discomfort, stomach or duodenal ulcers.

- ✔ Triggering an asthma attack. This uncommon (allergic) side-effect is more likely to occur if you also have nasal polyps.

- ✔ If you have diabetes and are taking drugs, such as insulin, that lower blood glucose, *high doses* of ASA may cause a further reduction in your blood glucose levels.

- ✔ *Tinnitus* (ringing in the ears). You're likely to experience this only if you're taking very high doses of ASA.

People with the following conditions shouldn't take ASA:

- ✔ Active stomach or duodenal ulcer.

- ✔ Serious, active bleeding, such as from an ulcer or a brain hemorrhage.

- ✔ Allergy to ASA *or other nonsteroidal anti-inflammatory drugs (NSAIDs)*.

 - ✔ Children, teenagers, or young adults with chickenpox, influenza, or flu-like illnesses. Taking ASA in these circumstances increases the risk of developing a serious neurological condition called Reye's syndrome. (It's safest for people of any age to avoid ASA if they have influenza.)

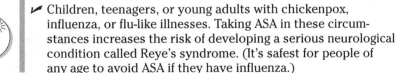

✔ Usually, within a week prior to having surgery. Whether you need to stop taking ASA depends on your individual circumstances. Be sure to find out from your doctor well in advance of scheduled surgery if and when you're to discontinue your ASA (and when you're to resume taking it).

Because ASA can cause bleeding and other complications during pregnancy, it's generally recommended it *not* be taken if you're pregnant. However, it's sometimes cautiously used in some special situations, such as in the treatment of certain blood pressure disorders of pregnancy. ASA is usually best avoided during breast-feeding. If you're pregnant or breastfeeding, we recommend you discuss it with your physician before taking this medicine.

Precautions to follow if you're taking ASA

Follow these precautions if you're taking ASA:

✔ If you're taking ASA to treat a fever, but the fever persists more than two to three days, it's wise to see a physician to have the cause of the fever determined.

✔ Because ASA can cause bleeding, check your stools for blood on a regular basis: if you see blood or if your stools are tarry and black (which can indicate a bleeding ulcer), seek prompt medical attention.

How to take ASA

Taking ASA with milk or food will help you avoid stomach irritation. Coated forms of ASA offer additional protection.

These are the usual ASA doses:

✔ For antiplatelet purposes, 81 mg to 325 mg taken once daily.

✔ For analgesic and anti-fever (*antipyretic*) purposes, 325 mg to 650 mg taken one to four times daily.

✔ For anti-inflammatory purposes, 650 mg to 975 mg taken three to four times daily.

 ℞ *Clopidogrel*

Plavix

Clopidogrel is a very effective antiplatelet drug and, for this reason, is used increasingly often. Sometimes it's used in combination with ASA, and sometimes it's used on its own. Precisely when to use the two together (and for how long to do so) as opposed to using one alone is still being sorted out.

Clopidogrel works by inhibiting the action of an enzyme called *adenosine diphosphate* (ADP). ADP stimulates platelets to clump together to form a clot; by inhibiting this enzyme, a clot is less likely to form.

How clopidogrel can help you

Clopidogrel can help you by preventing blood clots that cause strokes and heart attacks.

How clopidogrel might harm you

Possible side-effects from taking clopidogrel include:

✔ Bleeding.

✔ *Thrombotic thrombocytopenic purpura* (TTP). This is a very serious condition in which there is anemia, a low platelet count, fever, and kidney damage. Fortunately, it occurs only rarely.

✔ Abnormal liver tests.

✔ Skin rash.

People with the following conditions shouldn't take clopidogrel:

✔ A stomach or duodenal ulcer (if it's bleeding or if your doctor feels it's at risk of bleeding), brain hemorrhage, or other serious, active bleeding.

✔ Liver disease.

✔ Usually, within a week prior to having surgery. Whether you need to stop taking clopidogrel depends on your individual circumstances. Be sure to find out from your doctor well in advance of scheduled surgery if and when you're to discontinue your clopidogrel (and when you're to resume taking it).

The safety of clopidogrel in pregnancy is unknown. Breastfeeding isn't recommended if you're taking clopidogrel. If you're pregnant or breastfeeding, we recommend you discuss it with your physician before taking this medicine.

Precautions to follow if you're taking clopidogrel

Follow these precautions if you're taking clopidogrel:

✔ Because clopidogrel can cause bleeding, check your stools for blood on a regular basis: if you see blood or if your stools are tarry and black (which can indicate a bleeding ulcer), seek prompt medical attention.

✔ Don't take ASA unless prescribed by your doctor. (ASA is present in many over-the-counter products, so you need to carefully read the label of any such medicine you take.)

How to take clopidogrel

Clopidogrel is taken in a dose of 75 mg once daily, with or without food.

Avoid consuming grapefruit or grapefruit juice because it can affect the level of clipidogrel in your blood.

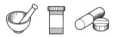

Antipsychotics

Antipsychotics are medications used to treat *psychoses* (psychoses are thinking disorders where one loses contact with reality). Some of these drugs are also used to prevent or treat nausea. Antipsychotics are usually grouped into older (*first generation* or *typical* antipsychotics) and newer (*second generation* or *atypical* antipsychotics) classes. First and second generation antpsychotics available in Canada are listed in Table 6-21.

Although the list is lengthy, the majority of people requiring antipsychotic medicine are treated with second generation drugs, of which there are very few. (For more on the use of these drugs, see Chapter 5.) The second generation antipsychotics are either "pines" (that is, clozapine, olanzapine, and quetiapine — these drugs have much in common) or risperidone. We focus our detailed discussion on two of the most commonly used second generation drugs: olanzapine and risperidone.

Table 6-21	Antipsychotics	
Class	*Generic Name*	*Trade Name(s)*
First generation ("typical") antipsychotics	Chlorpromazine	Novo-Chlorpromazine
	Flupenthixol	Fluanxol Depot, Fluanxol Tablets
	Fluphenazine	Apo-Fluphenazine, Fluphenazine Omega, Modecate Concentrate
	Haloperidol	Apo-Haloperidol, Apo-Haloperidol LA, Haloperidol Injection USP, Haloperidol LA, Haloperidol-LA Omega, Novo-Peridol

Class	Generic Name	Trade Name(s)
	Loxapine	Apo-Loxapine, Loxapac IM, Nu-Loxapine, PMS-Loxapine
	Methotrimeprazine	Apo-Methoprazine, Nozinan Injectable, Nozinan Syrup, Nozinan Tablets
	Perphenazine	Apo-Perphenazine, Trilafon
	Pimozide	Apo-Pimozide, Orap
	Prochlorperazine	Apo-Prochlorazine, Nu-Prochlor, Prochlorperazine Mesylate Injection, SAB-Prochlorperazine Suppository, Stemetil
	Thiothixene	Navane
	Trifluoperazine	Apo-Trifluoperazine
	Zuclopenthixol	Clopixol, Clopixol-Acuphase, Clopixol Depot
Second generation ("atypical") antipsychotics	Clozapine	Apo-Clozapine, Clozaril, Gen-Clozapine
	Olanzapine	Zyprexa, Zyprexa Zydis, Zyprexa IntraMuscular
	Quetiapine	Seroquel
	Risperidone	CO Risperidone, Novo-Risperidone, PMS-Risperidone, ratio-Risperidone, Risperdal Tablets, Risperdal Oral Solution, Risperdal M-Tab, Risperdal Consta, Sandoz Risperidone

 Olanzapine

Zyprexa, Zyprexa Zydis, Zyprexa IntraMuscular

Olanzapine, like other second generation antipsychotics, has largely replaced the older, first generation drugs.

The precise means by which olanzapine works isn't known; however, its effect appears to relate, at least in part, to its ability to block the action of two chemical messengers: dopamine and serotonin. It does this by preventing these messengers from stimulating their respective receptors.

How olanzapine can help you

Olanzapine can help you in the following ways:

✔ Controlling symptoms of schizophrenia.

✔ Controlling symptoms of bipolar disorder.

✔ Reducing nausea. This is incidental to its other purposes and isn't the primary reason this drug would be prescribed.

How olanzapine might harm you

Possible side-effects from olanzapine include:

✔ *Neuroleptic malignant syndrome.* This is a rare, serious, condition with symptoms including fever, rigid muscles, and confusion. It's more likely to occur if you also have Parkinson's disease.

✔ Weight gain.

✔ Decreased ability to regulate body temperature.

✔ Faintness due to low blood pressure. This is most likely to occur during the first few weeks of therapy.

✔ Diabetes or, if you already have diabetes, an increase in your blood glucose levels. This does not occur often.

✔ Elevated prolactin hormone levels. This can cause milky discharge from the breasts and can make your periods abnormally light or heavy.

✔ There is the theoretical risk that this drug can worsen breast cancer or pituitary tumours.

✔ *Priapism,* a persistent, painful erection (typically lasting several hours or more). This must be treated urgently, otherwise it can lead to permanent erectile dysfunction.

✔ Abnormal liver tests. Rarely, hepatitis.

✔ *Tardive dyskinesia.* This is a condition in which you have repetitive, involuntary movements. This occurs rarely.

✔ Increased risk of seizures. This is highly unlikely to be a problem unless you already have a seizure disorder.

✔ Increased risk of death *if* you're elderly and have dementia.

The safety of olanzapine in pregnancy is unknown. Breastfeeding isn't recommended if you're taking olanzapine. If you're pregnant or breastfeeding, we recommend you discuss it with your physician before taking this medicine.

Precautions to follow if you're taking olanzapine

Follow these precautions if you're taking olanzapine:

- ✔ If you have (or your doctor thinks you might have) liver malfunction, your doctor should check your liver tests (this is done with a simple blood test) before you start the medicine and periodically thereafter.

- ✔ Because you may not be able to properly rid yourself of excess heat, make sure you maintain adequate hydration (especially if you're exercising or in a hot environment).

- ✔ Notify your physician if you develop symptoms of high blood glucose (such as increased thirst, frequent urination, getting up at night to pass urine, unexpected weight loss, blurred vision).

- ✔ If you have diabetes, monitor your blood glucose reading more often — especially for the first few weeks after you start olanzapine. If your blood glucose levels rise, contact your doctor.

- ✔ To avoid fainting, when you rise from your chair or bed, stand for a moment and start walking only if you're sure you don't feel faint. If you do feel faint, sit (or, if necessary, lie) back down.

- ✔ This drug may make you drowsy, which would make it unsafe for you to perform activities — like driving — that require you to be alert and focused.

- ✔ Because alcohol may worsen drowsiness, it may be unwise to consume it. We recommend you check with your doctor to find out whether drinking (small amounts of) alcohol would be okay.

- ✔ Don't stop taking olanzapine without first speaking to your doctor. (In most people with psychoses, stopping antipsychotic medicine will allow the underlying condition to worsen.)

How to take olanzapine

The usual starting dose of olanzapine in the treatment of schizophrenia is 5 mg to 10 mg, and in the treatment of bipolar disorder it's 10 mg to 15 mg. The doses are then adjusted, under your doctor's supervision, based on your response. Your doctor may need to prescribe lower doses if you're elderly. Olanzapine is taken once daily and may be taken with or without food.

Risperidone

CO Risperidone, Novo-Risperidone, PMS-Risperidone, ratio-Risperidone, Risperdal Tablets, Risperdal Oral Solution, Risperdal M-Tab, Risperdal Consta, Sandoz Risperidone

Risperidone is a very commonly used antipsychotic medicine. (In 2005 there were almost 2.5 million prescriptions dispensed in Canada for this medicine.)

 By attaching to very specialized receptors (dopamine type 2 and serotonin type 2) in the brain, risperidone blocks the action of chemical messengers (*neurotransmitters*) such as dopamine and serotonin. With less stimulation by dopamine and serotonin of these receptors, certain psychotic symptoms are eased.

How risperidone can help you

Risperidone can help you in the following ways:

- ✔ Controlling symptoms of schizophrenia.

- ✔ Controlling symptoms of aggression due to severe dementia. It does not help other symptoms seen with dementia.

- ✔ Improving acute manic episodes of bipolar disorder.

- ✔ Reducing nausea. This is incidental to its other purposes and isn't the primary reason this drug would be prescribed.

How risperidone might harm you

Possible side-effects from risperidone include:

- ✔ Insomnia, agitation, headache, sleepiness, weight gain. These are the most common side-effects.

- ✔ Faintness due to low blood pressure. This is most likely to occur during the first few weeks of therapy.

- ✔ Elevated prolactin hormone levels. This can cause milky discharge from the breasts and can make your periods abnormally light or heavy.

- ✔ Decreased ability to regulate body temperature.

- ✔ Diabetes or, if you already have diabetes, an increase in your blood glucose levels. This does not occur often.

- ✔ *Priapism,* a persistent painful erection (typically lasting several hours or more). This must be treated urgently, otherwise it can lead to permanent erectile dysfunction.

✔ *Neuroleptic malignant syndrome.* This is a rare, serious, condition with symptoms including fever, rigid muscles, and confusion. It's more likely to occur if you also have Parkinson's disease.

✔ *Tardive dyskinesia.* This is a condition in which you have repetitive, involuntary movements.

✔ Increased risk of seizures. This is highly unlikely to be a problem unless you already have a seizure disorder.

✔ Increased risk of death *if* you're elderly and have dementia.

✔ There is the theoretical risk that this drug can worsen breast cancer or pituitary tumours.

The safety of risperidone in pregnancy is unknown; however, it's generally recommended it *not* be used. Risperidone is considered unsafe to take if you're breastfeeding. If you're pregnant or breastfeeding, we recommend you discuss it with your physician before taking this medicine.

Precautions to follow if you're taking risperidone

Follow these precautions if you're taking risperidone:

✔ Because you may not be able to properly rid yourself of excess heat, make sure you maintain adequate hydration (especially if you're exercising or in a hot environment).

✔ Notify your physician if you develop symptoms of high blood glucose (such as increased thirst, frequent urination, getting up at night to pass urine, unexpected weight loss, blurred vision).

✔ If you have diabetes, monitor your blood glucose reading more often — especially for the first few weeks after you start risperidone. If your blood glucose levels rise, contact your doctor.

✔ This drug may make you drowsy, which would make it unsafe for you to perform activities — like driving — that require you to be alert and focused.

✔ Because alcohol may worsen drowsiness, it may be unwise to consume it. We recommend you check with your doctor to find out whether drinking (small amounts of) alcohol would be okay.

✔ To avoid fainting, when you rise from your chair or bed, stand for a moment and start walking only if you're sure you don't feel faint. If you do feel faint, sit (or, if necessary, lie) back down.

✔ Don't stop taking risperidone without first speaking to your doctor. (In most people with psychoses, stopping antipsychotic medicine will allow the underlying condition to worsen.)

How to take risperidone

The usual starting dose in the treatment of schizophrenia is 1 mg to 2 mg per day (either taken in one dose or divided into two doses), and for bipolar disorder it's 2 mg to 3 mg taken once daily. The doses are then adjusted, under your doctor's supervision, based on your response to the medicine. Your doctor may need to prescribe lower doses if you're elderly.

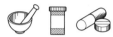

Antiretroviral Drugs

As we discuss in Chapter 5, antiretroviral drugs are used in the treatment of HIV/AIDS. (HIV is a retrovirus, and medicines to fight this are called *antiretroviral* drugs.)

The treatment of HIV/AIDS is complex. Many patients are prescribed three or more drugs to be taken in a special protocol called HAART (highly active antiretroviral treatment). Exactly which drugs to take and when they should be used are determined for each individual based on their own stage of illness.

A full discussion of these drugs is beyond the scope of this book; however, we list the antiretroviral therapies (ARTs) available in Canada in Table 6-22.

Table 6-22	Antiretroviral Drugs	
Class	*Generic Name*	*Trade Name(s)*
Nucleoside or nucleotide reverse transcriptase inhibitors (NRTIS)	Abacavir	Kivexa*, Trizivir*, Ziagen
	Didanosine	Videx, Videx EC
	Emtricitabine	Emtriva, Truvada*
	Lamivudine	3TC, Combivir*, Heptovir, Kivexa*, Trizivir*
	Stavudine	Zerit
	Tenofovir	Truvada*, Viread
	Zalcitabine	Hivid
	Zidovudine	Combivir*, Retrovir (AZT), Trizivir*

Class	Generic Name	Trade Name
Non-nucleoside reverse transcriptase inhibitors (NNRTIs)	Delavirdine	Rescriptor
	Efavirenz	Sustiva
	Nevirapine	Viramune
Protease inhibitors	Amprenavir	Agenerase Capsules, Agenerase Oral Solution
	Atazanavir	Reyataz
	Fosamprenavir	Telzir
	Indinavir	Crixivan
	Lopinavir	Kaletra*
	Nelfinavir	Viracept
	Ritonavir	Kaletra*, Novir, Novir SEC
	Saquinavir	Fortovase Roche, Invirase
	Tipranavir	Aptivus
Fusion inhibitor	Enfuvirtide	Fuzeon

This medicine is a combination of different drugs. Refer to the drug label to determine what they are.

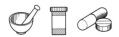

Antithyroid Agents

Antithyroid drugs are used to treat hyperthyroidism due to Graves' disease (and, occasionally, certain other forms of hyperthyroidism) when radioactive iodine therapy isn't considered appropriate. We discuss hyperthyroidism in Chapter 5. The antithyroid drugs available in Canada are listed in Table 6-23. Because they're so similar, we discuss them together.

Table 6-23	Antithyroid Agents
Generic Name	**Trade Name(s)**
Methimazole	Tapazole
Propylthiouracil	Propyl-Thyracil

Graves' disease causes the thyroid gland to produce excess quantities of thyroid hormone, which in turn can lead to symptoms such as weight loss, palpitations, tremor, excess sweating, and diarrhea. Methimazole and propylthiouracil block the thyroid's ability to produce thyroid hormone, and with less thyroid hormone in the body you will have fewer symptoms.

How antithyroid agents can help you

These drugs can help you by reducing your symptoms of hyperthyroidism.

How antithyroid agents might harm you

Possible side-effects from taking these drugs include:

✔ Skin rash, nausea, vomiting, joint pains. These occur uncommonly and quickly go away after the drug is stopped.

✔ Decreased numbers of white blood cells. This rarely occurs. A deficiency of white blood cells puts you at increased risk of infections.

Both methimazole and propylthiouracil can cause harm to a fetus (principally, thyroid malfunction); however, this risk is small and made smaller by taking the lowest possible dose of these drugs that keeps your thyroid levels in check. Typically, during pregnancy, propylthiouracil is used in preference to methimazole because it may be less likely to cause the baby to develop an unusual type of scalp defect (*cutis aplasia*).

Breastfeeding while taking either of these drugs is *generally* considered safe, but because the medicine may pass into the baby from your milk, speak to your doctor about whether you should take the medicine in this circumstance — and, if you do, whether the baby's thyroid hormone levels should be measured from time to time.

Precautions to follow if you're taking antithyroid agents

Follow these precautions if you're taking an antithyroid agent:

✔ You will need to have regular (every few weeks) blood tests to measure your thyroid hormone levels so that your doctor can determine whether your dose needs to be adjusted. This is especially so during the early stages of treatment.

✔ Because there is the (remote) possibility that methimazole or propylthiouracil will lower your white blood cell count and therefore put you at risk of an infection, seek immediate medical attention if you develop a fever, bad sore throat, yellow or greenish phlegm, or other symptoms suggesting you have an infection. (Your doctor should then order a blood test to check your white blood cell count.)

How to take antithyroid agents

The starting dose of methimazole varies from as little as 10 mg per day to as much as 60 mg per day depending on the severity of your hyperthyroidism. The starting dose of propylthiouracil ranges from 300 mg to 900 mg per day. The doses are then adjusted, under your doctor's supervision, based on your response. Your doctor may need to prescribe lower than usual doses if you have kidney failure. It's *usually* (there's no consensus) recommended that methimazole and propylthiouracil be taken with food.

One advantage to taking methimazole rather than propylthiouracil is that it's taken fewer times per day, so you'll have fewer doses to remember.

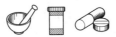

Antituberculosis Drugs

Antituberculosis drugs are sometimes referred to as *antimycobacterials*. This name is technically more accurate, as TB is but one member of a group of germs called mycobacteria. As we discuss in Chapter 5, combinations of these drugs are used to fight *active* TB, however isoniazid alone is used to treat *latent* TB. The drugs in Canada most commonly used to treat TB are listed in Table 6-24. They differ considerably from one another and offer complementary TB-fighting properties (hence the reason they're often used in combination). Isoniazid, by far the most commonly used of these drugs, is discussed in detail below.

Table 6-24	Antituberculosis Drugs
Generic Name	*Trade Name(s)*
Ethambutol	Etibi
Isoniazid	Isotamine, Rifater*
Pyrazinamide	Rifater*, Tebrazid
Rifampin	Rifadin, Rifater*, Rofact

* This medicine is a combination of different drugs. Refer to the drug label to determine what they are.

Isoniazid (INH)

Isotamine, Rifater*

Isoniazid is also known as INH, short for iso-nicotinic acid hydrazide. It's also short for inhaler and *L'Institut National d'Horticulture*. So, lest someone think you're having an asthma attack at a botany school in France, it's best to stick with the term "isoniazid."

Isoniazid attaches to and effectively kills tuberculosis germs. How it does this, however, isn't known.

How isoniazid can help you

Used with other antituberculosis drugs, isoniazid treats *active* tuberculosis. Taken on its own, it treats *latent* tuberculosis.

How isoniazid might harm you

Possible side-effects from taking isoniazid include:

- ✔ Nausea, vomiting.

- ✔ Hepatitis. This is the most worrisome side-effect. It's more likely to occur if you're older, have underlying liver disease, and/or consume alcohol (especially if in large quantities).

- ✔ Abnormal liver tests without hepatitis. Liver tests (on a blood sample) become mildly abnormal in 10 to 20 percent of people using this drug but usually return to normal even as the drug is continued. (With hepatitis, liver tests are usually severely abnormal.)

- ✔ Allergic reaction. Symptoms may include rash, fever, and swollen lymph glands. This rarely occurs.

- ✔ *Optic neuritis.* This is an inflammation of the *optic nerve* that connects the eye to the brain. Optic neuritis causes visual loss or blurring. This rarely occurs.

- ✔ *Peripheral neuropathy.* This is damage to nerves in the periphery of the body and typically causes a feeling of numbness in the toes. (See below.)

People with the following conditions shouldn't take isoniazid:

- ✔ Liver disease. There are exceptions to this.
- ✔ Previous severe reaction to this drug.

Isoniazid is generally considered safe to take during pregnancy. Its safety during breastfeeding is less proven. If you're pregnant or breastfeeding, we recommend you discuss it with your physician before taking this medicine.

Precautions to follow if you're taking isoniazid

Follow these precautions if you're taking isoniazid:

- ✔ Avoid alcohol.

- ✔ Your doctor may send you for blood tests to check your liver health prior to, then periodically during treatment. Whether this should be done routinely is controversial.

- ✔ If you start to feel generally unwell and develop a poor appetite, nausea, vomiting, dark urine, or yellowing of your skin or eyes (that is, jaundice), you may have developed hepatitis and should seek urgent medical attention.

- ✔ If you develop blurred or loss of vision, see an eye doctor right away.

- ✔ Peripheral neuropathy (see possible side-effects above) is more likely to occur if you're at risk of having a deficiency of vitamin B6. People at risk include those who are pregnant, malnourished, or drink large quantities of alcohol. To help you avoid peripheral neuropathy, your doctor may recommend you take vitamin B6 supplements (typically in a dose of 25 mg/day).

How to take isoniazid

The most common dose is 300 mg taken once daily. Take it on an empty stomach (one to two hours before eating or two or more hours after eating).

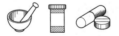

Antiviral Agents

Viruses are common causes of infections in adults. They cause the "common cold" and can be responsible for gastrointestinal illness such as the "stomach flu." Most of the time, the body's immune system can handle viral infections and no specific drug therapy is needed. However, in some situations medication can be very useful, such as in the treatment of influenza, shingles, and HIV/AIDS.

Table 6-25 lists many of the antiviral agents available in Canada. (We list antiretroviral drugs used to treat HIV/AIDS elsewhere in this chapter.) The various antiviral drugs vary significantly from one another in their properties (including when they're used); in this section we discuss acyclovir in detail, as it is in particularly common use.

Table 6-25	Antiviral Agents
Generic Name	**Trade Name(s)**
Acyclovir	Apo-Acyclovir, Gen-Acyclovir, Nu-Acyclovir, ratio-Acyclovir, Zovirax Cream, Zovirax Ointment, Zovirax Oral
Famciclovir	Famvir, Sandoz Famciclovir
Ganciclovir	Cytovene Capsules
Idoxuridine	Herplex-D
Oseltamivir	Tamiflu
Ribavirin	Pegasys RBV*, Pegetron*, Virazole
Trifluridine	Sandoz Trifluridine, Viroptic
Valacyclovir	Valtrex
Valganciclovir	Valcyte
Zanamivir	Relenza

* This medicine is a combination of different drugs. Refer to the drug label to determine what they are.

 Acyclovir

Apo-Acyclovir, Gen-Acyclovir, Nu-Acyclovir, ratio-Acyclovir, Zovirax Cream, Zovirax Ointment, Zovirax Oral

 Acyclovir enters into cells that have been infected by certain viruses and stops the virus from reproducing itself. Without being able to create more of itself, the virus eventually dies off.

How acyclovir can help you

Acyclovir can help you by treating the following viral illnesses:

- ✔ Genital herpes. This is caused by herpes simplex virus type 1 or type 2. Acyclovir can be used to improve symptoms of the initial episode and decrease the frequency and severity of future episodes.

> ✔ Shingles. This is caused by herpes zoster virus. Early use of acyclovir may speed the healing of the skin lesions and lessen their initial pain.
>
> ✔ Chicken pox when it occurs in adults.

Topical therapy isn't very effective, so oral therapy is typically preferred.

Acyclovir is also used in the treatment of certain other viral infections if they occur in adults at increased risk of severe infections because of a defective immune system.

How acyclovir might harm you

Possible side-effects from taking acyclovir include:

> ✔ Nausea, vomiting, diarrhea, malaise (that is, feeling generally unwell). These are the most common side-effects.
>
> ✔ Burning or itching of the skin (if using topical acyclovir).
>
> ✔ Low platelet count. This has been seen in people who have poor immune function.

When you shouldn't use acyclovir

The safety of acyclovir in pregnancy and breastfeeding is unknown. If you're pregnant or breastfeeding, we recommend you discuss it with your physician before taking either of these medicines.

Precautions to follow if you're taking acyclovir

If you have kidney failure, you will need a reduced dose, therefore, let your doctor know about anything that could potentially damage your kidneys, such as when you're given intravenous contrast (the "dye" given for some x-ray procedures) or start taking a new medicine, so that she can monitor your kidney function and adjust your acyclovir dose if necessary.

How to take acyclovir

Acyclovir cream and ointment are applied directly to the affected skin area four to six times per day for up to ten days.

The dose you're prescribed of the tablet or suspension forms of acyclovir depends on the reason it's being prescribed and your general health. The usual dose to treat a first attack of genital herpes is 200 mg five times per day taken for ten consecutive days. (To figure out when you will take it, divide up your waking hours into five equal time periods and take a dose at the beginning or, if you prefer, at the end of each of these periods.) Your doctor may need to prescribe lower than usual doses if you have kidney failure. You can take acyclovir with or without food.

Because acyclovir works best if it's started early in the infection, be sure to seek prompt medical attention when you notice symptoms.

Beta Blockers

Beta blockers, first prescribed more than 40 years ago, remain a key component of drug therapy for several heart problems, especially coronary artery disease where their use has been life-saving for untold numbers of people. Table 6-26 lists the oral beta blockers available in Canada.

Our bodies have two types of beta receptors: beta-1 receptors (found predominantly in the heart), and beta-2 receptors (found in the lungs, in the lining of blood vessels, and in some other organs). Beta-1 selective beta blockers preferentially block beta-1 receptors (and therefore are called *cardioselective* beta blockers). *Non-selective* beta blockers equally block both beta-1 and beta-2 receptors. Both beta-1 selective and non-selective beta blockers reduce stimulation of the heart and as a result the heart isn't required to work as hard. An important advantage that a beta-1 selective beta blocker has (compared to a non-selective beta blocker) is that — unless used in high doses — it will not worsen asthma or chronic obstructive airways disease (COPD).

Table 6-26	Oral Beta Blockers	
Class	*Generic Name*	*Trade Name(s)*
Beta-1 selective ("cardioselective")	Acebutolol	Apo-Acebutolol, Gen-Acebutolol, Gen-Acebutolol (Type S), Novo-Acebutolol, Nu-Acebutolol, Rhotral, Sandoz Acebutolol, Sectral
	Atenolol	Apo-Atenidone*, Apo-Atenol, CO Atenolol, Gen-Atenolol, Novo-Atenol, Nu-Atenol, PMS-Atenolol, RAN-Atenolol, ratio-Atenolol, Sandoz Atenolol, Tenoretic*, Tenormin
	Bisoprolol	Apo-Bisoprolol, Monocor, Novo-Bisoprolol, Sandoz Bisoprolol
	Metoprolol	Apo-Metoprolol, Apo-Metoprolol (Type L), Betaloc, Betaloc Durules, Gen-Metoprolol (Type L), Lopressor, Novo-Metoprolol, Nu-Metop, PMS-Metoprolol-L, Sandoz Metoprolol (Type L)

Class	Generic Name	Trade Name(s)
Non-selective	Carvedilol	Apo-Carvedilol, PMS-Carvedilol, RAN-Carvedilol, ratio-Carvedilol
	Labetalol	Apo-Labetalol, Trandate
	Nadolol	Apo-Nadol, Corgard, Novo-Nadolol
	Oxprenolol	Trasicor
	Pindolol	Apo-Pindol, Gen-Pindolol, Novo-Pindol, Nu-Pindol, Sandoz Pindolol, Viskazide*, Visken
	Propranolol	Apo-Propranolol, Inderal-LA, Novo-Pranol, Nu-Propranolol
	Sotalol	Apo-Sotalol, CO Sotalol, Gen-Sotalol, Novo-Sotalol, Nu-Sotalol, PMS-Sotalol, ratio-Sotalol, Sandoz Sotalol
	Timolol	Apo-Timol, Novo-Timol, Nu-Timolol, PMS-Timolol

* This medicine is a combination of different drugs. Refer to the drug label to determine what they are.

 ## Atenolol, Metoprolol

Apo-Atenidone*, Apo-Atenol, CO Atenolol, Gen-Atenolol, Novo-Atenol, Nu-Atenol, PMS-Atenolol, RAN-Atenolol, ratio-Atenolol, Sandoz Atenolol, Tenoretic*, Tenormin

Apo-Metoprolol, Apo-Metoprolol (Type L), Betaloc, Betaloc Durules, Gen-Metoprolol (Type L), Lopressor, Novo-Metoprolol, Nu-Metop, PMS-Metoprolol-L, Sandoz Metoprolol (Type L)

Because atenolol and metoprolol are so similar, we discuss them together.

How atenolol and metoprolol can help you

Atenolol and metoprolol can help you in the following ways:

- ✔ Controlling high blood pressure.
- ✔ Reducing the frequency of angina.
- ✔ Preventing another heart attack if you have already had one.
- ✔ Preventing certain heart rhythm problems.
- ✔ Controlling your heart rate if you have atrial fibrillation.

✔ Improving your prognosis if you have congestive heart failure. (Long-acting forms of metoprolol are the most proven for this use.)

✔ Preventing migraine headaches.

✔ Improving essential tremor.

Although cardioselective beta blockers such as atenolol and metoprolol may be used in the treatment of migraine headaches and essential tremor, traditionally, nonselective beta blockers (such as propranolol) are prescribed for these conditions.

As amazing as this list is, and despite the fact these drugs have been around for ages, we keep finding additional ways they can help.

How atenolol and metoprolol might harm you

Possible side-effects from taking atenolol and metoprolol include:

✔ Excessive slowing of the heartbeat and/or low blood pressure (which can lead to faintness).

✔ Making Raynaud's phenomenon worse.

✔ Fatigue. This isn't serious, but can be bothersome.

✔ Erectile dysfunction.

✔ Increasing your risk of developing type 2 diabetes.

✔ Masking symptoms of low blood glucose (*hypoglycemia*). This will be an issue only if you have diabetes and are on a medication such as glyburide or insulin that can cause low blood glucose.

✔ Worsening of asthma and chronic obstructive pulmonary disease (COPD). (This side-effect is more likely to occur if you're on high doses of atenolol or metoprolol and is far *less* likely to occur with either of these drugs than it is with use of a nonselective beta blocker such as propranolol.)

✔ Worsening of calf pains due to claudication (refer to Chapter 5).

Persons with the following conditions shouldn't take atenolol or metoprolol:

✔ A very slow heartbeat.

✔ Low blood pressure. (*How* low depends on your particular situation.)

✔ Uncontrolled congestive heart failure. (Note that these drugs can *improve* your prognosis if you have *controlled* heart failure; it's when heart failure is *uncontrolled* they shouldn't be taken.)

The safety of atenolol and metoprolol in pregnancy and breastfeeding isn't known for certain and, indeed, there are certain concerns regarding their use in these situations. It is, therefore, very important that if you're pregnant or breastfeeding you discuss it with your physician before taking either of these medicines.

Precautions to follow if you're taking atenolol or metoprolol

Follow these precautions if you're taking atenolol or metoprolol:

- ✔ Don't stop taking these medicines without first consulting your doctor.

- ✔ If you have asthma and you have just started taking atenolol or metoprolol, be on the lookout for any worsening of your condition and notify your physician promptly if this occurs.

- ✔ If you have diabetes and are being treated with drugs such as glyburide or insulin, which can cause hypoglycemia, be especially vigilant for symptoms of hypoglycemia (such as hunger, palpitations, sweating, and tremor).

How to take atenolol and metoprolol

Atenolol and metoprolol are usually started in a dose of between 50 mg and 100 mg per day. The doses are then adjusted, under the supervision of your doctor, based on how you're responding. Atenolol is taken once daily. Metoprolol is taken either once or twice daily depending on the particular brand that has been prescribed. You can take atenolol and metoprolol with or without food.

 ## Propranolol

Apo-Propranolol, Inderal-LA, Novo-Pranol, Nu-Propranolol

Propranolol was the first beta blocker available for use in Canada and is still in common use. We only wish the creators of this drug hadn't stuck that second 'r' in there; every time we say propranolol we feel like we need help from a Scottish diction coach.

How propranolol can help you

Propranolol can help you in the following ways:

- ✔ Improving hypertension.

- ✔ Reducing angina.

- ✔ Preventing another heart attack if you have already had one.

- ✔ Preventing certain heart rhythm problems.

- ✔ Controlling your heart rate if you have atrial fibrillation.

✔ Preventing migraine headaches.

✔ Improving essential tremor and tremor due to hyperthyroidism.

✔ Reducing the risk of bleeding from swollen blood vessels in the esophagus (*esophageal varices*) due to liver cirrhosis.

✔ Easing stage fright. (Certain performers such as some pianists take propranolol before playing. It seems to help "calm the nerves" and also seems to reduce anxiety-related tremor.)

How propranolol might harm you

Possible side-effects from taking propranolol include:

✔ Excessive slowing of the heart beat and/or low blood pressure (which can lead to faintness).

✔ Making Raynaud's phenomenon worse.

✔ Fatigue. This isn't serious, but can be bothersome.

✔ Erectile dysfunction.

✔ Increasing your risk of developing type 2 diabetes.

✔ Masking symptoms of low blood glucose (*hypoglycemia*). This will be an issue only if you have diabetes and are on a medication such as glyburide or insulin that can cause low blood glucose.

✔ Worsening of asthma.

✔ Worsening of calf pains due to claudication.

People with the following conditions shouldn't take propranolol:

✔ A very slow heartbeat.

✔ Low blood pressure. (*How* low depends on your particular situation.)

✔ Asthma or chronic obstructive pulmonary disease (COPD).

✔ Congestive heart failure.

The safety of propranolol in pregnancy and breastfeeding isn't known for certain and, indeed, there are certain concerns regarding their use in these situations. It is, therefore, very important that if you're pregnant or breastfeeding you discuss it with your physician before taking this medicine.

Precautions to follow if you're taking propranolol

Follow these precautions if you're taking propranolol:

✔ Don't stop taking propranolol without first consulting your
doctor.

✔ If you have diabetes and are being treated with drugs such as
glyburide or insulin, which can cause hypoglycemia, be especially vigilant for symptoms of hypoglycemia (such as hunger,
palpitations, sweating, and tremor).

How to take propranolol

Propranolol is taken daily either once (for the long-acting forms)
or twice (for the regular form). (The exception is if you're being
treated for severe symptoms due to hyperthyroidism, in which
case propranolol may be used four times daily.) The dose you
require varies considerably depending on the particular ailment
being treated. Typically, you would be started on a low dose and
the dose would then be adjusted, under your doctor's supervision,
based on how you're responding. Propranolol may be taken with
or without food.

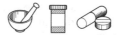

Biologic Response Modifiers

For a century, there has been hope that for each disease, a "magic
bullet" could be found — that is, a treatment that targets the specific, abnormal process in the body that allows a disease to occur.
We have taken a huge step forward with the discovery of biologic
response modifiers (or biologics). These proteins act on specific
pathways in the body that lead to certain diseases. At present we
have biologics to treat some cancers, some inflammatory and
autoimmune disorders, and to help prevent rejection of certain
transplanted organs.

Biologics are typically given by injection in an outpatient setting —
sometimes by a health care professional in a clinic and sometimes
by you at home. Although they're highly effective medicines, like
all drugs they have their downsides. Possible side-effects range
from the fairly minor (like irritation at the injection site) to the
more serious (such as increasing your risk of infection). The long-
term safety of these drugs isn't as yet known.

A detailed discussion of these highly specialized drugs is beyond
the scope of this book; however, the physician prescribing a biologic to you will be able to give you detailed information specific to
your situation.

Bisphosphonates

The most common use of oral bisphosphonates is for the prevention and treatment of osteoporosis. Until their recent availability, we had few therapeutic options for osteoporosis and those we did have were largely ineffective. Now, with the emergence of bisphosphonate therapy, we finally have an effective means to help prevent osteoporosis-related fractures (and therefore avoid the disability that all too often accompanies these).

Our bones contain two major types of cells responsible for the ongoing health of our skeleton. *Osteoblasts* are responsible for bone building, and *osteoclasts* are responsible for bone removal (a process called bone *resorption*). Bisphosphonates work by decreasing the number and activity of osteoclasts; as a result, we end up either maintaining the bone we have or, even better, we develop more and better bone.

In this section we look at the most commonly used bisphosphonates. Because alendronate and risedronate are so similar we discuss them together. We also look at etidronate, which has its own specific properties. We list the various orally administered bisphosphonates available in Canada in Table 6-27.

Table 6-27	Bisphosphonates
Generic Name	*Trade Name(s)*
Alendronate	Apo-Alendronate, CO Alendronate, Fosamax, Fosavance*, Gen-Alendronate, Novo-Alendronate, PMS-Alendronate
Clodronate	Bonefos, Clasteon, Ostac
Etidronate	CO-Etidronate, Didrocal*, Didronel, Gen-Etidronate
Risedronate	Actonel, Actonel Plus Calcium*

* This medicine is a combination of different drugs. Refer to the drug label to determine what they are.

 ## Alendronate, Risedronate

Apo-Alendronate, CO Alendronate, Fosamax, Fosavance*, Gen-Alendronate, Novo-Alendronate, PMS-Alendronate

Actonel, Actonel Plus Calcium*

Alendronate and risedronate reduce the risk of both vertebral (back) fractures and non-vertebral (hip and wrist) fractures in people with osteoporosis.

How alendronate and risedronate can help you

Alendronate and risedronate can help you in the following ways:

- Reducing your risk of a fracture if you have osteoporosis.

- Improving bone pain if you have a condition called Paget's disease of bone.

- Lowering the calcium level in your blood if it's high due to certain types of cancer.

How alendronate and risedronate might harm you

Possible side-effects from taking alendronate and risedronate include:

- Nausea, difficulty swallowing, esophageal and stomach ulcers, abdominal pain.

- Musculoskeletal pain (that is, pain in the bones, joints, muscles, and so on). This is typically felt as an ache similar to what you might feel if you were "coming down with the flu." Although not dangerous these pains are not pleasant, and sometimes stopping the medication is necessary in order for them to go away.

- *Osteonecrosis of the jaw* (death of the jaw bone). This is a rare complication and is much more likely to occur with intravenous bisphosphonate therapy, not oral use.

People with the following conditions shouldn't take alendronate or risedronate:

- A damaged esophagus (for example, if your esophagus is narrowed due to a stricture or has swollen blood vessels called *varices*).

- Severe kidney failure.

- Low blood calcium level. (When your low calcium level has been corrected you may then start taking the drug.)

- Being unable to sit or stand upright for at least a half-hour after taking a dose of the medication. (See below.)

 The safety of alendronate and risedronate in pregnancy and breastfeeding are unknown. If you're pregnant or breastfeeding, we recommend you discuss it with your physician before taking either of these medicines.

Precautions to follow if you're taking alendronate or risedronate

If you're prone to having a low blood calcium level, your doctor will need to monitor this level periodically.

How to take alendronate and risedronate

Alendronate and risedronate are very poorly absorbed if taken with or around the time of ingesting any other substance. Take these drugs first thing in the morning on an empty stomach and with 200 to 250 mL (6 to 8 ounces) of plain (not carbonated) water. Take no other food, beverages, or medicines for at least a half-hour after taking your dose.

To decrease the risk of the drug irritating your esophagus, stay upright (sitting, standing, or walking) for one half-hour after you take your dose so the medicine stays in the stomach.

When used to treat osteoporosis, the usual dose of alendronate is 10 mg daily or 70 mg taken once per week, and the usual dose of risedronate is 5 mg daily or 35 mg once per week. (The doses used in the treatment of Paget's disease of bone are more variable.)

For these drugs to work properly, you must consume sufficient amounts of calcium and vitamin D. If you're not getting enough in your diet, take calcium and vitamin D supplements.

℞ Etidronate

CO-Etidronate, Didrocal*, Didronel, Gen-Etidronate

Etidronate is effective at reducing the risk of having an osteoporosis-related vertebral (back) fracture, but isn't as good as other bisphosphonate drugs in helping you avoid an osteoporosis-related hip fracture. Of the various bisphosphonates, etidronate typically is the least likely to cause side-effects and is also the least expensive.

How etidronate can help you

Etidronate can help you in the following ways:

- ✔ Reducing your risk of a vertebral fracture if you have osteoporosis.

- ✔ Improving bone pain if you have a condition called Paget's disease of bone.

How etidronate might harm you

Possible side-effects from etidronate include:

- ✔ Abdominal pain, diarrhea. (Less frequently, constipation.)

- ✔ Musculoskeletal pain (that is, pain in the bones, joints, muscles, and so on). This is typically felt as an ache similar to what you might feel if you were "coming down with the flu." Although not dangerous these pains are not pleasant, and sometimes stopping the medication is necessary in order for them to go away.

People with advanced kidney failure shouldn't take etidronate.

 The safety of etidronate in pregnancy and breastfeeding is unknown. If you're pregnant or breastfeeding, we recommend you discuss it with your physician before taking this medicine.

Precautions to follow if you're taking etidronate

 If you're taking etidronate and one of your bones fractures with minimal or no obvious trauma, talk to your doctor about whether you might be better served by changing to a different bisphosphonate.

How to take etidronate

To be effective in the treatment of osteoporosis, etidronate should be taken in a special sequence with calcium: Take 400 mg of etidronate daily for 14 consecutive days, followed by 500 mg of *elemental* calcium daily for 76 consecutive days. After the completion of this 90-day protocol, start the same sequence over again.

 Etidronate and calcium come packaged together in a kit called Didrocal, which makes it easier to follow these directions.

Take etidronate two hours after your evening meal, with a glass of plain (not carbonated) water and with no other food, beverages, or other medicines for at least two hours after taking your dose.

 It's only the etidronate — not the calcium — pills that need to be taken two hours after dinner. In fact, you should take the calcium pills *with* food.

The doses of etidronate used in the treatment of Paget's disease of bone are more variable.

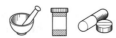

Calcium Channel Blockers

Calcium channel blockers (formerly called calcium channel antagonists) are primarily used in the treatment of cardiovascular diseases such as coronary artery disease and hypertension. Oral calcium channel blockers available in Canada are listed in Table 6-28. (Two others, nimodipine and flunarizine, have very specialized uses and thus are not discussed here.)

Certain cells within the heart and blood vessels have tiny pathways or openings (*channels*) that allow calcium to pass into these cells. Calcium channel blockers work by blocking this calcium channel; this, in turn, limits how much calcium can get into these cells. This reduction in calcium entering these cells causes the heart and blood vessels to alter their function, as we describe below.

Table 6-28	Calcium Channel Blockers	
Class	*Generic Name*	*Trade Name(s)*
Dihydropyridine	**Amlodipine**	Caduet*, Norvasc
	Felodipine	Plendil, Renedil, Sandoz Felodipine
	Nifedipine	Adalat XL, Apo-Nifed, Apo-Nifed PA, Nu-Nifed, Nu-Nifedipine-PA
Non-dihydropyridine	**Diltiazem**	Apo-Diltiaz, Apo-Diltiaz SR, Apo-Diltiaz CD, Cardizem, Cardizem CD, Gen-Diltiazem, Gen-Diltiazem CD, Novo-Diltiazem, Novo-Diltiazem CD, Novo-Diltiazem HCl ER, Nu-Diltiaz, Nu-Diltiaz-CD, ratio-Diltiazem CD, Sandoz Diltiazem CD, Sandoz Diltiazem D, Tiazac, Tiazac XC
	Verapamil	Apo-Verap, Apo-Verap SR, Covera-HS, Gen-Verapamil, Gen-Verapamil SR, Isoptin SR, Novo-Verapamil SR, Nu-Verap, Tarka*

* This medicine is a combination of different drugs. Refer to the drug label to determine what they are.

As Table 6-28 shows, there are two classes of calcium channel blocker: the dihydropyridine class and their rather uncreatively named counterpart, the non-dihydropyridine class. Drugs within each of these classes are quite similar. The main difference between the two classes is that the dihydropyridine group is

✔ Not as likely to cause the heartbeat to go too slow.

✔ Not effective at bringing an overly fast heartbeat (as, say, may happen if you have atrial fibrillation) under control.

✔ Less likely to cause congestive heart failure (if you have a damaged heart from, say, a previous heart attack).

Despite their name, calcium channel blockers have *no* effect on your blood calcium levels; also, they don't cause osteoporosis.

℞ *Amlodipine*

Caduet*, Norvasc

Amlodipine is a member of the *dihydropyridine* class of calcium channel blockers. It's, by far, the most commonly used calcium channel blocker in Canada, with more than 5 million prescriptions written for this drug in 2005.

How amlodipine can help you

Amlodipine can help you in the following ways:

✔ Controlling high blood pressure.

✔ Improving angina.

✔ Making you less prone to attacks of Raynaud's phenomenon. (There is, however, more evidence for the benefit of another calcium channel blocker — nifedipine — for this purpose.)

✔ Preventing migraine headaches. (There is, however, more evidence for the benefit of another calcium channel blocker — verapamil — for this purpose.)

How amlodipine might harm you

Possible side-effects from amlodipine include:

✔ *Peripheral edema* (ankle swelling) and headache. These are, by far, the most common side-effects. Although they can be bothersome, they aren't serious and typically go away promptly if the drug is discontinued.

✔ Worsening of angina. This happens rarely (the drug almost always *lessens* angina). If, shortly after starting amlodipine, you find your angina is worsening, seek prompt medical attention.

People with the following conditions shouldn't take amlodipine:

- ✔ Allergies to amlodipine or other dihydropyridine calcium channel blockers.

- ✔ Low blood pressure. (*How* low depends on your particular situation.)

 The safety of amlodipine in pregnancy and breastfeeding is unknown. If you're pregnant or breastfeeding, we recommend you discuss it with your physician before taking this medicine.

Precautions to follow if you're taking amlodipine

If you develop faintness it may mean your blood pressure has fallen too low. If this happens, inform your physician.

 If you're taking amlodipine to treat hypertension, consider obtaining a blood pressure machine for home use. Using it regularly will help you know if the therapy is working and, in the case of the aforementioned dizziness, will enable you to see if your blood pressure is too low.

How to take amlodipine

Amlodipine is taken once daily, starting with 5 mg. The dose is then adjusted, under your doctor's supervision, based on your response. The usual maintenance dose is 10 mg per day. You can take amlodipine with or without food.

  Avoid consuming grapefruit or grapefruit juice because it can affect the level of amlodipine in your blood.

℞ Diltiazem

Apo-Diltiaz, Apo-Diltiaz SR, Apo-Diltiaz CD, Cardizem, Cardizem CD, Gen-Diltiazem, Gen-Diltiazem CD, Novo-Diltiazem, Novo-Diltiazem CD, Novo-Diltiazem HCl ER, Nu-Diltiaz, Nu-Diltiaz-CD, ratio-Diltiazem CD, Sandoz Diltiazem CD, Sandoz Diltiazem D, Tiazac, Tiazac XC

Diltiazem is a member of the non-dihydropyridine class of calcium channel blockers. Its effectiveness and its good safety profile make it a justifiably popular prescription drug.

How diltiazem can help you

Diltiazem can help you in the following ways:

- ✔ Controlling high blood pressure.

- ✔ Improving *angina*.

✔ Controlling your heart rate if you have a heart rhythm problem called atrial fibrillation.

✔ Making you less prone to attacks of Raynaud's phenomenon. (There is, however, more evidence for the benefit of another calcium channel blocker — nifedipine — for this purpose.)

✔ Preventing migraine headaches. (There is, however, more evidence for the benefit of another calcium channel blocker — *verapamil* — for this purpose.)

How diltiazem might harm you

Possible side-effects from diltiazem include:

✔ Congestive heart failure. This is likely to occur only if you already have quite extensive heart damage (from, say, a previous heart attack).

✔ An overly slow heartbeat. If severe, this can make you feel faint.

✔ *Peripheral edema* (ankle swelling).

✔ Headache.

✔ Liver inflammation. This seldom occurs.

People with the following conditions shouldn't take diltiazem:

✔ Congestive heart failure.

✔ Very slow heartbeat.

✔ Low blood pressure. (*How* low depends on your particular situation.)

The safety of diltiazem in pregnancy and breastfeeding is unknown. If you're pregnant or breastfeeding, we recommend you discuss it with your physician before taking this medicine.

Precautions to follow if you're taking diltiazem

If you develop faintness it may mean your blood pressure has fallen too low. If this happens, inform your physician.

If you're taking diltiazem to treat hypertension, consider obtaining a blood pressure machine for home use. Using it regularly will help you know if the therapy is working and, in the case of the aforementioned dizziness, will allow you to see if your blood pressure is too low.

How to take diltiazem

Depending on the particular type of diltiazem you have been prescribed, you take it anywhere from once daily to three times daily. The usual *total* daily starting dose is between 90 mg and 180 mg.

It's possible that the level of diltiazem in your blood may be affected by consumption of grapefruit and grapefruit juice so we recommend avoiding these.

Whether you may take your diltiazem with food depends on the particular type of diltiazem you've been prescribed, so we recommend you check with your pharmacist.

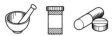

Cholesterol Absorption Inhibitors

There is, technically, only one drug (ezetimibe) in this group. But, because we don't think technicality should get in the way of practicality, Table 6-29 also includes *binding resins* — these also inhibit the absorption of cholesterol (albeit by a different means), but by convention are classified as, well, binding resins. With the advent of statins (which we discuss elsewhere in this chapter) and, latterly, etezimibe — both of which are generally well tolerated and effective — binding resins (which are not very potent and which can cause unpleasant gastrointestinal side-effects) are now seldom prescribed.

Table 6-29	Cholesterol Absorption Inhibitors	
Class	*Generic Name*	*Trade Name*
Binding resins	Cholestyramine Resin	PMS-Cholestyramine
	Colestipol	Colestid
Cholesterol absorption inhibitor	**Ezetimibe**	Ezetrol

 Ezetimibe

Ezetrol

Ezetimibe is typically used to treat high levels of LDL cholesterol in people who are not getting a sufficient response to — or are unable to tolerate — statin therapy. (For the lowdown on LDL cholesterol, see Chapter 5.)

The cholesterol in our food is absorbed into our body in the small intestine. Ezetimibe acts within the small intestine to block the absorption of cholesterol. This non-absorbed cholesterol is then excreted from the body in the stool.

How ezetimibe can help you

Ezetimibe can help you by improving your cholesterol and triglyceride levels. (Presumably this will lead to a reduced risk of a heart attack, but, unlike statin therapy, we don't yet have proof that ezetimibe reduces this risk.)

How ezetimibe might harm you

Possible side-effects from taking ezetimibe include:

- Headache.

- Abdominal pain, diarrhea.

- Abnormal liver tests. Taken on its own, ezetimibe is highly unlikely to cause this; however, if taken together with a statin, the risk is slightly increased compared to taking a statin alone.

- Inflammation of the pancreas (*pancreatitis*).

- Decreased platelet count.

- Muscle soreness, or damage (*rhabdomyolysis*).

Serious side-effects from ezetimibe seldom occur.

The safety of ezetimibe in pregnancy and breastfeeding is unknown. If you're pregnant or breastfeeding, we recommend you discuss it with your physician before taking this medicine.

Precautions to follow if you're taking ezetimibe

If you develop muscle pains or persisting abdominal pain, see your doctor promptly.

How to take ezetimibe

The dose of ezetimibe is 10 mg. You can take it with or without food and at any time during the day, but preferably at a similar time day to day. If you're also taking a binding resin, ezetimibe should be taken at least two hours before or four hours after this other medicine.

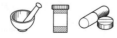

Contraceptive Therapy

In this section we look at prescription drug therapy for contraception (that is, preventing pregnancy). Over the past few years the number of such options has increased with the advent of contraceptive "rings" and injections. However, no contraceptive medicines are available for men (though, of course, condoms were still being sold the last time we were in a drugstore!) Table 6-30 lists the various contraceptive drugs available in Canada. (We don't include IUDs.)

Table 6-30	Contraceptive Therapy	
Class	*Generic Name*	*Trade Name(s)*
Oral contraceptive therapy (OCT or OC) ±	**Ethinyl Estradiol + Cyproterone Acetate**	Diane-35**
	Ethinyl Estradiol + Desogestrel	Marvelon, Ortho-Cept, Linessa 21, Linessa 28
	Ethinyl estradiol + Drospirenone	Yasmin (21 and 28)
	Ethinyl Estradiol + Ethynodiol Diacetate	Demulen 30
	Ethinyl estradiol + Levonorgestrel	Alesse 21, Alesse 28, Min-Ovral 21, Min-Ovral 28, Triphasil 21, Triphasil 28, Triquilar 21, Triquilar 28
	Ethinyl Estradiol + Norethindrone	Brevicon 0.5/35, Brevicon 1/35, Ortho 0.5/35, Ortho 1/35, Ortho 7/7/7, Select 1/35, Synphasic
	Ethinyl Estradiol + Norgestimate	Cyclen, Tri-Cyclen LO, Tri-Cyclen
	Ethinyl Estradiol + Norgestrel	Ovral 21, Ovral 28
Transdermal contraceptive patch	Ethinyl Estradiol + Norelgestromin	Evra
Transvaginal contraceptive ring	Ethinyl Estradiol + etonogestrel	NuvaRing

Class	Generic Name	Trade Name(s)
Injectable contra-ceptive therapy	**Medroxy-progesterone acetate**	Depo-Provera
Emergency contra-ceptive therapy	**Levonorgestrel**	Plan B

± *Oral contraceptive therapies are also known as combined oral contraceptives (COC).*

** *Although having contraceptive properties, Diane-35 is primarily used, as we discuss in Chapter 5, for the treatment of acne.*

There are also intrauterine contraceptive devices (IUDs) that contain progesterone.

Because oral contraceptives are so similar in terms of how they work, their side-effects, and so forth, we discuss them together.

Oral contraceptive therapies

The introduction of "The Pill" revolutionized birth control by giving women the opportunity to be in charge of their reproduction. Oral contraceptives, however, are not taken without some element of risk (although it's small).

Gonadotropins are hormones, produced in the brain, that travel in the blood stream to the ovaries, influencing the ovaries to release ova (eggs) into the fallopian tubes. The process of an ovum (ovum is singular; ova is plural) being released from the ovary is called *ovulation*. Within the fallopian tube, an ovum meets up with sperm (well, if the sperm happen to be there), and, if the sperm fertilizes the ovum, the fertilized ovum travels down into the uterus and attaches to the wall of the uterus, where the pregnancy continues.

Oral contraceptives work by lowering levels of the gonadotropins. With lower amounts of gonadotropins to stimulate the ovaries, ova are not released. And no ova, no pregnancy — just a bunch of lonely sperm hanging around with no place to go.

How oral contraceptives can help you

Oral contraceptives can help you in the following ways:

- ✔ Preventing pregnancy.
- ✔ Regulating your menstrual cycles, decreasing menstrual blood flow, and decreasing menstrual cramping.
- ✔ Decreasing the likelihood of developing ovarian cysts.

✔ Decreasing the risk of ovarian and uterine cancer.

✔ Treating severe acne — this is limited to preparations such as Alesse, Diane-35, and Tri-Cyclen.

How oral contraceptives might harm you

Possible side-effects from taking oral contraceptives include:

✔ Weight gain.

✔ Breast tenderness and enlargement.

✔ Nausea.

✔ Liver damage.

✔ Blood clots (which, in turn, can cause serious problems such as strokes, heart attacks, damage to the retina in the eye, deep vein thrombosis, and pulmonary emboli. We discuss these conditions in Chapter 5.)

Women with the following conditions shouldn't take oral contraceptives:

✔ Being both over age 35 *and* a smoker. If you smoke and are over 35, taking oral contraceptives becomes much riskier, with higher rates of serious complications such as heart attacks and strokes.

✔ Pregnancy or trying to become pregnant.

✔ Difficulty in remembering to take medication regularly.

✔ Serious liver disease.

✔ Previous blood clot or being at high risk for a blood clot.

✔ Uncontrolled high blood pressure.

✔ Previous heart attack or stroke or other serious cardiovascular disease.

✔ Migraine headache disorder if associated with other neurological symptoms (such as numbness or weakness of a limb).

✔ Undiagnosed, abnormal vaginal bleeding.

✔ Breast or uterine cancer.

Before you start taking oral contraceptives, you need to have a complete evaluation of your health by your doctor to assess your risk for side-effects.

Use of oral contraceptives is thought to be safe during breastfeeding; however, it may reduce the amount of breast milk you're producing. Before taking oral contraceptives in this circumstance we recommend you speak with your physician.

Precautions to follow if you're taking oral contraceptives

Follow these precautions if you're taking oral contraceptives:

✔ Oral contraceptives do *not* provide protection against getting (or giving) sexually transmitted diseases (including HIV/AIDS), so use of appropriate protection such as condoms remains essential.

✔ If you're to be immobilized for several weeks — for example, as a result of surgery — discontinuation of your contraceptive medication four to six weeks prior will help minimize your risk of *deep vein thrombosis* (that is, a blood clot in the veins of your leg) after surgery.

✔ You need to be meticulous about taking your medicine. Missing even a single dose of your oral contraceptive reduces its effectiveness.

If you miss any of your doses, make use of another form of contraception (such as a condom). The length of time you need to continue with this alternative contraception depends on a number of factors — ask your physician (or pharmacist) for advice specific to your circumstance.

How to take contraceptive medication

Most oral contraceptive medications come as 21- or 28-day packs.

✔ With the 21-day packs, all 21 pills are the active medication, and when they're finished you use no medication for the next seven days. You would then start another package of pills, so you keep a four-week cycle for your birth control medication.

✔ With the 28-day packs, the first 21 tablets are the active medication and when they're finished you then take the remaining 7 pills (which have no medication but are used to help you maintain a four-week cycle).

Take oral contraceptive medicine at the same time each day, with or without food.

Medroxy-progesterone acetate (Depo-Provera)

Depo-Provera is an injectable form of contraceptive. For some women, Depo-Provera is preferred to oral contraceptives as the user does not have to remember to take a contraceptive pill every day.

Gonadotropins are hormones, produced in the brain, that travel in the blood stream to the ovaries, influencing the ovaries to release ova (eggs) into the fallopian tubes. The process of an ovum (ovum is singular; ova is plural) being released from the ovary is called *ovulation.* Within the fallopian tube, an ovum meets up with sperm (well, if the sperm happen to be there), and, if the sperm fertilizes the ovum, the fertilized ovum travels down into the uterus and attaches to the wall of the uterus, where the pregnancy continues.

Depo-Provera works by lowering levels of the gonadotropins. With lower amounts of gonadotropins to stimulate the ovaries, ova are not released. And no ova, no pregnancy. (Which for women not seeking pregnancy may result in a standing *ova*tion.)

How medroxy-progesterone acetate (Depo-Provera) can help you

Depo-Provera can help you by preventing pregnancy. It's also used in the treatment of some cases of cancer of the uterus or kidney, and to lessen pain from endometriosis.

How medroxy-progesterone acetate (Depo-Provera) might harm you

Possible side-effects from taking Depo-Provera include:

✔ Menstrual irregularities. This occurs in most users during the first year of therapy, after which you become increasingly likely to start missing periods altogether.

✔ Weight gain.

✔ Abdominal or pelvic pain.

✔ Decreased interest in sexual activity (decreased *libido*).

✔ Osteoporosis.

When you shouldn't use medroxy-progesterone acetate (Depo-Provera)

Women with the following conditions shouldn't use Depo-Provera:

✔ Pregnancy or intending to become pregnant in the near future.

✔ Serious liver disease.

You may come across reputable sources of information that say medroxy-progesterone shouldn't be used by women who have had (or are at high risk for) blood clots. Nonetheless, many experts in the field feel it can be safely used in these circumstances.

It's considered safe to breastfeed while taking Depo-Provera.

Precautions to follow if you're using medroxy-progesterone acetate (Depo-Provera)

The effectiveness of Depo-Provera can be affected by other therapies (both prescription and non-prescription, including certain herbs). Be sure to review *all* your treatments with your pharmacist.

Depo-Provera does *not* provide protection against getting (or giving) sexually transmitted diseases (including HIV/AIDS). Using appropriate protection such as condoms remains essential.

How to use medroxy-progesterone acetate (Depo-Provera)

Depo-Provera is given by your health care provider as an injection into a muscle in the buttock or arm. The first injection is best given between the first and fifth day of your menstrual period to minimize the likelihood you're pregnant when starting the medication. The injections are then repeated every three months.

If there has been a delay between injections and it has been more than 13 weeks since your last dose, you may no longer be sufficiently protected from getting pregnant; therefore, another form of contraception will be required.

Levonorgestrel (Plan B)

Levonorgestrel is used as an emergency form of contraception; that is, if there has been sexual intercourse without effective contraception being used, or if the contraception being used failed (such as a condom breaking).

Levonorgestrel is available as a "behind-the-counter" medicine (that is; you can obtain it without a doctor's prescription). We discuss drug classification in Chapter 2.

How levonorgestrel (Plan B) works

Levonorgestrel works in several possible ways:

- Preventing *ovulation* (that is, release of an *ovum* — egg — from the ovary).

- Inhibiting the movement of an ovum and the sperm, making them less likely to meet and result in a fertilized egg.

- Preventing a fertilized egg from attaching to the lining of the uterus, where it would lead to continued pregnancy. (This particular mechanism isn't as proven as the previous two.)

How levonorgestrel (Plan B) can help you

Levonorgestrel can help you by preventing pregnancy.

How levonorgestrel (Plan B) might harm you

Possible side-effects from using levonorgestrel include:

- ✔ Nausea, vomiting, abdominal pain, fatigue, headache. One or more of these symptoms develop in up to 25 percent of people taking this drug.

- ✔ Menstrual irregularities.

When you shouldn't use levonorgestrel (Plan B)

Women with the following conditions shouldn't use levonorgestrel:

- ✔ Pregnancy (from previous intercourse).

- ✔ Vaginal bleeding if the cause is unknown.

It's *probably* safe to breastfeed after using levonorgestrel, however we recommend you discuss this with your physician.

Precautions to follow if you're using levonorgestrel (Plan B)

Levonorgestrel does *not* provide protection against getting (or giving) sexually transmitted diseases (including HIV/AIDS). Using appropriate protection such as condoms remains essential.

How to take levonorgestrel (Plan B)

Take one tablet as soon as possible after and within 72 hours of unprotected sexual intercourse, and then take a second tablet 12 hours after the first one. Each tablet contains 0.75 mg of levonorgestrel. You can take this medicine at any time during your menstrual cycle.

If you vomit within one hour of taking a dose, speak to your pharmacist or your doctor to see whether you should take an extra dose to make up for any medicine you may have lost when you vomited.

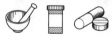

Corticosteroids

Corticosteroids are used to treat an incredibly wide variety of diseases, as we discuss below. These medicines act in a way that is similar to *cortisol,* which is the body's own, naturally occuring corticosteroid. Cortisol is a hormone produced by the *adrenal glands* (tiny little hat-shaped organs that sit on top of the kidneys). Cortisol is necessary for normal metabolism and to allow the body to respond to stress. Additionally, cortisol has powerful *anti-inflammatory* (the ability to reduce inflammation) and *immunosuppressive* (the ability to suppress the immune system) actions.

In your travels, you may come across the term glucocorticoid used interchangeably with corticosteroid. Although technically this isn't quite accurate (glucocorticoids are actually but *one type* of corticosteroid), the two words are typically used to refer to the same thing. Also, corticosteroids are *entirely different* from the notorious *anabolic* steroids that some body-builders and athletes (inappropriately) use.

Depending on the particular disease being treated, different forms of corticosteroid are given: drops, creams, pills, enemas ... if you can think of a way to give a drug you can be darn sure there's a corticosteroid that fits the bill. Whenever possible, your doctor will prescribe a form of corticosteroid that goes directly to the diseased area; that way, the risk of side-effects in other parts of the body is reduced.

This section is organized alphabetically by the route by which the corticosteroid medicine is given. Table 6-31 lists the different types of corticosteroids, alphabetically, by the headings we use in this section. (Inhaled corticosteroids are discussed in the "Inhaled Medicines to Treat Asthma and COPD" section of this chapter.) Corticosteroids act very similarly; as such, we discuss in detail those corticosteroids that are in particularly common use in Canada.

Table 6-31	Corticosteroids
Generic Name	**Trade Name(s)**
Nasal Corticosteroids	
Beclomethasone	Apo-Beclomethasone, Gen-Beclo AQ, Nu-Beclomethasone, ratio-Beclomethasone AQ, Rivanase AQ
Budesonide	Gen-Budesonide AQ, Rhinocort Aqua
Flunisolide	Apo-Flunisolide, ratio-Flunisolide, Rhinalar
Fluticasone	Flonase
Mometasone	Nasonex
Triamcinolone	Nasacort AQ

(continued)

Table 6-31 *(continued)*

Generic Name	Trade Name(s)
Ophthalmic (Eye) Corticosteroids	
Betamethasone	Garasone Ophthalmic *(solution and ointment)
Dexamethasone	Maxidex, Maxitrol*, PMS-Dexamethasone drops, Sandoz Opticort*, Sofracort*
Flunisolide	Apo-Flunisolide, ratio-Flunisolide
Fluorometholone	FML Forte
Hydrocortisone	Cortisporin*, Sandoz Cortimyxin Ophthalmic Ointment*
Prednisolone	Blephamide*, Pred Forte, Pred Mild, ratio-Prednisolone, Sandoz Prednisolone
Rimexolone	Vexol
Oral Corticosteroids	
Budesonide	Entocort Capsules
Cortisone	Cortisone Acetate
Dexamethasone	Apo-Dexamethasone, Dexasone, PMS-Dexamethasone elixir, PMS-Dexamethasone, ratio-Dexamethasone
Fludrocortisone±	Florinef
Hydrocortisone	Cortef
Methyprednisolone	Medrol
Prednisolone	Pediapred
Prednisone	Apo-Prednisone, Novo-Prednisone, Winpred
Triamcinolone	Kenalog in Orabase**, Oracort**
Otic (Ear) Corticosteroids	
Betamethasone	Garasone Otic*
Dexamethasone	Ciprodex*, PMS-Dexamethasone Drops, Sandoz Opticort*, Sofracort*, Tobradex*
Flumethasone	Locacorten Vioform*
Flunisolide	Apo-Flunisolide, ratio–Flunisolide
Hydrocortisone	Cortisporin ear/eye suspension*, Sandoz Cortimyxin Otic Solution*
Rectal Corticosteroids	
Budesonide	Entocort Enema

Generic Name	Trade Name(s)
Rectal Corticosteroids	
Hydrocortisone	Enemas: Cortenema, Hycort
	Suppositories and ointments: Proctodan HC*, Proctofoam HC*, Proctol*, Proctosedyl*, Sandoz Proctomyxin*
Topical Corticosteroids	
Amcinonide	Amcort, Cyclocort, ratio- Amcinonide, Taro-Amcinonide
Betamethasone	Betaderm, Diprolene Gycol, Diprosone, Dovobet*, Lotriderm*, Propaderm, ratio-Ectosone, ratio-Topilene, ratio- Topisalic*, ratio-Toposone, Sandoz Pentasone*, Taro- Sone, Valisone – G*, Valisone Scalp Lotion
Clobetasol	Clobetasol, Clobex preparations, Dermovate, Gen-Clobetasol, Novo-Clobetasol, ratio-Clobetasol
Clobetasone	Eumovate
Desonide	Desocort, PMS- Desonide
Desoximetasone	Topicort
Diflucortolone	Nerisone, Nerisalic*
Flumethasone	Locacorten Vioform*
Fluocinolone	Capex
Fluocinonide	Lyderm, Tiamol
Fluticasone	Cutivate
Halcinonide	Halog preparations
Halobetasol	Ultravate preparations
Hydrocortisone	Barriere-HC, Cipro HC*, Cortisporin Ointment*, Cortoderm, Emo-Cort, Hyderm, Hydrosone, HydroVal, Prevex HC, Sarna HC, Vioform Hydrocortisone, Westcort Preparations
Methyprednisolone	Medrol Acne Lotion*, NeoMedrol*
Mometasone	Elocom, ratio-Mometasone, Taro-Mometasone
Prednicarbate	Dermatop
Triamcinolone	Aristocort C, Aristocort R, ratio-Triacomb*, Triaderm, ViadermKC*

This medicine is a combination of different drugs. Refer to the drug label to determine what they are.

**These are "dental creams" for use within the mouth.*

± *Fludrocortisone is a mineralocorticoid type of corticosteroid.*

Nasal corticosteroids

Judging by the fact that every year in Canada there are millions of prescriptions written for nasal corticosteroids, one can reasonably conclude two things: first, those of us north of the 49th are having problems with nasal congestion, and second, facial tissue sales must be very brisk, indeed.

 ## Mometasone

Nasonex

Mometasone is the active ingredient in a commonly used, steroid-containing nose spray called Nasonex.

 Mometasone, when delivered by nasal spray, is absorbed into the tissues of the nose (known as the *nasal mucosa*), where it reduces the production of the chemical messengers that cause inflammation in the region. Taken as prescribed, it has very little, if any, effect on the rest of the body.

How mometasone nasal spray can help you

Mometasone nasal spray can help you by relieving runny nose, stuffiness, and congestion caused by seasonal allergies and some types of sinusitis.

How mometasone nasal spray might harm you

Side-effects from taking mometasone nasal spray rarely occur. Possible side-effects include:

- ✔ Headaches; stinging, burning, or bleeding in the nose.
- ✔ Upper respiratory infections.

People with the following conditions shouldn't take mometasone nasal spray:

- ✔ Ulcers in the nose.
- ✔ Recent surgery or injury/damage to your nose.
- ✔ Current infection, especially if affecting the nasal passages.
- ✔ Tuberculosis affecting the lungs.

 Mometasone nasal spray is likely safe to take during pregnancy and breastfeeding; however, if you're pregnant or breastfeeding, we recommend you discuss it with your physician before taking this medicine.

Precautions to follow if you're taking mometasone nasal spray

Eye infections caused by the herpes simplex virus can be made worse if this medicine gets into your eye. For this reason, if you have this type of infection, be sure to ask your doctor whether you should discontinue your mometasone until the eye infection is cured. If you continue the drug, be careful none of it gets into your eye.

Your doctor should examine your nostrils from time to time to assess the health of your nasal tissues.

How to take mometasone nasal spray

The usual starting dose of mometasone (if given as Nasonex) is two sprays in each nostril once daily, with the dose then adjusted, under your doctor's supervision, based on your response. We discuss the proper use of nose sprays in Chapter 4. Unlike fast-acting decongestant nose sprays (such as Otrivin or Dristan), mometasone nasal spray does not work immediately — it may take days or weeks before you receive full benefit.

If you have also been prescribed a decongestant, use the decongestant first and then take the mometasone.

Avoid prolonged exposure of this medication to direct light. It may be best to store it in the cardboard box in which it came.

Ophthalmic (eye) corticosteroids

Corticosteroid medication can be placed directly into the eye (in the form of eye drops) to reduce inflammation and to prevent scarring and, by so doing, to protect your sight. We discuss this form of therapy in this section.

 ## Prednisolone

Blephamide*, Pred Forte, Pred Mild, ratio-Prednisolone, Sandoz Prednisolone

Many steroid-containing eye drop products contain multiple ingredients. This discussion, however, looks only at one particular ingredient: the corticosteroid prednisolone.

Corticosteroid eye drops like prednisolone reduce the production of the chemical messengers that cause inflammation in the eye. Taken as prescribed, these eye drops have very little, if any, effect on the rest of the body.

How prednisolone eye drops can help you

Prednisolone eye drops can help you by relieving eye irritation and swelling (and, depending on the condition, reducing the likelihood of scarring) caused by allergies, autoimmune diseases (such as rheumatoid arthritis), and certain forms of eye injury or eye surgery.

How prednisolone eye drops might harm you

Possible side-effects from taking prednisolone eye drops include:

- Increased pressure within the eye (*raised intra-ocular pressure: IOP*). This can lead to or worsen glaucoma.
- Cataracts.
- Fungal infections of the eye.

Raised IOP can occur within two weeks of starting this medicine; however, it and the other side-effects listed above are more likely to occur with long-term use.

People with the following conditions shouldn't take prednisolone eye drops:

- Viral, fungal, or tuberculous infections of the eye.
- Untreated bacterial conjunctivitis.

Prednisolone eye drops are likely safe to take during pregnancy and breastfeeding, however we recommend before taking this medicine in these circumstances you discuss this with your physician.

Precautions to follow if you're taking prednisolone eye drops

Follow these precautions if you're taking prednisolone eye drops:

- Wearing contact lenses will increase your risk of an eye infection. We suggest you ask your doctor if you should discontinue using your contacts while taking this medicine.
- If you use these eye drops for 10 days or longer your eye doctor should monitor your intra-ocular pressure.
- Let your doctor know if you have previously had a herpes infection affecting your eye, because use of prednisolone eye drops may cause your old eye infection to re-emerge.

How to use prednisolone eye drops

The dose you require depends on the particular brand you're prescribed and the condition being treated. Prednisolone eye drops come in a liquid suspension and therefore must be shaken before use. We discuss the proper use of eye drops in Chapter 4.

If your doctor feels you may continue wearing contacts (see above), be sure to remove them before your dose and replace them no sooner than 15 minutes later.

Oral corticosteroids

Oral corticosteroids have revolutionized the treatment of an amazingly diverse group of diseases. Indeed, few, if any, other classes of drug have filled so many roles. Although oral corticosteroids are routinely life-enhancing and, indeed, life-saving, they can have very serious side-effects and are certainly not to be used lightly. Unlike corticosteroids that are placed in a specific part of the body (such as eye drops or ear drops), oral corticosteroids go to all regions of the body (hence, their greater risk of side-effects). The various oral corticosteroids are, in general, very similar.

℞ Prednisone

Apo-Prednisone, Novo-Prednisone, Winpred

Prednisone is in particularly common use in Canada and, thus, is the focus of this discussion.

Prednisone works by decreasing the amount of inflammation in the body and reducing the activity of the immune system. It accomplishes the former, in part, by lowering the number of inflammation-causing chemical messengers (such as cytokines) being produced by white blood cells.

How prednisone can help you

Prednisone can help you by alleviating symptoms and reducing damage to the body caused by an astounding number of serious conditions, including:

- ✔ Allergies (if severe).

- ✔ Lung diseases such as asthma, exacerbations of COPD, interstitial pneumonitis (a form of inflamed lung tissue), and sarcoidosis.

- ✔ Arthritis diseases such as rheumatoid arthritis, psoriatic arthritis, ankylosing spondylitis, and gout.

- ✔ *Connective tissue diseases* (special forms of arthritis conditions) such as lupus, polymyositis, dermatomyositis, vasculitis, polymyalgia rheumatica, and temporal arteritis.

- ✔ Skin diseases such as pemphigus, pemphigoid, and, if severe, dermatitis.

✔ Eye diseases such as iritis and optic neuritis.

✔ Blood diseases such as autoimmune thrombocytopenia and autoimmune hemolytic anemia.

✔ Bowel diseases such as Crohn's disease and ulcerative colitis.

✔ Neurologic diseases such as multiple sclerosis and brain tumours. (Corticosteroids are used to treat brain swelling due to brain tumours. Typically dexamethasone, rather than prednisone, is used in this situation.)

✔ Endocrine diseases such as Addison's disease and subacute thyroiditis.

✔ Cancers such as certain lymphomas and leukemias.

✔ Certain kidney diseases where large amounts of protein are lost into the urine (*nephrotic syndrome*).

✔ Organ transplants. Prednisone is used to help minimize rejection.

As you look through this list of ailments, you will almost certainly recognize diseases you have some familiarity with, either because you have had one of these conditions or because you know someone who has. We can only imagine the number of people whose lives have been made better — indeed, whose continued existence has been made possible — because of corticosteroid therapy like prednisone. Regrettably, though, these drugs are not without their *very* significant downsides. We discuss these next.

How prednisone might harm you

Possible side-effects from taking prednisone include:

✔ Increased appetite, weight gain (especially around the waist), a rounded appearance to the face (*cushingoid facies*). With long-term therapy you may develop stretch marks on your abdomen (*striae*).

✔ Diabetes or, if you already have diabetes, an increase in your blood glucose levels.

✔ Adrenal gland malfunction. Long-term therapy can make your adrenal glands unable to make cortisol (the body's own natural equivalent of prednisone).

✔ Mood changes and insomnia; rarely, hallucinations or psychosis.

✔ High blood pressure, elevated cholesterol levels, atherosclerosis (which can lead to heart disease), fluid retention.

✔ Increased risk of infection and, if you have an infection, loss of some of the usual clues that might alert you to this. (If you *already have* an infection, let your doctor know this before you start taking prednisone.)

✔ Easy bruising, thinning of the skin, slow healing of cuts and other wounds.

✔ Glaucoma and cataracts.

✔ Weakness of arm and leg muscles, osteoporosis, damage to the hip joint (*avascular necrosis*).

You may find this list intimidating. We sure do. Prednisone is much more likely to cause these side-effects, however, if it's used in high doses and for long periods of time. The moral of the story: prednisone can be a wondrous drug, but it can also do significant harm and thus needs to be used in the lowest dose and for the shortest period of time necessary.

If you're taking appropriate doses of prednisone (or another type of corticosteroid) to treat Addison's disease you're not at risk of these side-effects, because you will be simply taking the amount of hormone your body would normally produce.

People with the following conditions shouldn't be started on prednisone:

✔ Serious, internal, fungal infections.

✔ Ameba infections. If you're at high risk for this (such as if you were recently in the tropics) or if you have unexplained diarrhea, have a test for ameba infection before you start prednisone.

Prednisone is generally very safe for pregnant women, however there is evidence of an increased risk of cleft palate in the newborn. Prednisone is considered safe to take during breastfeeding. If you're pregnant or breastfeeding, we recommend you discuss it with your physician before taking this medicine.

Precautions to follow if you're taking prednisone

Follow these precautions if you're taking prednisone:

✔ **Never** stop taking your prednisone — especially if you have been on it for a long time — unless directed to do so by your doctor. Long-term prednisone therapy, as we discuss above, can cause the adrenal glands to stop making cortisol (your own body's equivalent to prednisone). In this circumstance, suddenly stopping prednisone can lead to life-threatening consequences. (The other reason to have your prednisone dose slowly decreased is to reduce the risk of the disease under treatment flaring.)

✔ If you have diabetes, make sure you have a blood glucose meter and check your blood glucose reading more often — especially for the first few weeks after you start prednisone. If your blood glucose levels rise, contact your physician. If you don't have diabetes, be aware of the symptoms of high blood glucose (in particular, thirst, frequent urination, getting up at night to pass urine, unexpected weight loss, blurred vision) and seek medical attention if these occur.

✔ Bone density testing (this is a test for osteoporosis) should be done when starting prednisone therapy if the duration of treatment is expected to be more than three months. A second test is recommended 6 to 12 months later depending on the dose of prednisone you have been using.

✔ If it's expected that you will be on prednisone for more than three months, be sure to ask your doctor if you should be taking calcium and vitamin D supplements to minimize the (negative) impact of prednisone on your bone health.

✔ Your blood pressure should be checked regularly — especially if you already have hypertension.

If you're going to be taking prednisone for more than a few weeks, getting (and using) your own blood pressure cuff would be a good idea. That way you will quickly be alerted to a risk in your pressure.

How to take prednisone

Prednisone is available as 1 mg, 5 mg, and 50 mg tablets. The dose you require depends on many things including the disease being treated and how active the disease is. Prednisone is taken anywhere from several times per day to once every second day. (One advantage to taking prednisone every second day is that this reduces the risk of side-effects.)

Prednisone is best taken with meals and many people find that taking it earlier in the day makes it less likely they will run into problems sleeping (see the list of side-effects above).

Otic (ear) corticosteroids

Corticosteroid medicine that's applied directly to the ear often comes premixed with other ingredients such as an antibiotic. The corticosteroid is helpful to reduce inflammation, and the antibiotic is helpful to eradicate infection.

℞ *Dexamethasone*

Ciprodex*, PMS-Dexamethasone Drops, Sandoz Opticort*, Sofracort*, Tobradex*

Dexamethasone ear drops work directly on the tissues of the external ear (not the middle or inner ear), where they reduce inflammation.

How dexamethasone ear drops can help you

Dexamethasone ear drops can help you by treating skin rashes in the external ear due to inflammation caused by eczema or other forms of dermatitis.

 Some dexamethasone-containing drops also contain an antibiotic and so may be useful in treating *otitis externa* (swimmer's ear) caused by a bacterial infection.

How dexamethasone ear drops might harm you

If used for a short time — as is customary — side-effects are not expected.

When you shouldn't use dexamethasone ear drops

People with the following conditions shouldn't take dexamethasone ear drops:

- ✔ Middle ear infections (*otitis media*).
- ✔ Fungal, viral, or tuberculous ear infections.
- ✔ Untreated, severe, bacterial ear infections.

 Dexamethasone ear drops are likely safe for use by pregnant or breastfeeding women; however, if you're pregnant or breastfeeding, we recommend you discuss it with your physician before taking this medicine.

Precautions to follow if you're using dexamethasone ear drops

If you notice stinging or burning in the ear, discontinue using dexamethasone ear drops until you first see your doctor to make sure you don't have a perforated ear drum.

How to use dexamethasone ear drops

The dose you require depends on the particular problem being treated and the specific form of medicine you're prescribed. We discuss the proper use of ear drops in Chapter 4.

Rectal corticosteroids

Corticosteroids are given rectally to treat certain diseases of the rectum and large bowel. The advantage of this route of administration compared to oral therapy is that the medicine is directed to precisely where the problem is and there are fewer side-effects from treatment.

 ## Budesonide

Entocort Enema

Corticosteroid enemas are very effective in the treatment of ulcerative colitis when it affects the end part of the colon and the rectum. Budesonide enemas act directly on the lining of the bowel to decrease inflammation.

How budesonide enemas can help you

Budesonide enemas can help you by relieving symptoms such as diarrhea and rectal bleeding when due to ulcerative colitis affecting the end part of the colon and the rectum.

How budesonide enemas might harm you

Side-effects from using budesonide enemas are typically minor. The most common side-effects are flatulence, nausea, and diarrhea. Occasionally, a rash develops.

When you shouldn't use budesonide enemas

Budesonide enemas shouldn't be used if you have any of a number of other, serious bowel problems including an obstruction, infection, or abscess.

 The safety of budesonide enemas in pregnancy and breastfeeding is unknown. If you're pregnant or breastfeeding, we recommend you discuss it with your physician before taking this medicine.

Precautions to follow if you're taking budesonide enemas

We recommend you not stop this medicine without first discussing this with your physician.

How to take budesonide enemas

Budesonide enemas come packaged in two parts: a tablet containing the budesonide, and a liquid. Place the tablet in the bottle and then shake the bottle for at least 10 seconds until the tablet dissolves. Refer to Chapter 4 for more details on enema use.

Topical corticosteroids

Topical corticosteroids are used to treat certain skin diseases.

 ## Topical hydrocortisone

Barriere-HC, Cipro HC*, Cortisporin Ointment*, Cortoderm, Emo-Cort, Hyderm, Hydrosone, HydroVal, Prevex HC, Sarna HC, Vioform Hydrocortisone, Westcort Preparations

Topical hydrocortisone, like other topical corticosteroids, works by reducing inflammation in the area being treated.

How topical hydrocortisone can help you

Topical hydrocortisone can help you by improving skin rashes caused by or related to inflammation and/or allergies.

How topical hydrocortisone might harm you

Side-effects from short-term use of standard doses of topical hydrocortisone are not expected. Using it long-term — especially in high doses — can damage your skin (most commonly, this takes the form of thinning of the skin). The skin on your face is particularly susceptible to injury.

Other, more potent, topical corticosteroids may be more effective at treating some skin diseases, but also carry a greater risk of serious side-effects than does topical hydrocortisone, including the risk that your adrenal glands will be affected. (We discuss this above under "Oral Corticosteroids.")

When you shouldn't use topical hydrocortisone

You shouldn't use topical hydrocortisone if you have any of a number of different types of skin infection. Before prescribing this medicine, your doctor will need to examine your skin to determine whether any of these might be present.

 Topical hydrocortisone isn't expected to be a danger if taken by a pregnant or breastfeeding woman; however, if you're pregnant or breastfeeding we recommend you discuss it with your physician before taking this medicine.

Precautions to follow if you're using topical hydrocortisone

Be sure to take this medicine only as prescribed: overuse may put you at risk of side-effects (see above).

How to use topical hydrocortisone

Hydrocortisone is available as a cream, a lotion, or a special scalp preparation. The % sign on the label tells you the strength of the specific preparation and usually is between 1 and 2.5 percent. Apply the minimum amount of medication that will appropriately cover the area being treated. We discuss use of topical medicines in Chapter 4.

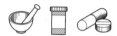

Diuretics

Diuretics are sometimes called "water pills" because of their tendency to make you pass more urine. Nonetheless, diuretics have other roles, the most important of which is helping control blood pressure. Diuretics available in Canada are listed in Table 6-32.

Several classes of diuretics exist:

- ✔ Loop diuretics are used primarily to reduce excess fluid in the body, as might occur if you have congestive heart failure, kidney failure, or, sometimes, simple ankle swelling (even if not due to anything serious). Furosemide, by far the most commonly used loop diuretic, is discussed in detail below.

- ✔ Potassium-sparing diuretics have the special property of not causing the body to become depleted of potassium. Drugs within this class are very similar to one another. We discuss the prototypical potassium-sparing diuretic — spironolactone — in detail below.

- ✔ Thiazide diuretics (with the notable exception of metolazone, which is used for similar purposes as loop diuretics) are quite similar to one another and are used primarily to help control blood pressure. Hydrochlorothiazide, the most commonly used of this class, is discussed in detail below.

Table 6-32	Diuretics	
Class	**Generic Name**	**Trade Name(s)**
Loop	Bumetanide	Burinex
	Ethacrynic Acid	Edecrin
	Furosemide	Apo-Furosemide, Lasix, Lasix Special, Novo-Semide
Potassium-sparing	Amiloride	Apo-Amiloride, Apo-Amilzide*, Gen-Amilazide*, Moduret*, Novamilor*, Nu-Amilzide*
	Spironolactone	Aldactazide 25*, Aldactazide 50*, Aldactone, Novo-Spiroton, Novo-Spirozine*
	Triamterene	Apo-Triazide*, Novo-Triamzide*, Nu-Triazide*
Thiazide	Chlorthalidone	Apo-Atenidone*, Apo-Chlorthalidone, Tenoretic*
	Hydrochlorothiazide (HCT)	Accuretic*, Aldactazide 25*, Aldactazide 50*, Apo-Amilzide*, Apo-Hydro, Apo-Triazide*, Atacand Plus*, Avalide*, Diovan-HCT*, Gen-Amilazide*, Hyzaar*, Hyzaar DS*, Inhibace Plus*, Micardis Plus*, Moduret*, Novamilor*, Novo-Hydrazide, Novo-Spirozine*, Novo-Triamzide*, Nu-Amilzide*, Nu-Triazide*, PMS-Hydrochlorothiazide, Prinzide*, Teveten Plus*, Vaseretic*, Viskazide*, Zestoretic*
	Indapamide	Apo-Indapamide, Coversyl Plus*, Gen-Indapamide*, Lozide, Novo-Indapamide, Nu-Indapamide, PMS-Indapamide, Preterax*
	Metolazone	Zaroxolyn
Carbonic anhydrase inhibitor	Acetazolamide	Apo-Acetazolamide

*This medicine is a combination of different drugs. Refer to the drug label to determine what they are. (As you can see, there is an extraordinarily lengthy list of drugs that are available in combination with diuretics. The main reason for this is that so many people with hypertension require more than one drug to control their blood pressure; by taking a combination pill containing two different drugs you're able to minimize the number of different pills you have to take. We discuss the treatment of hypertension in Chapter 5.)

Furosemide

Apo-Furosemide, Lasix, Lasix Special, Novo-Semide

Furosemide is an old drug still in common use because of its proven effectiveness in helping the body rid itself of excess fluid arising from diseases such as heart or kidney failure.

Furosemide acts on the kidneys (in special areas called the *loop of Henle*; hence the reason why furosemide is called a *loop* diuretic), causing sodium and water to be lost from the body into the urine.

How furosemide can help you

Furosemide can help you in the following ways:

- Reducing edema. This is its main role. Furosemide is particularly valuable in eliminating fluid buildup caused by congestive heart failure, liver disease, and kidney disease.

- Improving high blood pressure. Furosemide isn't typically used to treat hypertension unless you also have kidney failure or edema.

How furosemide might harm you

Possible side-effects from taking furosemide include:

- Low potassium (due to loss of potassium in the urine). This commonly occurs and can cause symptoms such as weakness and leg cramps and, infrequently, heart rhythm problems. (See the "Precautions" section below.)

- Sodium imbalance. This isn't usually a major problem.

- Dehydration. If severe, this can lead to faintness (due to low blood pressure) and can cause or worsen kidney failure.

- Gout. This typically occurs only if you're predisposed to this condition.

- Abnormal lipid (cholesterol and triglyceride) levels.

- Elevated blood glucose levels in people with diabetes.

- *Tinnitus* (ringing in the ears) and hearing loss. These occur rarely (and, when they do, it's usually in people who have severe kidney failure and are on a high dose of furosemide).

People with the following conditions shouldn't take furosemide:

✔ A very low potassium level in the blood.

✔ Dehydration.

✔ Low blood pressure. (*How* low depends on your particular situation.)

Furosemide is a sulfa-based drug, so if you've reacted to some other sulfa drug you're at risk of also reacting to furosemide. (Incidentally, many doctors are not aware of this.) Nonetheless, most people with a history of a sulfa drug reaction do *not* react to furosemide. You and your doctor need to determine whether the potential benefits of taking furosemide outweigh the potential risk of having an allergic reaction.

The safety of furosemide in pregnancy and breastfeeding is unknown. If you're pregnant or breastfeeding, we recommend you discuss it with your physician before taking this medicine.

Precautions to follow if you're taking furosemide

Follow these precautions if you're taking furosemide:

✔ You will need periodic blood tests to check your sodium, potassium, and kidney function.

✔ Monitor your blood pressure regularly.

✔ If you're taking furosemide because of edema, your weight should be closely monitored. (Your weight may reflect the amount of fluid in your body and thus may influence the dose you require.)

✔ If you have diabetes, it's wise to test your blood glucose a bit more often for the first few weeks after you start furosemide. If your blood glucose levels rise, contact your physician.

✔ You will likely need to take potassium supplements. If these have not been prescribed, we suggest you ask your doctor if they would be appropriate for you.

How to take furosemide

Furosemide is typically taken once or twice daily. The usual starting dose of furosemide is between 20 mg and 80 mg per day, with the dose subsequently adjusted, under the supervision of your doctor, based on how you're responding. Higher doses are generally required if you have kidney failure. Furosemide works best if taken on an empty stomach; however, if it upsets your stomach you may take it with food or milk.

Because furosemide is a diuretic, you may wish to make sure you have access to a bathroom for the first few hours after taking your dose. Similarly, taking a dose no closer than six hours before bedtime will help you avoid having to get up during the night to pass urine.

R⃥ *Spironolactone*

Aldactazide 25*, Aldactazide 50*, Aldactone, Novo-Spiroton, Novo-Spirozine*

We think it's kind of neat when a medicine that's been around for ages and has largely been ignored suddenly regains popularity after a new and important role for it is discovered. (Sort of reminds us how popular we became with our kids when they discovered we controlled the car keys.) This is what recently happened with spironolactone, as we discuss in this section.

Spironolactone acts on the kidneys, causing sodium and water to be lost from the body into the urine. The loss of sodium and water from the body results in lower blood pressure and improvement of *edema* (fluid retention). Unlike loop and thiazide diuretics (which we discuss elsewhere in this section), spironolactone does not cause potassium loss from the body into the urine; this is why it's called a *potassium-sparing* diuretic.

How spironolactone can help you

Spironolactone can help you in the following ways:

- ✔ Improving high blood pressure.

- ✔ Reducing edema.

- ✔ Reducing *ascites*. Ascites is a fluid buildup in the abdomen often due to cirrhosis of the liver.

- ✔ Not causing potassium deficiency (unlike loop and thiazide diuretics, which may cause potassium deficiency).

- ✔ Lowering the likelihood you will die of heart disease *if you already have a severely damaged heart.* It's this wonderful benefit that has renewed its popularity.

- ✔ Improving *hirsutism* (excess hair) and acne. It does this because it has some *anti-androgen* properties (that is, it opposes the action of male hormones such as testosterone).

How spironolactone might harm you

Possible side-effects from spironolactone include:

✔ High potassium levels (*hyperkalemia*) in the blood. If severe, this can cause life-threatening heart rhythm problems. You're at particular risk of developing high potassium levels if you have kidney failure and/or are also taking other drugs (such as angiotensin converting enzyme — ACE — inhibitors or angiotensin receptor blockers: ARBs) that tend to cause potassium retention.

✔ Erectile dysfunction, breast enlargement, menstrual irregularities.

✔ Nausea, vomiting, diarrhea. These occur infrequently.

People with the following conditions shouldn't take spironolactone:

✔ Kidney failure (unless very mild).

✔ High potassium levels in the blood.

Spironolactone is a sulfa-based drug, so if you've reacted to some other sulfa drug you're at risk of also reacting to spironolactone. (Incidentally, many doctors are not aware of this.) Nonetheless, most people with a history of a sulfa drug reaction do *not* react to spironolactone. You and your doctor need to determine whether the potential benefits of taking spironolactone outweigh the potential risk of having an allergic reaction.

The safety of spironolactone in pregnancy and breastfeeding is unknown, but because of safety concerns it's generally recommended it *not* be taken in these circumstances. If you're pregnant or breastfeeding, we recommend you discuss it with your physician before taking this medicine.

Precautions to follow if you're taking spironolactone

Follow these precautions if you're taking spironolactone:

✔ You need periodic blood tests to check your sodium, potassium, and kidney function.

✔ Your blood pressure needs to be monitored regularly.

✔ If you're taking spironolactone because of edema, closely monitor your weight. (Your weight may reflect the amount of fluid in your body and thus may influence the dose you require.)

✔ Don't use salt substitutes. These typically contain potassium and put you at risk of dangerously high blood potassium levels. Additionally, your doctor may advise you to avoid potassium-rich foods such as bananas and nuts.

How to take spironolactone

Spironolactone is typically taken once or twice daily. The usual starting dose of spironolactone is between 12.5 mg and 100 mg per day, with the dose subsequently adjusted, under your doctor's supervision, based on how you're responding. Spironolactone should be taken with food.

Because spironolactone is a diuretic, you may wish to make sure you have access to a bathroom for the first few hours after taking your dose. Similarly, taking a dose no closer than six hours before bedtime will help you avoid having to get up during the night to pass urine.

℞ Hydrochlorothiazide

Accuretic*, Aldactazide 25*, Aldactazide 50*, Apo-Amilzide*, Apo-Hydro, Apo-Triazide*, Atacand Plus*, Avalide*, Diovan-HCT*, Gen-Amilazide*, Hyzaar*, Hyzaar DS*, Inhibace Plus*, Micardis Plus*, Moduret*, Novamilor*, Novo-Hydrazide, Novo-Spirozine*, Novo-Triamzide*, Nu-Amilzide*, Nu-Triazide*, PMS-Hydrochlorothiazide, Prinzide*, Teveten Plus*, Vaseretic*, Viskazide*, Zestoretic*

Ah, hydrochlorothiazide. What a drug! Safe, well tolerated, effective, inexpensive, and gets along well with friends (in the sense of other drugs that is). Even better, recent medical studies have shown this old warhorse to be just as good as many newer, much more expensive drugs.

Hydrochlorothiazide, being the mouthful it is, is often abbreviated as HCT or, sometimes, HCTZ.

Hydrochlorothiazide acts on the kidneys, causing sodium and water to be lost from the body into the urine.

How hydrochlorothiazide can help you

Hydrochlorothiazide can help you in the following ways:

- ✔ Improving high blood pressure. This is its most common role.

- ✔ Reducing edema. It's not as effective in this role as *loop diuretics.*

- ✔ Lowering your risk of having calcium-containing kidney stones. (It does this by reducing the amount of calcium in the urine.)

- ✔ Controlling *diabetes insipidus* (this is a rare disease in which your fluid balance is out of control and you're prone to dehydration).

How hydrochlorothiazide might harm you

Possible side-effects from taking hydrochlorothiazide include:

- Low potassium.

- Sodium imbalance. This seldom happens.

- Gout. This typically occurs only if you're predisposed to this condition.

- Abnormal lipid (cholesterol and triglyceride) levels.

- Diabetes or, if you already have diabetes, making your blood glucose levels go up.

- High calcium levels in your blood (*hypercalcemia*).

- Nausea, vomiting, diarrhea. These occur infrequently.

- Muscle cramps.

- *Photosensitive skin rash.* (That is, a rash that occurs upon sun exposure.)

- Erectile dysfunction.

Many of these side-effects are more likely to occur if you're on higher doses of hydrochlorothiazide. (See "How to take hydrochlorothiazide" below.)

Hydrochlorothiazide is a sulfa-based drug, so if you've reacted to some other sulfa drug you're at risk of also reacting to hydrochlorothiazide. (Incidentally, many doctors are not aware of this.) Nonetheless, most people with a history of a sulfa drug reaction do *not* react to hydrochlorothiazide. You and your doctor will need to determine if the potential benefits of taking hydrochlorothiazide outweigh the potential risk of you having a reaction.

The safety of hydrochlorothiazide in pregnancy is unknown, but because of safety concerns it's generally recommended it *not* be taken. The safety of hydrochlorothiazide during breastfeeding is also unknown but it's generally considered safe. We recommend before taking this medicine if you're pregnant or breastfeeding, you discuss this with your physician.

Precautions to follow if you're taking hydrochlorothiazide

Follow these precautions if you're taking hydrochlorothiazide:

- You need periodic blood tests to check your sodium, potassium, and kidney function.

- Your blood pressure needs to be monitored regularly.

✔ Use sunscreen and protective clothing to help you avoid getting a photosensitive skin rash (see above).

✔ If you have diabetes, it would be wise to test your blood glucose a bit more often for the first few weeks after you start hydrochlorothiazide. If your blood glucose levels rise, contact your physician.

How to take hydrochlorothiazide

The usual starting dose of hydrochlorothiazide is 6.25 mg to 25 mg taken once daily with the dose subsequently adjusted, under your doctor's supervision, based on how you're responding. Doses higher than 25 mg per day don't usually provide additional benefit and are more likely to lead to side-effects. Hydrochlorothiazide may be taken with or without food; if it's upsetting your stomach, you may find relief by taking it with food or milk.

Hydrochlorothiazide tablets are typically 25-mg strength. If you've been prescribed a 6.25-mg dose, they need to be broken into quarters. This isn't an easy task, so you may want to ask your pharmacist to do it for you.

Because hydrochlorothiazide is a diuretic, you may wish to make sure you have access to a bathroom for the first few hours after taking your dose. Similarly, taking a dose no closer than six hours before bedtime will help you avoid having to get up during the night to pass urine. In any event, after about two weeks of use most people find they aren't needing to pass more urine than they did before they started the drug. (Despite this, the medicine continues to provide the benefits we discuss above.)

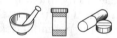

Dopamine Agonists

Dopamine agonists have different roles depending on which member of this drug family is being used. We discuss dopamine agonist therapy for Parkinson's disease in the "Antiparkinsonian Drugs" section of this chapter. In this section we look at those dopamine agonists whose main role is the treatment of health issues related to high prolactin hormone levels (*hyperprolactinemia*).

The pituitary gland's normal responsibilities include making prolactin hormone and growth hormone. Certain pituitary tumours can make too much hormone and can also be big enough to press on surrounding healthy brain tissue; both of these things can be dangerous. Dopamine agonists act directly on the cells in the pituitary gland that make prolactin and growth hormone and decrease their production of these hormones.

Table 6-33 lists those dopamine agonists available in Canada to treat high prolactin levels. These two drugs (bromocriptine and cabergoline) are very similar to one another; their main differences are that bromocriptine is *much* cheaper and, at the same time, much more likely to make you feel nauseated. No justice here, we'd say.

Table 6-33	Dopamine Agonists
Generic Name	*Trade Name(s)*
Bromocriptine	Apo-Bromocriptine, Parlodel, PMS-Bromocriptine
Cabergoline	Dostinex

 Bromocriptine

Apo-Bromocriptine, Parlodel, PMS-Bromocriptine

Bromocriptine is a highly effective and safe drug. Its use, as we discuss in Chapter 5, has spared many people from neurosurgery.

How bromocriptine can help you

Bromocriptine can help you in the following ways:

✔ Shrinking certain types of pituitary tumours.

✔ Reducing an abnormally high *prolactin* level, which helps to:

- Improve *libido* (sex drive).
- Restore and regulate a woman's periods.
- Restore fertility.
- Stop breast milk production.
- Prevent osteoporosis.

✔ Reducing an abnormally high *growth hormone* level in people with pituitary tumours that are over-producing this hormone; this in turn helps prevent excess growth (*gigantism*), and abnormal bone thickening in adults (*acromegaly*).

✔ Improving symptoms of parkinsonism.

How bromocriptine might harm you

Possible side-effects from taking bromocriptine include:

- ✔ Nausea, vomiting, constipation, diarrhea. Of all side-effects, nausea is the most common.

- ✔ Faintness (especially upon first arising from a bed or from a chair). This is more likely to occur soon after starting the medicine.

- ✔ Headaches, dizziness, sleepiness. These occur in only a small percentage of people.

- ✔ High blood pressure; inflammation of the lungs or tissue around the heart. These rarely occur.

People with the following conditions shouldn't take bromocriptine:

- ✔ Uncontrolled hypertension (high blood pressure).

- ✔ Pregnant women who have high blood pressure brought on with the pregnancy.

- ✔ Coronary artery disease or other severe diseases of the circulation.

- ✔ Women who are breastfeeding.

As the safety of bromocriptine during pregnancy isn't proven, the *usual* practice is to discontinue it when pregnancy takes place. As this drug is commonly taken to enhance fertility it's crucial you speak with your physician *before* you get pregnant to find out what should be done with your drug in the event you do get pregnant.

Precautions to follow if you're taking bromocriptine

Follow these precautions if you're taking bromocriptine:

- ✔ Until you're sure the medicine isn't causing you to feel faint, pause for a moment after you get up from bed or from a chair to make sure you're not lightheaded before you walk away. If you feel dizzy, sit or lie back down.

- ✔ For women not seeking pregnancy, appropriate contraception should be used.

- ✔ This drug may make you drowsy, which would make it unsafe for you to perform activities — like driving — that require you to be alert and focused.

- ✔ Alcohol should be avoided.

- ✔ If you're being treated for a large pituitary tumour (*macroadenoma*), don't discontinue the drug suddenly. Also, seek urgent medical attention if you find your vision suddenly worsens.

How to take bromocriptine

The dose you take depends on the condition being treated. The starting dose for most conditions is 1.25 mg to 2.5 mg per day with the dose then adjusted, under the supervision of your doctor, based on how you're responding. When starting bromocriptine, you should take it at bedtime and with food. If you're tolerating it well you may take it at another time (preferably still with food).

Avoid consuming grapefruit or grapefruit juice because it can affect the level of bromocriptine in your blood.

If, despite following these measures, you continue to have bothersome nausea, we suggest you ask your doctor about possibly switching you to cabergoline. Cabergoline is much less likely to cause nausea (but is much more expensive).

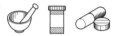

Gastrointestinal Tract Motility Modifiers and Related Drugs

Drugs within this group act on the gastrointestinal tract and affect how it propels food along its 20-plus feet. Gastrointestinal tract motility modifiers — *geesh,* what a mouthful — and related drugs available in Canada are listed in Table 6-34. Domperidone and metoclopramide act on the upper portion of the gut (and hence are used primarily for stomach problems), whereas trimebutine, pinaverium, and tegaserod act primarily on the lower portion of the gut (and so are used to treat conditions such as irritable bowel syndrome — we discuss irritable bowel syndrome and its treatment in Chapter 5). In this section we take a detailed look at domperidone — a particularly commonly used drug in this family.

Table 6-34	Gastrointestinal Tract Motility Modifiers and Related Drugs	
Class	**Generic Name**	**Trade Name(s)**
Upper gastrointestinal tract motility modifiers±	**Domperidone**	Apo-Domperidone, Gen-Domperidone, Novo-Domperidone, Nu-Domperidone, PMS-Domperidone, RAN-Domperidone, ratio-Domperidone

(continued)

Table 6-34 *(continued)*

Class	Generic Name	Trade Name(s)
	Metoclopramide	Apo-Metoclop, Nu-Metoclopramide
Lower gastrointestinal tract motility regulator	Trimebutine	Apo-Trimebutine, Modulon
Gastrointestinal calcium antagonist	Pinaverium	Dicetel
Serotonin receptor partial agonist	Tegaserod	Zelnorm

± These drugs are also known as "dopamine antagonists."

 ## Domperidone

Apo-Domperidone, Gen-Domperidone, Novo-Domperidone, Nu-Domperidone, PMS-Domperidone, RAN-Domperidone, ratio-Domperidone

Domperidone is a helpful drug to treat nausea and vomiting. It's also generally very well tolerated, with a low likelihood of causing side-effects.

 Domperidone blocks *dopamine* receptors located in the stomach. This action results in more forceful and more coordinated contractions of the stomach, which in turn helps it to empty its contents into the intestine. Domperidone also blocks dopamine stimulation of the *chemoreceptor trigger zone* (CTZ) in the brain; this action helps ease nausea and vomiting.

How domperidone can help you

Domperidone can help you in the following ways:

- ✔ Easing nausea and vomiting, especially if caused by migraine headaches or as a side-effect from drugs used to treat Parkinson's disease.

- ✔ Improving the ability of the stomach to empty its contents into the small intestine. This may ease symptoms (such as nausea, vomiting, bloating, and overly quick fullness with eating) seen with disorders like *gastritis, diabetic gastroparesis,* and *anorexia nervosa,* where the stomach has been damaged and, as a result, has a hard time emptying.

- ✔ Reducing heartburn due to *gastro-esophageal reflux disease* (GERD).

How domperidone might harm you

Possible side-effects from taking domperidone include:

- ✔ In women, loss of periods, breast tenderness, and milky discharge (*galactorrhea*).
- ✔ Erectile dysfunction.
- ✔ Headache, dry mouth, abdominal cramps, diarrhea, elevated liver tests.
- ✔ Abnormal heart rhythm. This is a very dangerous side-effect; however it occurs very rarely.

Most people don't experience any side-effects from this medicine.

People with the following conditions shouldn't take domperidone:

- ✔ Pituitary tumours that are making prolactin hormone.
- ✔ Bleeding from the stomach.
- ✔ Blockage of the bowel (*bowel obstruction*).

 The safety of domperidone in pregnancy and breastfeeding is unknown. If you're pregnant or breastfeeding, we recommend you discuss it with your physician before taking this medicine.

 Some breast cancers are thought possibly to be stimulated by prolactin hormone. In *theory* — there is no proof of this — because domperidone increases prolactin levels it could worsen breast cancer. If you have or have had breast cancer, we recommend you discuss this with your doctor.

Precautions to follow if you're taking domperidone

If you develop palpitations while taking domperidone, we recommend you seek prompt medical attention.

How to take domperidone

The usual starting dose of domperidone is 10 mg taken 15 to 30 minutes before meals and at bedtime. The dose is then adjusted, under your doctor's supervision, based on your response.

 Avoid consuming grapefruit or grapefruit juice because it might (it's not yet known but is suspected) affect the level of domperidone in your blood.

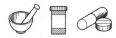

Eye Drops to Treat Glaucoma

As we discuss in Chapter 5, the mainstay of glaucoma treatment is with eye drops. Eye drops available in Canada to treat glaucoma are listed in Table 6-35. Each class listed in this table has its own special properties that enables it often to be used in combination. In this section we look in detail at one of the most commonly used members of each class.

Remember these important points if you're taking prescription eye drops to treat glaucoma:

- ✔ Your eye drops to treat glaucoma will work more effectively if, after you put a drop in your eye, you gently press with a finger for a few minutes over the inside corner of your eye. Doing this will reduce the amount of medicine that drains down the tear duct and keeps the eye drop medicine in the eye longer so it will have more time to do its job. Doing so also reduces absorption of the drug into your body and so will minimize side-effects.

- ✔ Many prescription eye drops may contain a preservative (benzalkonium chloride) that can damage soft contact lens. For this reason, be sure to remove your contacts before using your eye drops and don't reinsert them for at least 15 minutes.

- ✔ If you're taking more than one type of eye drop, take them at least five minutes apart.

Table 6-35	Eye Drops to Treat Glaucoma	
Class	*Generic Name*	*Trade Name(s)*
Adrenergic agonists	Apraclonidine	Iopidine
	Brimonidine	Alphagan, Alphagan P, Apo-brimonidine, Combigan*, PMS-Brimonidine Tartrate, ratio-brimonidine
Beta blockers	Betaxolol	Betoptic S
	Levobunolol	Apo-Levobunolol, Betagan, Novo-Levobunolol, PMS-Levobunolol, ratio-Levobunolol
	Timolol	Apo-Timop, Combigan*, Cosopt*, Cosopt Preservative-Free*, DuoTrav*, Gen-Timolol, PMS-Timolol, Sandoz Timolol, Timoptic, Timoptic-XE, Xalacom*

Class	Generic Name	Trade Name(s)
Carbonic anhydrase inhibitors	Brinzolamide	Azopt
	Dorzolamide	Cosopt*, Cosopt Preservative-Free*, Trusopt
Cholinergic agonists	**Pilocarpine**	Isopto Carpine, Pilopine HS
	Carbachol	Isopto Carbachol, Miostat
Prostaglandin analogs	Bimatoprost	Lumigan
	Latanoprost	Xalacom*, Xalatan
	Travoprost	DuoTrav*, Travatan

* This medicine is a combination of different drugs. Refer to the drug label to determine what they are.

 # Brimonidine

Alphagan, Alphagan P, Apo-brimonidine, Combigan*, PMS-Brimonidine Tartrate, ratio-brimonidine

Brimonidine is a helpful drug to treat glaucoma; however, it has a tendency to cause allergic reactions (confined to the eye). It's typically used in combination with other eye drops.

 Brimonidine attaches to *alpha adrenergic* receptors in the eye. By *activating* these receptors, less *aqueous humour* fluid is made and more leaves the eye. Like shutting off the tap and opening the drain in your bathtub, the net result is less fluid. This leads to a lowering of your *intra-ocular pressure* (IOP).

How brimonidine can help you

Lowering your IOP will improve your glaucoma and pose less of a threat to your vision. Here's lookin' at you, kid.

How brimonidine might harm you

Possible side-effects from brimonidine include:

- Dry mouth.
- Local eye irritation: Your eyes may be sore, red, and/or itchy. It may feel like you have some grit in your eye when you do not.

✔ Blood pressure elevation. This does not occur often. It's more likely to be an issue if you have hypertension to start with.

✔ Headache and/or dizziness.

You shouldn't take brimonidine if you have taken a drug from the monoamine oxidase (MAO) inhibitor family within the past 14 days, nor should you start taking an MAO inhibitor within 14 days of stopping brimonidine. Doing so could cause dangerously high blood pressure.

The safety of brimonidine in pregnancy and breastfeeding is unknown. Similarly, its safety if you have kidney or liver disease is also unknown. If you're pregnant or breastfeeding, we recommend you discuss it with your physician before taking this medicine.

Precautions to follow if you're taking brimonidine

Contact a physician in the unlikely event you develop (or have a worsening of) any of the following symptoms:

✔ Depression.

✔ Dizziness.

✔ Chest pains.

✔ Weakness of an arm or leg.

✔ Raynaud's phenomenon (we discuss this condition in Chapter 5).

How to take brimonidine

Brimonidine is typically used in a dose of one drop given into the affected eye approximately every 12 hours.

If you're also taking another type of eye drop, use this other eye drop *first* then wait at least five minutes before taking brimonidine.

℞ Timolol

Apo-Timop, Combigan*, Cosopt*, Cosopt Preservative-Free*, DuoTrav*, Gen-Timolol, PMS-Timolol, Sandoz Timolol, Timoptic, Timoptic-XE, Xalacom*

Timolol is a member of the beta blocker family of drugs. It's available in oral form to treat heart disease and high blood pressure (which we discuss elsewhere in this chapter), and as an eye drop, which we discuss here.

Timolol in the eye drop medicine attaches to beta adrenergic receptors in the eye and, by doing so, reduces the amount of aqueous humour made within the eye. (Timolol eye drops may also help this fluid leave the eye.) With less fluid in the eye, intra-ocular pressure (IOP) is reduced.

How timolol eye drops can help you

Lowering your IOP will improve your glaucoma and pose less of a threat to your vision.

How timolol eye drops might harm you

Possible side-effects from timolol eye drops include:

- Sore red eyes.
- Dizziness.
- Shortness of breath, wheezing.

You should generally not take timolol eye drops if you have

- Asthma or chronic obstructive pulmonary disease (COPD).
- A very slow heartbeat.
- Certain disorders of the heart's electrical system.
- Congestive heart failure.

The safety of timolol eye drops in pregnancy and breastfeeding is unknown. Similarly, its safety if you have kidney or liver disease is unknown. If you're pregnant or breastfeeding, we recommend you discuss it with your physician before taking this medicine.

Precautions to follow if you're taking timolol eye drops

Keep a lookout for the development of shortness of breath or faintness — especially if you have a history of heart problems. If these symptoms develop be sure to promptly inform your physician.

How to take timolol eye drops

Timolol eye drops are typically started in a dose of one drop of 0.25 % solution into the affected eye twice per day, then, if necessary, the dose is increased, under your doctor's supervision, to one drop of 0.5% solution (also given twice daily). If your glaucoma responds well, your doctor may later advise you to reduce the dose to one drop daily.

Dorzolamide

Cosopt*, Cosopt Preservative-Free*, Trusopt

Dorzolamide is a member of the carbonic anhydrase group of drugs. This type of eye drop is usually used together with an eye drop from another class; however, it may be used alone if you're unable to tolerate other eye drops (for example, if you cannot take timolol eye drops because you have asthma).

By blocking the action of an enzyme (*carbonic anhydrase*) in the eye, dorzolamide decreases the amount of aqueous humour fluid that is made. With less fluid in the eye, intra-ocular pressure (IOP) is reduced.

How dorzolamide can help you

Lowering your IOP will improve your glaucoma and pose less of a threat to your vision.

How dorzolamide might harm you

Possible side-effects from taking dorzolamide include:

- ✔ Symptoms of eye irritation such as burning, stinging, redness, itching, tearing.
- ✔ A bitter taste in the mouth.

You shouldn't take dorzolamide if you're also taking an oral form of carbonic anhydrase inhibitor (such as acetazolamide). Because we don't have adequate safety information about the use of dorzolamide if you have kidney failure, it's generally recommended it not be used in this situation.

The safety of dorzolamide in pregnancy and breastfeeding is unknown. Similarly, its safety if you have kidney or liver disease is unknown. If you're pregnant or breastfeeding, we recommend you discuss it with your physician before taking this medicine.

Precautions to follow if you're taking dorzolamide

Because dorzolamide has a sulfur base, if you're allergic to other sulfur-based drugs, you may also be prone to having an allergic reaction to this medicine. Be sure to let your doctor know if you've had a previous problem with a sulfur-based drug and, if you're taking dorzolamide, be on the lookout for a skin rash or difficulty breathing and stop the drug immediately (and get in touch with your physician) if these develop.

How to take dorzolamide

When used alone, the usual dose of dorzolamide is one drop of 2% solution inserted into the affected eye three times daily. If dorzolamide is being used in addition to another type of eye drop, the usual dose is one drop of 2% solution taken two times daily.

 ## Pilocarpine

Isopto Carpine, Pilopine HS

Pilocarpine is typically used only when other eye drops to treat glaucoma have not been sufficiently effective.

 Pilocarpine stimulates certain receptors in the eye and by doing so causes a tiny muscle (called the *ciliary* muscle) to contract. When this muscle contracts, it widens the channel through which aqueous fluid can exit from the eye. (Sort of like activating a wall switch that causes your garage door to open and your teenage daughter to exit with your car, your credit card, and your peace of mind.) With less fluid in the eye, intra-ocular pressure (IOP) is reduced.

How pilocarpine can help you

Lowering your IOP will improve your glaucoma and pose less of a threat to your vision.

How pilocarpine might harm you

Possible side-effects from taking pilocarpine include:

- ✔ Blurred vision (especially if you have cataracts), impaired night vision. This happens quite often.
- ✔ Headaches. These tend to go away as you continue the medicine.

You shouldn't take pilocarpine if you have inflammation within the front chamber of the eye (this is something your doctor will assess before prescribing this medicine).

 The safety of pilocarpine in pregnancy and breastfeeding is unknown. If you're pregnant or breastfeeding, we recommend you discuss it with your physician before taking this medicine.

Precautions to follow if you're taking pilocarpine

Because pilocarpine can impair your night vision, you may not be able to see sufficiently well at night to drive. As such, before you consider getting behind the wheel you need to determine how much the medicine is affecting your night vision.

Pilocarpine will make your pupil small. This is normal and not a cause for concern.

How to take pilocarpine

Pilocarpine is typically taken as one to two eye drops four times daily, or once daily as a gel. If you're taking both the eye drop *and* the gel, use the drop first and wait at least five minutes before inserting the gel.

Latanoprost

Xalacom*, Xalatan

Latanoprost is a member of the prostaglandin analog class of eye drops. Because medications from this class work well and are typically very safe to use they're a popular choice for the treatment of glaucoma.

Latanoprost works by helping aqueous fluid leave the eye. With less fluid in the eye, intra-ocular pressure (IOP) is reduced.

How latanoprost can help you

Lowering your IOP will improve your glaucoma and pose less of a threat to your vision.

How latanoprost might harm you

Possible side-effects from latanoprost include:

- ✔ Eye irritation: You may experience blurred vision, a burning or stinging feeling, redness, itching, or a feeling like you have some grit in your eye when you do not.

- ✔ Eyelash changes: Your eyelashes may become thicker, longer, and/or greater in number. Also, they may start to angle the wrong way (which can lead to eye irritation). These changes typically go away after you stop taking the drug.

- ✔ Increased pigmentation: Occasionally, the iris, eyelids and/or eyelashes become more deeply pigmented. If you stop the drug, this discolouration will not progress; however, although the eyelids and eyelashes may return to normal, the changes to the iris will not.

If you're using lantoprost in only one eye, if increased pigmentation does occur it may make your eyes look different from one another.

The safety of latanoprost in pregnancy and breastfeeding is unknown. If you're pregnant or breastfeeding, we recommend you discuss it with your physician before taking this medicine.

Precautions to follow if you're taking latanoprost

Because the long-term implications of increased pigmentation of the eye are not known, be sure to have your eyes examined regularly while you're taking latanoprost.

How to take latanoprost

Latanoprost is taken as one drop once daily administered in the evening. Don't exceed this dose; doing so can actually make the drug work less well.

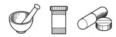

Fibrates (Fibric Acid Derivatives)

As we discuss in Chapter 5, fibrates (or *fibric acid derivatives*) are medicines used to treat lipid abnormalities; in particular, high triglycerides. The three members of this class share much in common. We discuss the most commonly used of these drugs — fenofibrate — in detail below. Fibrates available in Canada are listed in Table 6-36.

Table 6-36	Fibrates
Generic Name	*Trade Name(s)*
Bezafibrate	Bezalip SR
Fenofibrate	Apo-Fenofibrate, Apo-Feno-Micro, Apo-Feno-Super, Gen-Fenofibrate Micro, Lipidil EZ, Lipidil Supra, Novo-Fenofibrate Micronized, Nu-Fenofibrate, PMS-Fenofibrate Micro, ratio-Fenofibrate MC
Gemfibrozil	Apo-Gemfibrozil, Gen-Gemfibrozil, Lopid, Novo-Gemfibrozil, Nu-Gemfibrozil, PMS-Gemfibrozil

Fenofibrate

Apo-Fenofibrate, Apo-Feno-Micro, Apo-Feno-Super, Gen-Fenofibrate Micro, Lipidil EZ, Lipidil Supra, Novo-Fenofibrate Micronized, Nu-Fenofibrate, PMS-Fenofibrate Micro, ratio-Fenofibrate MC

When certain receptors in the body (the *peroxisome proliferator activated receptor alpha* receptors — thankfully, this is abbreviated as PPAR alpha receptors) are stimulated by fenofibrate, it changes the way the body handles the production and destruction of certain lipids. We look at these changes next.

How fenofibrate can help you

Fenofibrate can help you in the following ways:

- Decreasing triglyceride levels.
- Decreasing LDL cholesterol levels.
- Increasing HDL cholesterol levels.

How fenofibrate might harm you

Possible side-effects from taking fenofibrate include:

- Nausea, abdominal pain, diarrhea, constipation.
- Muscle aching (most commonly in the arms or legs).
- Muscle damage (*rhabdomyolysis*). Fortunately, this occurs only rarely.
- Abnormal liver tests. Only infrequently does significant liver injury develop.
- Gallstones.
- Anemia. This occurs infrequently and is typically mild.

People with the following conditions shouldn't take fenofibrate:

- Liver disease.
- Severe kidney failure.
- Gallbladder disease.
- Pregnancy, breastfeeding.

Precautions to follow if you're taking fenofibrate

Follow these precautions if you're taking fenofibrate:

✔ Have a blood test to check your liver function and hemoglobin level from time to time. This is something your doctor can order.

✔ If you develop muscle pains see your doctor promptly.

How to take fenofibrate

Your dose of fenofibrate depends on which form of the product you're prescribed. Your doctor may need to prescribe lower than usual doses if you have kidney failure. It's taken once daily, preferably around the same time each day, and may be taken with or without food.

As it can take six to eight weeks before the full effect of fenofibrate on your cholesterol and triglyceride levels is seen, it's usually inappropriate to have these levels measured sooner than that.

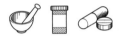

Histamine (H1) Agonist

There is but one member of this drug family available in Canada; it's noted in Table 6-37.

Table 6-37	Histamine (H1) Agonist
Generic Name	**Trade Names**
Betahistine	Novo-Betahistine, Serc

 ## Betahistine

Novo-Betahistine, Serc

Betahistine is one of the very few drugs available to treat dizziness due to Meniere's disease. We discuss this disease in Chapter 5.

 Dizziness due to Meniere's disease is related to an imbalance in the amount of fluid in the inner ear. Betahistine appears to help treat this condition by improving this fluid balance. It's theorized that by activating histamine (type 1) receptors in the inner ear, betahistine improves blood flow within the ear and that this, in turn, reduces the amount of fluid (and, therefore, pressure) within the balance mechanism resulting in improvement in dizziness. Of course, it was once theorized that the earth was flat . . .

How betahistine can help you

Betahistine can help you if you have Meniere's disease by

- Decreasing the *frequency* of attacks.

- Decreasing the *severity* of attacks by reducing the amount of vertigo (a form of dizziness in which you feel you or your environment is moving — for a more detailed definition, think teenage years plus case of 24) and tinnitus (ringing in the ears).

How betahistine might harm you

Possible side-effects from taking betahistine include:

- Rash, itching.

- Nausea.

- Headache.

- Worsening of asthma or chronic obstructive pulmonary disease (COPD). (This isn't proven.)

- Redevelopment of stomach or duodenal ulcers.

People with the following conditions shouldn't take betahistine:

- Using antihistamines.

- *Pheochromocytoma.* This is a rare disease in which one has very high levels of *epinephrine* (adrenaline).

- Stomach or duodenal ulcer (present or previous).

 The safety of betahistine in pregnancy and breastfeeding is unknown. If you're pregnant or breastfeeding, we recommend you discuss it with your physician before taking this medicine.

Precautions to follow if you're taking betahistine

Follow these precautions if you're taking betahistine:

- If you have asthma or COPD and, after starting betahistine, your breathing worsens, stop taking the betahistine and consult your doctor.

- If you experience an attack of Meniere's, continue to take the medicine because it may make the episode less severe.

How to take betahistine

The usual starting dose is 8 mg to 24 mg taken two to three times daily. Betahistine should be taken with food as this will minimize stomach upset.

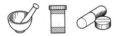

Immunosuppressive Drugs

Many diseases, including rheumatoid arthritis and inflammatory bowel disease, involve significant overactivity of the immune system leading to inflammation and, subsequently, to damage of tissues. Immunosuppressive drugs are helpful to treat these conditions because they *suppress* (that is, reduce the activity of) the *immune* system. As a result, they help bring these diseases under control and can minimize the occurrence of flares.

An additional benefit is that these drugs allow prednisone — a steroid drug that is excellent at treating inflammation but often causes side-effects when used in higher doses — to be used in lower doses. (Immunosuppressive drugs are called *steroid-sparing agents* because of this property.) The immunosuppressive drugs available in Canada are listed in Table 6-38. These drugs differ markedly from one another, and a detailed discussion of each of them is beyond the scope of this book. In this section we look in depth at two of the most commonly used immunosuppressive drugs.

Table 6-38	Immunosuppressive Drugs
Generic Name	*Trade Name(s)*
Azathioprine±	Apo-Azathioprine, Imuran, Novo-Azathioprine
Cyclophosphamide±	Cytoxan, Procytox
Cyclosporine±	Neoral, Sandoz Cyclosporine
Gold±	Sodium Aurothiomalate, Myochrysine
Hydroxychloroquine±	Apo-Hydroxychloroquine, Gen-Hydroxychloroquine, Plaquenil

(continued)

Table 6-38 *(continued)*

Generic Name	Trade Name(s)
Leflunomide±	Apo-Leflunomide, Arava, Novo-Leflunomide, Sandoz Leflunomide
Methotrexate±	Apo-Methotrexate, Methotrexate, Methotrexate Tablets USP, ratio-Methotrexate
Mycophenolate	Cellcept, Myfortic
Pimecrolimus	Elidel
Sirolimus	Rapamune
Sulfasalazine±	Salazopyrin, Salazopyrin En-tabs
Tacrolimus	Prograf, Protopic

± These drugs are also categorized as disease-modifying antirheumatic drugs (DMARDs). We discuss this further in the "Rheumatoid Arthritis" section in Chapter 5.

℞ *Azathioprine*

Apo-Azathioprine, Imuran, Novo-Azathioprine

Azathioprine works by decreasing the number and/or the activity of white blood cells called *lymphocytes.* This action reduces the amount of inflammation present in the body and, as a result, less tissue damage occurs.

How azathioprine can help you

Azathioprine (often in combination with other medications) is helpful in the treatment of many different conditions, including:

- Arthritis diseases where there is significant inflammation. Examples include rheumatoid arthritis, systemic lupus erythematosis, and polymyositis.

- Inflammatory bowel disease.

- Myasthenia gravis. This is a rare neurological disease in which the muscles are weak.

- Organ transplantation (for example, heart, kidney, liver, lung). In this circumstance, azathioprine helps to prevent rejection of the transplanted organ.

How azathioprine might harm you

Possible side-effects from taking azathioprine include:

- ✔ Bone marrow *suppression*. This results in fewer red blood cells (causing anemia), white blood cells (increasing the risk of infection), and platelets (increasing the risk of bleeding).

- ✔ Decreased appetite, nausea, vomiting, abdominal pain, malaise (that is, feeling generally unwell), fever. These symptoms are most likely to occur soon after starting the drug and quickly go away upon stopping it.

- ✔ Slightly increased risk of cancer.

The safety of azathioprine in pregnancy and breastfeeding is unknown, but because of safety concerns it's generally recommended it *not* be taken in these circumstances. If you're pregnant or breastfeeding, we recommend you discuss it with your physician before taking this medicine.

Precautions to follow if you're taking azathioprine

If you're taking azathioprine, it's important to have your blood counts and liver function checked regularly. These tests are especially important in the early stages of treatment or if your dose has been recently increased.

How to take azathioprine

Azathioprine is usually taken once daily and is started in a dose determined by your body weight. The dose is then adjusted, under your doctor's supervision, based on your response. Your doctor may need to prescribe lower than usual doses if you have kidney failure. You can take azathioprine with or without food.

It may take two to eight weeks from the time you start azathioprine before you notice any improvement in your symptoms.

℞ *Methotrexate*

Apo-Methotrexate, Methotrexate, Methotrexate Tablets USP, ratio-Methotrexate

In this section we look at methotrexate therapy in doses used to treat diseases related to inflammation. (Higher doses are given to treat some types of cancer. See below.)

How methotrexate works

Methotrexate reduces the amount of inflammation present in the body, and as a result, less tissue damage occurs. How, exactly, it accomplishes this isn't known but it may be because of one or more of the following actions:

✔ Decreasing the number and/or the activity of white blood cells called lymphocytes.

✔ Inhibiting the action of an enzyme called dihydrofolate reductase. (This results in a decreased ability of cancer cells to form new cells and hence is the action that allows this drug to help treat cancer.)

✔ Decreasing the number of inflammation-causing substances in the blood such as tumor necrosis factor (TNF) and interleukins.

How methotrexate can help you

Methotrexate (often in combination with other medications) is helpful in the treatment of many different conditions, including:

✔ Arthritis diseases where there is significant inflammation. Examples include rheumatoid arthritis, systemic lupus erythematosis, and polymyositis.

✔ Inflammatory bowel disease.

✔ Psoriasis. Methotrexate is only used for severe psoriasis that has not responded to topical therapy.

✔ Some types of cancer.

How methotrexate might harm you

Possible side-effects from taking methotrexate include:

✔ Fatigue, nausea, vomiting. These are common side-effects and are usually mild.

✔ Mouth ulcers.

✔ Decreased blood counts. This has the potential to cause anemia, infections, or bleeding. Serious blood abnormalities, however, seldom occur with the doses used to treat inflammatory diseases.

✔ Abnormal liver tests.

✔ Cough, shortness of breath.

✔ Fever.

✔ Skin rash.

People with the following conditions shouldn't take methotrexate:

- ✔ Alcoholism (alcohol dependence).
- ✔ Liver disease from alcohol use.
- ✔ Severe liver, kidney, bone marrow, or blood disease.
- ✔ For couples trying to get pregnant, neither the male nor the female should take methotrexate.
- ✔ Pregnancy or breastfeeding.

Precautions to follow if you're taking methotrexate

Follow these precautions if you're taking methotrexate:

- ✔ Have your blood counts and liver function checked regularly. These tests are especially important in the early stages of treatment or if your dose has been recently increased.
- ✔ If you have a serious infection, you may need to stop taking methotrexate until the illness has been treated.
- ✔ Do not consume alcohol. Drinking alcohol will increase the risk of methotrexate damaging your liver.

How to take methotrexate

When used as an immunosuppressive drug, methotrexate is taken once per week, usually in a dose of 7.5 mg to 25 mg taken with or without food (however, be consistent in whether you take it with food or without food). Your doctor may need to prescribe lower than usual doses if you have kidney failure. It can be taken in tablet form — each of which is 2.5 mg — or by injection into a muscle or under the skin (which your health care provider can show you how to do). The full effectiveness of methotrexate may not be seen until two to four months from the time you start treatment.

Taking methotrexate just before bedtime may help lessen side-effects such as nausea and fatigue.

When taking methotrexate to treat arthritis, it's generally safe to also take nonsteroidal anti-inflammatory drugs (NSAIDs); however, before taking an NSAID, it's best to first discuss this with your doctor. Also, folic acid is sometimes prescribed to help reduce the risk of side-effects; we suggest you ask your doctor whether taking folic acid supplements is appropriate for you.

Inhaled Medicines to Treat Asthma and Chronic Obstructive Pulmonary Disease (COPD)

Over the past few years a number of new types of inhaled medicine have become available to treat asthma and chronic obstructive pulmonary disease (COPD). Using inhaled medicine rather than pills for breathing disorders has several advantages, the most important of which is that the medicine gets sent directly to where it's needed rather than going throughout the body. This translates into fewer side-effects.

These new treatments are administered with special devices that work in a variety of ways. Having a fondness for sports cars (though currently driving vans), we love the cool names for some of these new products: Spincaps, Turbuhaler, Diskus — sounds like they'd be right at home on a Porsche! Inhaled medicines available in Canada to treat asthma and COPD are listed in Table 6-39. Drugs within a class are very similar. In this section we look in detail at the most commonly used drug within a class.

Table 6-39   Inhaled Medicines to Treat Asthma and COPD

Class	Generic Name	Trade Name(s)
Short-acting beta-2 agonists	**Salbutamol**	Airomir, Apo-Salvent, Apo-Salvent CFC Free, Combivent Inhalation Aerosol*, Combivent Inhalation Solution*, Gen-Combo Sterinebs*, Gen-Salbutamol Respirator Solution, Gen-Salbutamol Sterinebs P.F., Nu-Salbutamol Solution, ratio-Salbutamol HFA, Sandoz Salbutamol, Ventodisk Diskhaler, Ventolin Diskus, Ventolin HFA, Ventolin Nebules P.F., Ventolin Oral Liquid, Ventolin Respirator Solution
	Fenoterol	Berotec Inhalation Aerosol, Berotec Inhalation Solution, Duovent UDV*
	Terbutaline	Bricanyl Turbuhaler
Long-acting beta-2 agonists	**Salmeterol**	Advair Diskus*, Advair Inhalation Aerosol*, Serevent, Serevent Diskhaler Disk, Serevent Diskus
	Formoterol	Foradil, Oxeze Turbuhaler, Symbicort Turbuhaler*

Class	Generic Name	Trade Name(s)
Short-acting anticholinergic agent	**Ipratropium**	Apo-Ipravent, Atrovent HFA Inhalation Aerosol, Atrovent Inhalation Aerosol, Atrovent Inhalation Solution, Combivent Inhalation Aerosol*, Combivent Inhalation Solution*, Duovent UDV*, Gen-Combo Sterinebs*, Gen-Ipratropium, Novo-Ipramide, Nu-Ipratropium, ratio-Ipratropium, Ratio-Ipratropium UDV
Long-acting anticholinergic agent	**Tiotropium**	Spiriva
Corticosteroids	Beclomethasone	Qvar
	Budesonide	Pulmicort Nebuamp, Pulmicort Turbuhaler, Rhinocort Turbuhaler, Symbicort Turbuhaler*
	Fluticasone	Advair Diskus*, Advair Inhalation Aerosol*, Flovent HFA, Flovent Diskus
	Ciclesonide	Alvesco
Mast cell stabilizer	Sodium cromoglycate	Apo-Cromolyn, Nu-Cromolyn

* This medicine is a combination of different drugs. Refer to the drug label to determine what they are.

 ## Salbutamol

Airomir, Apo-Salvent, Apo-Salvent CFC Free, Combivent Inhalation Aerosol*, Combivent Inhalation Solution*, Gen-Combo Sterinebs*, Gen-Salbutamol Respirator Solution, Gen-Salbutamol Sterinebs P.F., Nu-Salbutamol Solution, ratio-Salbutamol HFA, Sandoz Salbutamol, Ventodisk Diskhaler, Ventolin Diskus, Ventolin HFA, Ventolin Nebules P.F., Ventolin Oral Liquid, Ventolin Respirator Solution

From the time it first became available, salbutamol has been a mainstay in the treatment of asthma and wheezing due to chronic obstructive pulmonary disease (COPD). It's a generally very effective medicine and has fairly few side-effects — a nice combination indeed.

The air passages (*bronchi*) within the lungs have numerous cells called *smooth muscle cells*. On the surface of these cells are many beta-2 receptors that, when stimulated by salbutamol, make the muscles in the bronchi relax. As a result, the bronchi open wider (a process called *bronchodilation*), which allows air to more easily flow through them.

How salbutamol can help you

Salbutamol can help you by relieving an attack of wheezing and preventing exercise-induced asthma (if taken before exercise).

How salbutamol might harm you

Possible side-effects from taking salbutamol include:

- Anxiety and tremor. These are the most common side-effects, and tend to be mild.

- Headache, muscle cramps, insomnia, nausea, and dizziness. These occur infrequently.

- Abnormal heart rhythm. Although, particularly with high doses, palpitations may be experienced, serious heart rhythm problems rarely occur. People with known heart disease are more at risk.

- Low blood potassium levels. This is a rare side-effect and is usually related to very-high-dose therapy.

- Making your wheezing worse, not better. (Whether this actually happens is a subject of controversy.)

- Worsening of diabetes blood glucose control. This is usually related to very-high-dose therapy.

You shouldn't take salbutamol if you're prone to heart rhythm disorders in which the heart beats too quickly.

Salbutamol is generally considered safe to take during pregnancy and breastfeeding. If you're pregnant or breastfeeding, we recommend you discuss it with your physician before taking this medicine.

Precautions to follow if you're taking salbutamol

Follow these precautions if you're taking salbutamol:

- Salbutamol's main value is in the treatment of attacks of wheezing. If you're wheezing *regularly* (especially if this is more than three days per week), ask your doctor about being treated with additional, *preventive* medicines.

✔ Carry it with you at all times. You never know when you might unexpectedly need it.

✔ If you're having an attack of wheezing that isn't responding to salbutamol, seek urgent medical attention. Failure to do so can be life-threatening.

How to take salbutamol

Salbutamol is taken using a variety of different inhaler devices. We discuss these devices in Chapter 4. The dose you're prescribed depends on the particular device you're using and the strength of the product you're taking.

℞ Salmeterol

Advair Diskus*, Advair Inhalation Aerosol*, Serevent, Serevent Diskhaler Disk, Serevent Diskus

Salmeterol is a fairly new drug and, though it appears to be a very helpful tool in the treatment of asthma and COPD, there have been recent safety concerns regarding this medicine. (Some people using salmeterol have had rapid deterioration in their condition; whether this was due to the drug or their underlying breathing disorder isn't known.) It will take more time before we know for certain if these concerns are warranted.

The air passages (*bronchi*) within the lungs have numerous cells called *smooth muscle cells*. On the surface of these cells are many beta-2 receptors that, when stimulated by salmeterol, make the muscles in the bronchi relax. As a result, the bronchi open wider (a process called *bronchodilation*), which allows air to more easily flow through them.

How salmeterol can help you

Salmeterol can help you by preventing attacks of wheezing.

How salmeterol might harm you

Possible side-effects from taking salmeterol include:

✔ Headache, tremor, palpitations. These are seldom serious.

✔ Abnormal heart rhythm. This is an uncommon complication and is most likely to occur if you have heart disease.

✔ Making your wheezing worse, not better. (Whether this actually happens is a subject of controversy.)

People with the following conditions shouldn't take salmeterol:

- ✔ Wheezing that is infrequent and quickly resolves with occasional use of short-acting beta-2 agonist therapy (such as salbutamol).

- ✔ Asthma that has not yet been treated with optimal doses of an inhaled corticosteroid. (It's not dangerous to do so, it's simply ill-advised because salmeterol is thought to be inferior therapy in this situation.)

- ✔ Heart problems where the heart is prone to beating overly quickly.

The safety of salmeterol in pregnancy is unknown. It's *probably* safe to take if you're breastfeeding. If you're pregnant or breastfeeding, we recommend you discuss it with your physician before taking this medicine.

Precautions to follow if you're taking salmeterol

Follow these precautions if you're taking salmeterol:

- ✔ Salmeterol is intended for use to *prevent* attacks of wheezing. It's of no value for — and should not be used for — the treatment of active wheezing (that is, wheezing that is already present).

- ✔ *Always* have available a short-acting beta-2 agonist medicine like salbutamol to treat wheezing.

How to take salmeterol

Salmeterol is taken using a variety of different inhaler devices. We discuss these devices in Chapter 4. The dose you're prescribed depends on the particular device you're using and the strength of the product you're taking.

℞ Ipratropium

Apo-Ipravent, Atrovent HFA Inhalation Aerosol, Atrovent Inhalation Aerosol, Atrovent Inhalation Solution, Combivent Inhalation Aerosol*, Combivent Inhalation Solution*, Duovent UDV*, Gen-Combo Sterinebs*, Gen-Ipratropium, Novo-Ipramide, Nu-Ipratropium, ratio-Ipratropium, Ratio-Ipratropium UDV

Ipratropium is an inhaled form of anticholinergic medicine and is used to treat asthma and COPD.

The air passages (*bronchi*) within the lungs have numerous cells called *smooth muscle cells*. When these cells are stimulated by a chemical messenger (*acetylcholine*) the bronchial muscles contract, which makes the airways narrow. Ipratropium works by blocking the action of acetylcholine (hence, it's considered an anticholinergic drug); this results in wider airways (a process called *bronchodilation*), which in turn allows more air to flow through the bronchi.

How ipratropium can help you

Ipratropium can help you by relieving and preventing attacks of wheezing.

Ipratropium is of more value in the treatment of COPD than of asthma and is more effective at *preventing* wheezing than treating it when it's already present.

How ipratropium might harm you

Possible side-effects from ipratropium include coughing, headache, nausea, vomiting, and dry mouth. Most people don't experience any side-effects.

You may find some relief from a dry mouth by taking sips of water or by sucking on hard candy or chewing sugarless gum. Also, having a persistent dry mouth can increase your risk of cavities, so be sure to look after your teeth well and have regular dental care.

It's *probably* safe to take ipratropium if you're pregnant. Its safety during breastfeeding is unknown. If you're pregnant or breastfeeding, we recommend you discuss it with your physician before taking this medicine.

Precautions to follow if you're taking ipratropium

Follow these precautions if you're taking ipratropium:

- ✔ Infrequently, ipratropium can worsen symptoms related to glaucoma, prostatism, and myasthenia gravis (a rare neurological condition in which the muscles are weak). If you have one of these conditions and you observe your symptoms to worsen after starting ipratropium, speak to your physician.

- ✔ Avoid having ipratropium get into your eyes. (It may cause eye pain or worsening of glaucoma.)

- ✔ Because ipratropium isn't very effective for the treatment of wheezing attacks, be sure to *always* have available a short-acting beta-2 agonist medicine such as salbutamol to treat wheezing.

How to take ipratropium

Ipratropium is taken using a variety of different inhaler devices. We discuss these devices in Chapter 4. The dose you're prescribed depends on the particular device you're using and the strength of the product you're taking.

 ℞ **Tiotropium**

Spiriva

Tiotropium is a quite new drug. It's similar to ipratropium, but is longer lasting.

 The air passages (*bronchi*) within the lungs have numerous cells called *smooth muscle cells*. When these cells are stimulated by a chemical messenger (*acetylcholine*) the bronchial muscles contract, which makes the airways narrow. Tiotropium works by blocking the action of acetylcholine (hence, it's considered an *anticholinergic* drug); this results in wider airways (a process called *bronchodilation*), which in turn allows more air to flow through the bronchi.

How tiotropium can help you

Tiotropium can help you by preventing wheezing if you have COPD.

How tiotropium might harm you

Possible side-effects from tiotropium include dry mouth and constipation. Most people don't experience any side-effects.

 You may find some relief from a dry mouth by taking sips of water or by sucking on hard candy or chewing sugarless gum. Also, having a persistent dry mouth can increase your risk of cavities, so be sure to look after your teeth well and have regular dental care.

 The safety of tiotropium in pregnancy and breastfeeding is unknown. If you're pregnant or breastfeeding, we recommend you discuss it with your physician before taking this medicine.

Precautions to follow if you're taking tiotropium

Follow these precautions if you're taking tiotropium:

  ✔ Infrequently, tiotropium can worsen symptoms related to glaucoma, prostatism, and myasthenia gravis (a rare neurological condition in which the muscles are weak). If you have one of these conditions and you observe your symptoms to worsen after starting tiotropium, speak to your physician.

- ✔ Avoid having tiotropium get into your eyes. (It may cause eye pain or worsening of glaucoma.)

- ✔ Because tiotropium isn't effective for the treatment of wheezing attacks, be sure to *always* have available a short-acting beta-2 agonist medicine such as salbutamol to treat wheezing.

How to take tiotropium

Tiotropium is administered once daily using a HandiHaler (gotta love the name!). We suggest you ask your pharmacist to demonstrate how this device is to be used. It doesn't matter what time of day you take your dose of tiotropium, but choose the same time each day.

 Fluticasone

Advair Diskus*, Advair Inhalation Aerosol*, Flovent HFA, Flovent Diskus

Fluticasone is a member of the *corticosteroid* family of drugs. In this section we discuss the inhaled forms of this medicine. Inhaled corticosteroid therapy is a cornerstone in the treatment of asthma and also has a role to play in the treatment of chronic obstructive pulmonary disease (COPD).

When the air passages (*bronchi*) within the lungs become inflamed, they become narrowed. This makes it more difficult to move air into and out of the lungs and results in wheezing and shortness of breath. By reducing this inflammation, fluticasone allows the airways to widen; this in turn allows air to move through the bronchi more easily.

How fluticasone can help you

Fluticasone can help you by *preventing* wheezing if you have asthma. Fluticasone is likely to offer a similar (but less powerful) benefit if you have COPD (this is somewhat controversial).

How fluticasone might harm you

Possible side-effects from fluticasone include:

- ✔ Yeast infections within the mouth and throat (a condition called *thrush*). This is a common but often avoidable side-effect.

- ✔ Sore throat and hoarseness. These are fairly common, though not serious side-effects.

- ✔ Adrenal gland malfunction. This is more likely to occur if fluticasone is used in very high doses.

✔ Cataracts and glaucoma. This is an uncommon side-effect and is more likely to occur after long-term use.

✔ Osteoporosis. This is an uncommon side-effect and is more likely to occur after long-term use of high doses.

You shouldn't take fluticasone if you have an untreated respiratory tract infection due to bacteria, tuberculosis, or fungi (with the exception of simple oral yeast infections, which can be treated with appropriate antibiotics without interrupting fluticasone therapy).

 The safety of fluticasone in pregnancy and breastfeeding is unknown. If you're pregnant or breastfeeding, we recommend you discuss it with your physician before taking this medicine.

Precautions to follow if you're taking fluticasone

Follow these precautions if you're taking fluticasone:

✔ Don't stop the drug without first speaking to your doctor. If the drug is to be stopped, it may need to be gradually weaned, not suddenly discontinued.

✔ To help avoid mouth yeast infections, sore throat, and hoarseness:

- Use a spacer device when taking your medicine. (We discuss these in Chapter 4.)

- Rinse your mouth well and gargle with water immediately after taking a dose of fluticasone.

✔ If you have either glaucoma or a family history of glaucoma, be sure to see an eye doctor regularly to be tested for this condition.

✔ If you have been a long-term user of high doses of fluticasone, your bone density (a test for osteoporosis) should be measured from time to time.

 ✔ Because fluticasone isn't effective for the treatment of wheezing attacks, be sure to *always* have available a short-acting beta-2 agonist medicine such as salbutamol to treat wheezing.

How to take fluticasone

Fluticasone is taken using a variety of different inhaler devices. We discuss these devices in Chapter 4. The dose you're prescribed depends on the particular device you're using and the strength of the product you're taking.

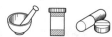

Insulin

Until not too long ago, the only insulin available to treat people with diabetes was obtained from the pancreases of pigs and cows. Nowadays, however, virtually all the insulin we use is manufactured in laboratories. Table 6-40 lists the insulins available in Canada. The classification of insulin is confusing, as some classes are based on how quickly an insulin starts to work (for example, "rapid-acting" and "fast-acting"), and others on how long it lasts (for example, "long-acting"). Even worse, we find the terms "rapid-acting" and "fast-acting" hopelessly confusing. Rapid? Fast? Who's got the better arm: the guy with the rapid pitch or the guy with the fast pitch? We don't know, either. Even worse, sometimes "fast-acting" insulin is also called "short-acting" insulin. The solution: stick with the generic or trade names when you're discussing your insulin therapy; that way, you and your health care providers will all be on the same page.

Figure 6-1 illustrates when each insulin starts to work, when it has its peak action, and when its effect wears off. In the case of premixed insulins (see Table 6-40), an injection will act on your body the same way as if you had injected each insulin in the mixture separately. We take a closer look at premixed insulins in the accompanying sidebar.

Table 6-40	Insulins	
Class	**Generic Name**	**Trade Name(s)**
Rapid-acting	**Aspart**	NovoRapid
	Lispro	Humalog
Fast-acting	**Regular**	Humulin-R, Novolin ge Toronto
Intermediate-acting±	**NPH**	Humulin-N, Novolin ge NPH
Long-acting	**Detemir**	Levemir
	Glargine	Lantus
Premixed		Humalog Mix25
		Humalog Mix50
		Humulin 30/70
		Novolin ge (30/70, 40/60, 50/50)
		NovoMix 30

± Another intermediate-acting insulin — "lente" — is no longer being supplied to the Canadian market and existing supplies will soon be gone. (It won't be missed; it had no advantage over NPH insulin and had the disadvantage of not being compatable with insulin pen devices.)

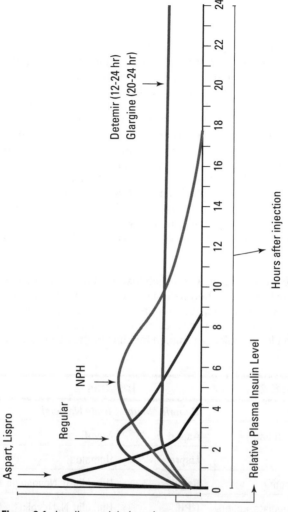

Figure 6-1: Insulins and their actions.

Pork-based insulins, though no longer manufactured in Canada and though rarely used, are still available.

Because the various insulins available share much in common (differing primarily in how long they take to have their peak effect and how long they last in the body), we discuss them together.

People with diabetes who require insulin therapy can usually obtain very good blood glucose control using various combinations of these medicines. None of these therapies makes having diabetes easy, mind you. *Easier,* yes, but certainly not *easy.*

Insulin is injected, using a tiny needle, under the skin. It's absorbed from the area it is injected and travels to various cells in the body where it attaches to insulin receptors. Insulin binds to insulin receptors on fat and muscle cells, causing these cells to extract glucose from the blood. Insulin also causes the liver to release less glucose into the blood.

How insulin can help you

Insulin can help you in the following ways:

- ✔ Lowering the levels of glucose in your blood. This provides you with more energy, makes you feel generally better, and reduces your risk of diabetes complications including blindness, kidney failure, erectile dysfunction, and heart attacks.

- ✔ Allowing glucose to enter into your muscle cells. This provides your muscles with more fuel so they can work more effectively.

How insulin might harm you

Possible side-effects from taking insulin include:

- ✔ *Hypoglycemia* (low blood glucose). This is, by far, the most common side-effect. Most of the time it's mild, but it can be severe to the point of causing you to lose consciousness.

- ✔ Injection site problems. The most common of these is *lipohypertrophy* (fat accumulation in the area where the insulin is injected). Occasionally, soreness and even inflammation can occur. Rarely, an allergic reaction develops.

- ✔ *Peripheral edema* (ankle swelling). This occasionally occurs shortly after starting insulin — especially if your blood glucose levels were exceptionally high prior to treatment. It tends to go away on its own soon thereafter.

There are virtually no situations in which insulin, as a class of drug, must absolutely not be taken. If you have had a bad skin reaction to a specific type of insulin (for example, red, inflamed, skin from injecting detemir insulin) then you should not take that particular type of insulin. If you have an allergy to insulin — this is extraordinarily rare with the newer, human insulins — special allergy treatments may be required to enable you to continue to take insulin.

Aspart, lispro, regular, and NPH insulins are considered safe to take during pregnancy and breastfeeding. The safety of detemir and glargine insulins during pregnancy and breastfeeding isn't known.

Precautions to follow if you're taking insulin

Follow these precautions if you're taking insulin:

✔ Monitor your blood glucose regularly; this will help you to determine if you're giving the correct doses. Regularly review your blood glucose levels with your health care team members. This is especially important during periods of illness, when your insulin requirements may change markedly.

✔ Rotate your injection sites to help you avoid lipohypertrophy (see above).

✔ If you're prone to hypoglycemia (from your insulin), get a glucagon emergency kit and have your pharmacist show your sufficiently mature family members how to use it. If you're incapacitated from an episode of severe hypoglycemia, being given an injection of glucagon will help bring your glucose level back up to a safe level.

✔ Alcohol use will make you more prone to hypoglycemia. Limiting alcohol consumption to a maximum of one drink per day (for a woman) and one to two drinks per day (for a man) is recommended.

Always make sure you have immediate access to a sugar source in the event you experience hypoglycemia. Immediate access isn't in the trunk of your car!

How to take insulin

At present, insulin is available in Canada only by injection and is typically given by using an insulin *pen*. (Inhaled insulin is newly approved for use in the United States; however, its long-term safety isn't yet proven.) We strongly believe that the only way to safely and effectively learn how to administer and adjust insulin is by being taught by a diabetes educator, not by reading a book (even *this* book). We discuss insulin therapy further in Chapter 5.

Premixed insulins

Premixed insulins are mixtures of other insulins in ratios as follows:

- Humalog Mix25 is 25% lispro and 75% lispro protamine*

- Humalog Mix50 is 50% lispro and 50% lispro protamine*

- Humulin 30/70 is 30% regular and 70% NPH

- Novolin 30/70 is 30% regular and 70% NPH

- Novolin 40/60 is 40% regular and 60% NPH

- Novolin 50/50 is 50% regular and 50% NPH

- NovoMix 30 is 30% aspart and 70% protaminated aspart*

* Lispro protamine and protaminated aspart both act similarly to NPH insulin.

If ever you need to buy insulin in the United States, it's important to be aware that in the U.S. they reverse the order of the numbers: 30/70 insulin in Canada is called 70/30 insulin in the U.S. Hmm, we wonder if the U.S. would consider reversing the results of the 2006 Stanley Cup finals?

The most commonly used of these premixed insulins is 30/70. This can work well for some people with type 2 diabetes, but because you would be unable to adjust each of the insulins separately (because the two insulins are already mixed together) there is less flexibility and less room to fine-tune the dose to suit your body's needs.

There is no such thing as a "standard" dose of insulin. You should be taking the dose of insulin that allows you the best control of your blood glucose levels. You may require 20 units per day and your next-door neighbour 200 units per day. This does not in any way mean that one of you is healthier or on a better or safer dose. Your neighbour wears size 12 shoes and you wear size 9 shoes. So what? You wear the shoe size that fits. And you take the insulin dose that works. Period.

Warning: Shameless plug ahead! For more information, we heartily recommend people with diabetes read *Diabetes For Canadians For Dummies* (which — by total coincidence, we assure you — happens to be co-authored by one Ian Blumer, MD).

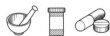

Leukotriene Antagonists

Leukotriene antagonists are newer drugs that have quickly found a role in the treatment of asthma. Table 6-41 lists the leukotriene antagonists available in Canada. We feel that the people who came up with the trade names for these two drugs surely deserve entry into a marketing hall of fame. Accolades for Accolate? Singular air of success about Singulair? Ah, a rose would smell as sweet by any other name, but when it comes to making drug names memorable ... well, maybe that's an entirely different matter.

Leukotrienes are substances that, when released from certain blood cells, act on leukotriene receptors on the bronchial tree and cause the bronchi to narrow. This results in wheezing (that is, an asthma attack). Leukotriene antagonists work by attaching to these same receptors and blocking leukotrienes from attaching. As a result leukotrienes are prevented from triggering an asthma attack.

Leukotriene antagonists are very similar. In this section we look in detail at the commonly used drug montelukast (which, as we note in Chapter 5, was discovered in Canada).

Table 6-41	Leukotriene Antagonists
Generic Name	*Trade Name*
Montelukast	Singulair
Zafirlukast	Accolate

 ## Montelukast

Singulair

Montelukast is approved in Canada for the prevention of asthma attacks, however its role will likely expand over the next few years as additional information on the potential benefits of this drug become available.

How montelukast can help you

Montelukast can help you in the following ways:

- Preventing asthma attacks.
- Preventing exercise-induced asthma.
- Improving seasonal (environmental) allergies.

How montelukast might harm you

Most people taking montelukast don't experience any side-effects. Possible side-effects from taking montelukast include:

- ✔ Headache.
- ✔ Abdominal pain, diarrhea.
- ✔ Rash.
- ✔ Flu-like illness with rash, numb arms and legs, joint pains, and sinus congestion.

The safety of montelukast in pregnancy and breastfeeding is unknown. If you're pregnant or breastfeeding, we recommend you discuss it with your physician before taking this medicine.

Precautions to follow if you're taking montelukast

If you develop a flu-like illness while taking montelukast (see above), seek prompt medical attention.

Because montelukast isn't effective for the treatment of wheezing attacks, be sure to *always* have available a short-acting beta-2 agonist medicine such as salbutamol to treat wheezing.

How to take montelukast

Montelukast is taken in a dose of 10 mg, with or without food, every evening. This drug should be continued daily, without interruption, even if you develop a flare of your asthma.

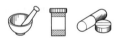

Lithium

As we discuss in Chapter 5, lithium is used primarily in the treatment of bipolar disorder. It was first discovered that lithium could help treat this condition more than 50 years ago. Table 6-42 lists the various lithium products available in Canada.

Table 6-42	Lithium
Generic Name	*Trade Names*
Lithium	Apo-Lithium Carbonate, Apo-Lithium Carbonate SR, Carbolith, Duralith, Lithane, PMS-Lithium Carbonate, PMS-Lithium Citrate

Lithium

Apo-Lithium Carbonate, Apo-Lithium Carbonate SR, Carbolith, Duralith, Lithane, PMS-Lithium Carbonate, PMS-Lithium Citrate

Although the precise way in which lithium helps control bipolar disorder isn't known, it appears to work by maintaining stable levels of certain chemical messengers (*neurotransmitters*) in the brain.

How lithium can help you

Lithium can help you if you have bipolar disorder by treating acute episodes of mania and by helping prevent future attacks. Less common uses are in the treatment of depression, post-traumatic stress disorder, and to help prevent attacks of an uncommon (and highly unpleasant) type of headache called "cluster headaches."

How lithium might harm you

Possible side-effects from taking lithium include:

- Nausea, abdominal discomfort, dizziness or feeling "dazed," muscle weakness. These symptoms are most likely soon after starting treatment.

- Increased thirst and passing increased amounts of urine.

- Tremor of the hands.

- Thyroid malfunction including hypothyroidism and goiter (that is, a swollen thyroid).

People with the following conditions generally shouldn't take lithium (because they're at increased risk of developing toxic levels of lithium):

- Serious cardiovascular disease.

- Serious kidney disease.

- Dehydration or being at risk of dehydration because of diuretic therapy.

If your bipolar disorder must be treated with lithium and you have one or more of the preceding conditions, treatment may still be possible (depending on the severity of the condition) under very close medical supervision.

Lithium can harm a fetus and thus, whenever possible, this drug isn't used during pregnancy or in women using insufficient contraception. Its use may also be unsafe during breastfeeding. If you're pregnant or breastfeeding, we recommend you discuss it with your physician before taking this medicine.

Precautions to follow if you're taking lithium

Follow these precautions if you're taking lithium:

> ✔ Have consistent amounts of sodium and water in your diet. Stay well hydrated.

> ✔ Seek medical attention if you develop fatigue, muscle weakness, incoordination, drowsiness, tremor, vomiting, diarrhea. These symptoms may indicate the level of lithium in your body is too high.

> ✔ Don't stop the drug without first speaking to your doctor.

> ✔ Lithium may make you drowsy, which would make it unsafe for you to perform activities — like driving — that require you to be alert and focused.

> ✔ Because alcohol may worsen drowsiness, it may be unwise to consume it. We recommend you check with your doctor to find out whether drinking (small amounts of) alcohol would be okay.

Your doctor will need to do blood tests from time to time to measure the level of lithium in your blood and to monitor your kidney and thyroid function.

How to take lithium

The starting dose of lithium will vary depending on the condition being treated; however, it's typically 200 mg to 600 mg three times daily. This dose is then adjusted a few days later, based on how you're responding to the medicine and what the lithium level is in your blood. After your dose has been stable for a time, your doctor may recommend you take your lithium once daily (rather than three times daily).

Lithium may be taken with or without food, however taking it with meals will help prevent it from making you feel nauseated. Extended-release lithium should not be crushed or chewed.

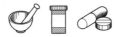

Menopausal Hormone Therapy

Menopausal hormone therapy (MHT), also known as *hormone replacement therapy* (HRT), *estrogen and progesterone therapy* (EPT), or *ovarian hormone therapy* (OHT), refers to the use of estrogen with or without progesterone in women who no longer produce their own estrogen and progesterone from the ovaries due to age-related changes, illness, or surgery.

Estrogen and progesterone are the most significant sex hormones in women and are made mainly by the ovaries. These hormones continue to be produced until mid-life (late 40s to early 50s) unless your ovaries have been damaged or surgically removed prior to that. When these hormones stop being produced, women no longer have menstrual periods (a not necessarily unwelcome event) and also commonly develop hot flushes, night sweats, sleep disturbances, and changes in bone density (definitely unwelcome events). By using menopausal hormone therapy (MHT), a woman replaces the missing estrogen and/or progesterone, and as a result these problems are eased. This can, however, be associated with some risk, as we discuss below.

MHT preparations available in Canada are listed in Table 6-43. Because these various drugs share so much in common we discuss them as a group.

Table 6-43	Menopausal Hormone Therapy	
Class	*Generic Name*	*Trade Name(s)*
Estrogens	**17 beta estradiol**	Tablet: Estrace
		Patch: Climara, Estraderm, Estradot,
		Gel: Estrogel
		Vaginal Ring: Estring
		Vaginal Cream: Vagifem
	Estropipate	Ogen
	Conjugated estrogens	Tablets: CES, Premarin
		Vaginal: Premarin Vaginal Cream

Class	Generic Name	Trade Name(s)
Progesterone/ progestins**	**Medroxy-Progesterone acetate (MPA)**	Tablets: Apo-Medroxy, Gen-Medroxy, novo-Medrone, Provera, Provera-Pak, ratio-MPA
		Injection: Depo-Provera
	Progesterone	Tablet: Prometrium±
Combined estrogen/ progestin	**17 Beta estradiol + Norethindrone acetate**	Patch: Estalis, Estalis Sequi, Estracomb
	Ethinyl estradiol and Norethindrone acetate	femHRT
	Conjugated Estrogen + Medroxyprogesterone acetate	Tablets: Premplus, Premplus Cycle

** Progestins are synthetic forms of progesterone.

± See the warning below regarding peanut allergies.

How menopausal hormone therapy can help you

Menopausal hormone therapy can help you in the following ways:

- ✔ Lessening symptoms of menopause including decreasing the frequency and severity of hot flushes and night sweats, improving sleep patterns, stabilizing your mood if this has been adversely affected by menopausal changes, reducing vaginal dryness, and helping maintain interest in sexual activity (that is, assisting your libido).

- ✔ Reducing your risk of osteoporosis by maintaining/improving bone quality and quantity. This helps minimize your risk of having an osteoporosis-related fracture.

- ✔ Decreasing the risk of colon cancer.

How menopausal hormone therapy might harm you

Possible side-effects from taking menopausal hormone therapy include:

- ✔ Breast cancer (especially with long-term use).

- ✔ Coronary artery disease.

- ✔ Weight gain.

✔ Headaches. (In particular, if you're prone to migraines you're at risk of these being more frequent.)

✔ Blood clots (which, in turn, can cause serious problems such as strokes, heart attacks, damage to the retina in the eye, deep vein thrombosis, and pulmonary emboli. We discuss these conditions in Chapter 5.)

Although taking MHT increases your risk of serious side-effects, the great majority of people using MHT don't develop these complications. Nonetheless, these risks are real and MHT should be taken only if you and your doctor, after careful review of your particular situation, determine that the potential benefits clearly outweigh the risks.

Women with the following conditions shouldn't take menopausal hormone therapy:

✔ Breast or uterine cancer.

✔ Coronary artery disease (CAD) or having a high risk of CAD. (Risk is determined by looking at a number of factors including your family history, whether you have high blood pressure, high cholesterol, and so on).

✔ Previous blood clots.

✔ Vaginal bleeding if the cause isn't known. (Vaginal bleeding is never normal in a woman who is past menopause.)

✔ Liver disease.

✔ Being premenopausal (that is, you have not yet reached menopause), pregnant, or breastfeeding.

Precautions to follow if you're taking menopausal hormone therapy

Follow these precautions if you're taking menopausal hormone therapy:

✔ Estrogen should be used in the lowest possible dose and for the shortest period of time necessary to keep your symptoms controlled. (This will reduce your risk of complications.)

✔ Perform a monthly breast self-examination and have a professional breast examination at least once a year.

✔ Unless you've had a hysterectomy, if you're taking MHT it should include *both* estrogen and progesterone (or progestin). Taking estrogen alone increases the risk of developing cancer of the uterus.

Prometrium brand of progesterone (see Table 6-43) contains peanut oil and should not be used if you have a peanut allergy.

How to take menopausal hormone therapy

The way in which MHT is taken varies *considerably* depending on the specific prescription you're given and, in particular, whether you have been prescribed estrogen, progesterone, or both. For this reason, your pharmacist should review with you how you're to take your particular MHT prescription.

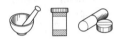

Narcotic ("Opioid") Analgesics

Narcotic analgesics (also called "opioids") are used for pain relief when non-narcotic analgesics such as acetaminophen are insufficient. Some narcotics (like codeine or hydrocodone) are also used to suppress a cough. Narcotic analgesics (excluding those given by injection) available in Canada are listed in Table 6-44. Narcotics share many properties in common including their ability to ease pain and, if used improperly, their risk of addiction. In this section we look in detail at the particularly commonly used drug, oxycodone.

Table 6-44	Narcotic Analgesics
Generic Name	*Trade Name(s)*
Butorphanol	Apo-Butorphanol, PMS-Butorphanol
Codeine±	Codeine Contin, ratio-Codeine, Codeine, Fiorinal-C*, ratio-Codeine, Tylenol with Codeine*
Fentanyl	Duragesic 12, Duragesic 25, Duragesic 50, Duragesic 75, Duragesic 100, RAN-Fentanyl Transdermal System
Hydrocodone	Dalmacol*, Dimetane Expectorant-DC*, Hycodan, Hycomine*, Hycomine-S*, Novahistex DH*, Novahistine DH*, ratio-Calmydone*, ratio-Coristex-DH*, Tussionex*
Hydromorphone	Dilaudid, Hydromorph Contin, Hydromorph·IR, PMS-Hydromorphone
Methadone	Metadol

(continued)

Table 6-44 (continued)

Generic Name	Trade Name(s)
Morphine	Kadian, M-Eslon, M.O.S., M.O.S.-SR, M.O.S.-Sulfate, MS Contin, MS·IR, PMS-Morphine Sulfate SR, ratio-Morphine, ratio-Morphine SR
Oxycodone	Endocet*, Endodan*, OxyContin, Oxy·IR, Percocet*, Percocet-Demi*, Percodan*, PMS-Oxycodone-Acetaminophen*, ratio-Ocycocet*, ratio-Oxycodan*, Supeudol
Pentazocine	Talwin Tablets
Propoxyphene	Darvon-N

* This medicine is a combination of different drugs. Refer to the drug label to determine what they are.

± Codeine is also found (in combination with other drugs like ASA or acetaminophen, and caffeine) in dozens of other products.

 ℞ *Oxycodone*

Endocet*, Endodan*, OxyContin, Oxy·IR, Percocet*, Percocet-Demi*, Percodan*, PMS-Oxycodone-Acetaminophen*, ratio-Ocycocet*, ratio-Oxycodan*, Supeudol

Oxycodone is available either alone or in combination with other drugs (typically acetaminophen or ASA). Oxycodone is in very common use, with more than 3 million prescriptions dispensed in Canada in 2005.

 Although the precise way in which oxycodone causes pain relief isn't known, it likely works in part by its action on opioid receptors in the brain and spinal cord, and also by altering levels of chemical messengers (*neurotransmitters*) such as acetylcholine and dopamine.

How oxycodone can help you

Oxycodone can help you by relieving your pain.

 Oxycodone is only to be used for moderate to severe pain that cannot be controlled with non-narcotic analgesics such as acetaminophen or ibuprofen.

How oxycodone might harm you

Possible side-effects from taking oxycodone include:

- ✔ Nausea, vomiting, constipation, sleepiness/sedation, headache, dry mouth, sweating, weakness. These are the most common side-effects.

- ✔ Low blood pressure. This can cause faintness.

- ✔ *Respiratory depression* (that is, insufficient breathing to keep up with your body's needs).

- ✔ Addiction and drug withdrawal symptoms. We discuss these below.

People with the following conditions shouldn't take oxycodone:

- ✔ Acute asthma (that is, an asthma attack) or an acute exacerbation of COPD.

- ✔ Respiratory depression.

- ✔ Alcohol intoxication or alcohol withdrawal.

- ✔ Decreased mental alertness.

- ✔ Recent head injury (unless you have been checked by your doctor and it's believed safe to take the drug).

- ✔ You shouldn't take oxycodone if you have taken a drug from the monoamine oxidase (MAO) inhibitor family within the past 14 days, nor should you start taking an MAO inhibitor within 14 days of stopping oxycodone.

It can be unsafe to take oxycodone for an extended period of time during pregnancy and/or to take it in high doses at the end of pregnancy. There are also safety concerns when this drug is taken during breastfeeding. If you're pregnant or breastfeeding, we recommend you discuss it with your physician before taking this medicine.

Precautions to follow if you're taking oxycodone

Follow these precautions if you're taking oxycodone:

- ✔ Don't stop the drug without first speaking to your doctor. Suddenly stopping the drug can bring on withdrawal symptoms including aching, loss of appetite, anxiety, nausea, insomnia, palpitations, and fever. (Gradually withdrawing the medicine will minimize these symptoms.)

- ✔ If you're prescribed another drug that can also be sedating, your oxycodone dose may need to be reduced.

✔ This drug may make you drowsy, which would make it unsafe for you to perform activities — like driving — that require you to be alert and focused.

✔ Because alcohol may worsen drowsiness, it may be unwise to consume it. We recommend you check with your doctor to find out whether drinking (small amounts of) alcohol would be okay.

How to take oxycodone

The dose of oxycodone you require will vary widely depending on factors such as your general health, the other drugs you're taking, and the particular form of oxycodone you're prescribed.

These are the important points about *inappropriate* use of oxycodone:

✔ Taking an overdose can be *fatal*.

✔ Using oxycodone in excessive amounts or for longer than necessary can lead to *addiction*.

✔ If oxycodone is injected into a vein, you may develop infections, lung damage, and/or heart damage.

Taking oxycodone in *appropriate* quantities and for an appropriate length of time for pain control does *not* result in addiction.

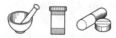

Nitrates

Nitrates are various forms of nitroglycerin used in the treatment of angina. (We discuss angina in Chapter 5.) One of the earliest people to be prescribed nitroglycerin was Alfred Nobel (founder of the Nobel Prize), an irony that was not lost on the man who had used nitroglycerin to create dynamite: "Isn't it the irony of fate that I have been prescribed nitroglycerin, to be taken internally!" he wrote in 1896. Table 6-45 lists the nitrates available in Canada.

Nitroglycerin causes tiny muscles that line blood vessel walls to relax. When these muscles relax, the blood vessels widen (a process called *vasodilation*) in much the same way that if you relax the muscles of a clenched fist, your hand opens. It's not known if the most important part of this is dilatation of the arteries in the heart (which would allow more oxygen to get directly to the heart muscle), dilatation of the arteries elsewhere in the body (which would allow the heart to use less effort to pump blood through the body), or dilatation of the veins (which would result in less blood flowing back to the heart and thus require it to perform less work).

There are fast-acting nitrates (taken sublingually — that is, under the tongue — as a spray) and there are longer-acting nitrates (available orally or as a patch; the latter is more commonly used). Fast-acting nitrates are taken in two situations:

- ✔ To *treat* an angina attack (that is; when you have developed symptoms of angina).

- ✔ To *prevent* an angina attack. If you know that you will likely develop angina if you perform an activity (such as walking up a hill or having sexual intercourse), taking a fast-acting nitrate *immediately before* the activity will help prevent an attack from occurring.

Long-acting nitrates, on the other hand, are taken exclusively to prevent angina attacks.

When you have an episode of angina, sit down and take a dose of *fast-acting* nitroglycerin under your tongue. If your attack isn't relieved within five minutes, take another dose. If your attack isn't relieved within another five minutes, take a third dose. If within the next five minutes your attack is still not relieved, call an ambulance. In baseball, it's three strikes and you're out. With angina, it's three sprays and you're in (to hospital, that is).

Table 6-45	Nitrates
Generic Name	*Trade Name(s)*
Nitroglycerin	**Sublingual**: Gen-Nitro, Nitrolingual Pump Spray, Nitrostat, Rho-Nitro Pumpsray
	Topical: Minitran, Nitro-Dur, Nitrol, Transderm-Nitro, Trinipatch
Isosorbide Dintrate	Apo-ISDN
Isosorbide-5-mononitrate	Imdur

Topical Nitroglycerin

Minitran, Nitro-Dur, Nitrol, Transderm-Nitro, Trinipatch

Topical nitroglycerin is usually given in the form of a patch and provides a continual release of medicine from the patch into the body.

How topical nitroglycerin can help you

Topical nitroglycerin can help you by preventing attacks of angina and allowing you to perform greater amounts of activity before an attack of angina occurs.

Topical nitroglycerin will *not* abort an angina attack. It's a *preventive* medicine only. As we discuss above, treat an attack of angina with *sublingual* (fast-acting) nitroglycerin.

How topical nitroglycerin might harm you

Possible side-effects from topical nitroglycerin include:

- ✔ Headache. This is a frequent side-effect and can be treated with plain analgesics such as acetaminophen. If your headache persists, discuss this with your physician.

- ✔ Faintness (especially upon first arising from a bed or from a chair).

- ✔ Skin irritation. This is usually mild and goes away within a few hours of removing the patch.

People with the following conditions shouldn't take topical nitroglycerin:

- ✔ An allergy to the adhesive.

- ✔ Increased pressure within the brain (*raised intracranial pressure*).

- ✔ Increased intra-ocular pressure (as is seen with glaucoma).

- ✔ Severe anemia.

- ✔ Use of phosphodiesterase type 5 inhibitors (for example sildenafil, trade name Viagra). Combined use of a phosphodiesterase type 5 inhibitor and nitrates can result in a life-threatening drop in your blood pressure. Therefore, if you require nitroglycerin medication you need to discontinue use of drugs such as sildenafil. We discuss these drugs elsewhere in this chapter.

The safety of topical nitroglycerin in pregnancy and breastfeeding is unknown. We recommend before taking this medicine in these circumstances, you discuss this with your physician.

Precautions to follow if you're taking topical nitroglycerin

Follow these precautions if you're taking topical nitroglycerin:

- ✔ If you have a home defibrillator, make sure whomever in your household may be the one to use the device knows to remove the topical nitroglycerin before shocking you. (Otherwise, it could burn your skin.)

- ✔ Remove it prior to MRI scans. (Some patches contain metal.)

- ✔ If you develop faintness while taking topical nitroglycerin, be sure to immediately sit and, if necessary, lie down. This will help you avoid fainting.

- ✔ Don't stop the drug without first speaking to your doctor. (Suddenly stopping the drug may make your angina worse.)

How to take topical nitroglycerin

Your dose depends on your specific situation; however, in general, if topical nitroglycerin is being administered in the form of Nitro-Dur (which is a patch) it's started in a dose of 0.2 (mg/hr). It's worn daily for a maximum of 12 to 14 hours, at which point it should be removed. (Wearing it longer than this will make it less effective). It should be applied each day at a similar time.

 The best stretch of time to wear topical nitroglycerin is when you're most likely to experience angina attacks. For most people this is during the daytime, but for some people it's overnight. We recommend you discuss this with your doctor.

You can apply topical nitroglycerin to most convenient places on your body, but not toward (or on) your hands or feet. The arms and chest are the preferred locations. Vary the site you use to help minimize skin irritation from the patch.

 In order for a patch to stick, you may need to first shave the area where you're going to be putting it. Also, be sure to wash your hands thoroughly after touching the patch.

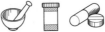

Nonsteroidal Anti-Inflammatory Drugs (NSAIDs)

Nonsteroidal anti-inflammatory drugs (NSAIDs) are used to treat a variety of conditions, especially those that cause inflammation and pain. Given that all of us have pain at least some of the time (and some of us have pain pretty well all of the time), it's perhaps not surprising that NSAIDs are some of the most commonly used medicines in the world.

We list the various NSAIDs available in Canada in Table 6-46. (In your travels, you may come across ASA being listed as an NSAID. In high doses it does have an anti-inflammatory action, however ASA is so vastly different from NSAIDs in most every other way that it needs to be considered as an entirely different class of drug. For this reason, we discuss ASA elsewhere in this chapter.)

Table 6-46	Nonsteroidal Anti-inflammatory Drugs
Generic Name	*Trade Name(s)*
Celecoxib	Celebrex
Diclofenac	Apo-Diclo, Apo-Diclo Rapide, Apo-Diclo SR, Arthrotec*, Novo-Difenac, Novo-Difenac-K, Novo-Difenac SR, Nu-Diclo, Nu-Diclo SR, Pennsaid, PMS-Diclofenac, PMS-Diclofenac SR, Sandoz Diclofenac, Sandoz Diclofenac Rapide, Sandoz Diclofenac SR, Voltaren, Voltaren Ophtha, Voltaren Rapide
Diflunisal	Apo-Diflunisal, Novo-Diflunisal, Nu-Diflunisal
Etodolac	Apo-Etodolac
Floctafenine	Apo-Floctafenine
Flurbiprofen	Ansaid, Apo-Flurbiprofen, Froben, Froben SR, Novo-Flurprofen, Nu-Flurbiprofen, Ocufen
Ibuprofen**	Advil, Apo-Ibuprofen, Motrin, Novo-Profen, Nu-Ibuprofen, Robax Platinum*
Indomethacin	Apo-Indomethacin, Novo-Methacin, Nu-Indo
Ketoprofen	Apo-Keto, Apo-Keto-E, Apo-Keto SR, Nu-Ketoprofen-SR
Ketorolac	Acular, Acular LS, Apo-Ketorolac, Apo-Ketorolac Ophthalmic Solution, Novo-Ketorolac, ratio-Ketorolac, Toradol
Lumiracoxib	Prexige

Generic Name	Trade Name(s)
Mefenamic Acid	Apo-Mefenamic, Nu-Mefenamic
Meloxicam	Apo-Meloxicam, CO Meloxicam, Gen-Meloxicam, Mobicox, Novo-Meloxicam, PMS-Meloxicam, ratio-Meloxicam
Nabumetone	Apo-Nabumetone, Gen-Nabumetone, Novo-Nabumetone, Sandoz Nabumetone
Naproxen	Anaprox, Anaprox DS, Apo-Napro-Na, Apo-Napro-Na DS, Apo-Naproxen, Apo-Naproxen EC, Apo-Naproxen SR, Gen-Naproxen EC, Naprosyn, Novo-Naprox, Novo-Naprox-EC, Novo-Naprox SR, Novo-Naprox Sodium, Novo-Naprox Sodium DS, Nu-Naprox
Oxaprozin	Apo-Oxaprozin, Daypro
Piroxicam	Apo-Piroxicam, Gen-Piroxicam, Novo-Pirocam, Nu-Pirox
Sulindac	Apo-Sulin, Novo-Sundac, Nu-Sulindac
Tenoxicam	Apo-Tenoxicam
Tiaprofenic Acid	Apo-Tiaprofenic, Novo-Tiaprofenic, Nu-Tiaprofenic, Surgam, Surgam SR

* This medicine is a combination of different drugs. Refer to the drug label to determine what they are.

** This is a partial list. (Ibuprofen is available over-the-counter under a variety of trade names).

Because NSAIDs are so similar in terms of how they work, their side-effects, and so forth, we discuss them together.

We all have naturally occurring substances within our bodies called *prostaglandins*. Prostaglandins cause inflammation. NSAIDs work by reducing the amount of prostaglandin. They do this by blocking the action of an enzyme (*cyclo-oxygenase*) that promotes production of prostaglandins. Less cyclo-oxygenase, less prostaglandin; less prostaglandin, less inflammation; less inflammation, less pain. Voila!

How NSAIDs can help you

NSAIDs can help you in the following ways:

- Reducing pain, stiffness, and swelling in your muscles and joints.
- Lowering fever.
- Easing dental pain, headaches, and menstrual pains.

Of the NSAIDs, ibuprofen is particularly effective at helping relieve dental pain.

How NSAIDs might harm you

Possible side-effects from taking NSAIDs include:

- ✔ Indigestion, heartburn, and stomach ulcers. These are less likely to occur with celecoxib than other NSAIDs. Your risk of an ulcer is greater if you're elderly, if you smoke, and/or if you drink excess quantities of alcohol.

- ✔ Heart attack and stroke.

- ✔ High blood pressure.

- ✔ Kidney failure.

- ✔ Abnormal liver tests. This is seldom serious.

People with the following conditions shouldn't take NSAIDs:

- ✔ Allergies to ASA or other NSAIDs. (If you have nasal polyps and/or asthma, you may be at especially high risk of being allergic to NSAIDs.)

- ✔ Serious liver disease.

- ✔ Serious kidney disease.

- ✔ Inflammatory bowel disease (such as ulcerative colitis).

- ✔ High levels of potassium in the blood.

- ✔ Coronary artery disease (CAD), especially if you have had recent heart bypass surgery. (Because of increasing evidence that taking NSAIDs if you have CAD may increase the risk of heart attack, it's often recommended to avoid all NSAIDs — except ASA — if you have this condition. If you have CAD and must take an NSAID, take the lowest possible dose for the shortest possible time.)

It's generally recommended that you don't take NSAIDs during pregnancy and breastfeeding. If you're pregnant or breastfeeding, we recommend you discuss it with your physician before taking NSAIDs.

Precautions to follow if you're taking NSAIDs

Follow these precautions if you're taking NSAIDs:

- ✔ Your blood pressure should be checked periodically.

- ✔ Blood tests to measure your hemoglobin level (that is, to see if you have anemia), kidney function, and liver function are typically done about 6 to 12 weeks after starting NSAID therapy.

✔ Check your stools for blood on a daily basis: if you see red blood or if your stools are tarry and black (which can indicate bleeding within the gut), seek urgent medical attention.

Because some NSAIDs are now available as over-the-counter medications it can be easy to forget to mention to your doctor that you're taking this type of drug. As a result, your doctor may end up prescribing another NSAID for you for an unrelated condition. Taking two different NSAIDs increases your risk of side-effects, so be sure to let your doctor know *all* the drugs you're taking — prescription *and* non-prescription.

How to take NSAIDs

Oral NSAIDs are best swallowed whole and taken with a meal to help minimize stomach upset. NSAIDs also come as suppositories and as eye drops. We discuss how to take suppositories and eye drops in Chapter 3.

Topical NSAIDs (almost always in the form of drops) can be used for localized discomfort by applying the drops directly on the skin over the painful area, but should not be put directly on cuts or other skin wounds.

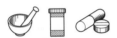

Oral Hypoglycemic Agents

If you have type 2 diabetes, the medicines you take by mouth to keep your blood glucose levels under control are called *oral hypoglycemic agents* (OHAs). And like all, ahem, agents, they go by a few aliases, including "oral antihyperglycemic agents" or "oral antidiabetic agents." (And, speaking of agents, can someone explain to us why it is that that most famous agent of all, the incomparable 007, always uses his real name when introducing himself? Wouldn't a *secret* agent use a *secret* name?)

What all OHAs have in common is that they help to lower your blood glucose ("blood sugar") levels, and by doing so they reduce your risk of developing diabetes complications including eye damage (*retinopathy*), kidney damage (*nephropathy*), and nerve damage (*neuropathy*). Some OHAs have additional benefits, which we mention when we discuss the individual drugs. Most people with type 2 diabetes require more than one type of OHA. We list the various oral hypoglycemic agents available in Canada in Table 6-47. In Chapter 5, we discuss the general approach to OHA therapy, including the benefits of using one class versus another.

Table 6-47	Oral Hypoglycemic Agents	
Class	*Generic Name*	*Trade Name(s)*
Alpha glucosidase inhibitor	**Acarbose**	Glucobay**
Biguanide	**Metformin**	Apo-Metformin, Avandamet*, CO Metformin Coated, Gen-Metformin, Glucophage, Glumetza, Novo-Metformin, Nu-Metformin, PMS Metformin, RAN-Metformin, ratio-Metformin, Sandoz Metformin FC
Non-sulfonylurea insulin secretagogues	Nateglinide	Starlix
	Repaglinide	GlucoNorm
Sulfonylureas	Chlorpropamide	Apo-Chlorpropamide, Novo-Propamide
	Gliclazide	Apo-Gliclazide, Diamicron, Diamicron MR, Gen-Gliclazide, Novo-Gliclazide, Sandoz Gliclazide
	Glimepiride	Amaryl, Avandaryl*, CO Glimepiride, Novo-Glimepiride, ratio-Glimepiride, Sandoz Glimepiride
	Glyburide	Apo-Glyburide, Diabeta, Gen-Glybe, Novo-Glyburide, Nu-Glyburide, PMS-Glyburide, ratio-Glyburide, Sandoz Glyburide
	Tolbutamide	Apo-Tolbutamide
Thiazolidinediones (TZDs)	**Pioglitazone**	Actos
	Rosiglitazone	Avandamet*, Avandaryl*, Avandia

* This medicine is a combination of different drugs. Refer to the drug label to determine what they are.

** This drug was, until recently, called Prandase.

℞ *Acarbose*

Glucobay

Acarbose is very safe to take, but it's not very potent and can have some unpleasant side-effects; as such, it's typically not used as often as some other OHAs.

By blocking the action of an enzyme (alpha-glucosidase) in the small intestine, acarbose slows down the absorption of sugars from the bowel into the blood stream; this results in better blood glucose control.

How acarbose can help you

Acarbose can help you in the following ways:

- ✔ Lowering your blood glucose levels: This in turn reduces your risk of developing diabetes complications.
- ✔ Preventing (or delaying the onset of) diabetes if you have pre-diabetes. (Pre-diabetes is a condition where your blood glucose levels are increased compared with normal, but not to a level where diabetes is diagnosed. Having pre-diabetes puts you at high risk of eventually developing diabetes.)

How acarbose might harm you

Possible side-effects from taking acarbose include:

- ✔ Abdominal discomfort, diarrhea, and flatulence: The flatulence can be plentiful, so this drug is best suited to those people who are "loud and proud." These symptoms tend to improve as time goes by.
- ✔ Skin rash.
- ✔ Hepatitis.

Serious side-effects very rarely occur.

People with the following conditions shouldn't take acarbose:

- ✔ Type 1 diabetes.
- ✔ Chronic, serious bowel diseases including inflammatory bowel disease, ulcers within the large bowel, or a very large bowel hernia.

The safety of acarbose in pregnancy and breastfeeding is unknown. If you're pregnant or breastfeeding, we recommend you discuss it with your physician before taking this medicine.

Precautions to follow if you're taking acarbose

Consuming lots of *sucrose* (table sugar) when taking acarbose makes you more likely to develop unpleasant gastrointestinal side-effects like bloating, flatulence, and diarrhea.

If you experience hypoglycemia (because of insulin or some other OHA you're taking) while on acarbose, you need to treat this with glucose (as is contained, for example, in Dextrosol tablets), not sucrose (as is contained in colas, table sugar, and fruit juice).

How to take acarbose

The usual starting dose of acarbose is 50 mg taken once daily. The dose is subsequently slowly increased, under the supervision of your doctor, based on how you're responding. The usual maintenance dose is 50 to 100 mg taken three times daily. Acarbose should be taken with the first bite of your meal.

If you skip a meal, you can omit your dose.

℞ Glyburide

Apo-Glyburide, Diabeta, Gen-Glybe, Novo-Glyburide, Nu-Glyburide, PMS-Glyburide, ratio-Glyburide, Sandoz Glyburide

Glyburide is a very effective drug to help you manage your diabetes. It's inexpensive and quite potent and, because it has been around for many years, we know a good deal about its pros and cons. In most respects, all the members of the sulfonylurea class of oral hypoglycemic agent are pretty similar.

Glyburide stimulates the pancreas to produce more insulin. Insulin, in turn, helps your body move glucose from your blood into your muscle cells, where it can be used as fuel, or, if in excess supply, into your fat cells, where it can be used as storage in the form of fat.

How glyburide can help you

By lowering your blood glucose levels, glyburide will reduce your risk of developing diabetes complications.

How glyburide might harm you

Possible side-effects from taking glyburide include:

✔ Hypoglycemia: Glyburide can lower your blood glucose too much, leading to hypoglycemia. Symptoms of hypoglycemia include sweatiness, palpitations, anxiety, and hunger.

✔ Weight gain: Glyburide often leads to some weight gain. Fortunately this tends to be small and, by paying close attention to your diet and by exercising regularly, you can minimize this.

✔ Nausea and heartburn: These are seldom particularly bothersome.

✔ *Photosensitive skin rash.* (That is, a rash that occurs upon sun exposure.) Other forms of skin rash may also be experienced.

People with the following conditions shouldn't take glyburide:

✔ Type 1 diabetes.

✔ Severe liver disease.

✔ Serious kidney disease.

Recent evidence suggests it's *probably* safe to take glyburide during pregnancy and breastfeeding, but this remains uncertain. If you're pregnant or breastfeeding, we recommend you discuss it with your physician before taking this medicine.

Precautions to follow if you're taking glyburide

Follow these precautions if you're taking glyburide:

✔ Glyburide is a sulfa-based drug, so if you've reacted to some other sulfa drug you're at risk of also reacting to glyburide. (Incidentally, many doctors are not aware of this.) Nonetheless, most people with a history of a sulfa drug reaction do *not* react to glyburide. You and your doctor will need to determine if the potential benefits of taking glyburide outweigh the potential risk of you having a reaction.

✔ Use sunscreen and protective clothing to help avoid getting a photosensitive skin rash (see above).

✔ Occasionally, people cannot tolerate alcohol if they're taking glyburide, developing flushing, nausea, and palpitations after having a drink. Makes the whole idea of a nice glass of Chardonnay quite a turn-off.

How to take glyburide

The usual starting dose of glyburide is 2.5 mg to 5.0 mg taken once daily just prior to or during your breakfast (you *do* eat breakfast, don't you?). The dose is subsequently increased, under your doctor's supervision, based on your response. Doses beyond 7.5 mg taken twice daily seldom provide additional benefit.

Metformin

Apo-Metformin, Avandamet*, CO Metformin Coated, Gen-Metformin, Glucophage, Glumetza, Novo-Metformin, Nu-Metformin, PMS Metformin, RAN-Metformin, ratio-Metformin, Sandoz Metformin FC

Although metformin has been around for ages, it has not only managed to survive the test of time — it's thrived from it. Metformin is considered the pre-eminent OHA. Nonetheless, like a temperamental movie star, it needs to be dealt with cautiously.

Metformin lowers blood glucose levels by reducing the amount of glucose the liver releases into the blood; its other, less powerful action is on muscle and fat cells, where it helps these cells to more efficiently extract glucose from the blood.

How metformin can help you

Metformin can help you in the following ways:

- ✔ Lowering your blood glucose levels. This in turn will reduce your risk of developing diabetes complications.

- ✔ Reducing your risk of having a heart attack or stroke (if you have diabetes). The way in which metformin provides this nice benefit isn't clear.

- ✔ Not causing weight gain. Unlike almost all other OHAs, metformin does not cause weight gain (a not unimportant point given that the vast majority of people with type 2 diabetes are overweight to start with).

- ✔ Improving fertility. Metformin has been found to increase a woman's fertility if she has polycystic ovary syndrome.

- ✔ Preventing (or delaying the onset of) diabetes if you have pre-diabetes. (Pre-diabetes is a condition where your blood glucose levels are increased compared with normal, but not to a level where diabetes is diagnosed. Having pre-diabetes puts you at high risk of eventually developing diabetes.)

How metformin might harm you

Possible side-effects from taking metformin include:

- ✔ Nausea, abdominal cramping, diarrhea. These occur commonly.

- ✔ Vitamin B12 deficiency: Metformin can make it harder for your gut to properly absorb vitamin B12 from food you've eaten.

✔ Lactic acidosis: This life-threatening disorder causes symptoms of malaise (that is, feeling generally unwell), nausea, vomiting, headache, muscle pain, and confusion, and can lead to shock (as in dangerously low blood pressure; not shock as in emotional upset or surprise).

People with the following conditions shouldn't take metformin:

✔ Kidney failure.

✔ Liver disease.

✔ Congestive heart failure.

Recent evidence suggests it's probably safe to take metformin during pregnancy and breastfeeding, but this remains uncertain. If you're pregnant or breastfeeding, we recommend you discuss it with your physician before taking this medicine.

Precautions to follow if you're taking metformin

Follow these precautions if you're taking metformin:

✔ Have your vitamin B12 level checked from time to time. If your level is low, taking oral vitamin B12 supplements will typically correct the situation.

✔ Because metformin may increase some women's fertility (see earlier in this section), if you're a woman of child-bearing age and are not wanting to get pregnant, you need to use appropriate birth control measures.

✔ *Intravenous contrast* ("intravenous dye") used for some types of x-rays can, rarely, cause kidney failure. This, in turn, can increase your risk of developing lactic acidosis from metformin therapy. Therefore, you need to discontinue your metformin for a brief period of time before and after receiving this contrast. We recommend you check with your doctor well in advance of the scheduled x-ray to find out her specific instructions regarding what you should do with your metformin.

How to take metformin

Stomach upset, abdominal cramps, and diarrhea are minimized if you take metformin with food and if you start metformin in a very low dose of 250 to 500 mg once daily with the dose then slowly increased, under your doctor's supervision, depending on your response. Maintenance doses beyond 1.5 g per day (taken as 500 mg three times daily or 750 mg twice daily) seldom provide additional benefit. (A newer form of metformin — Glumetza — can be taken once daily.)

Pioglitazone, Rosiglitazone

Pioglitazone: Actos

Rosiglitazone: Avandamet*, Avandaryl*, Avandia

Because pioglitazone and rosiglitazone are so similar, we discuss them together. These two drugs are members of a fairly new class of medicine, the thiazolidinediones (TZDs). These new drugs on the block are being used increasingly often to help manage type 2 diabetes.

TZDs attach to and stimulate peroxisome proliferator activated receptor gamma receptors. (Fortunately, this is abbreviated as *PPAR gamma* receptors. Still a mouthful, mind you.) When these receptors are stimulated, they enhance the action of the insulin your pancreas makes. As a result, glucose is more readily able to pass from the blood into fat and muscle cells. Also, the liver releases less glucose into the blood. These collective actions result in lower glucose levels in the blood. Because TZDs enable your own insulin to work better, they're said to reduce insulin resistance.

How TZDs can help you

TZDs can help you in the following ways:

- ✔ Lowering your blood glucose levels. This in turn reduces your risk of developing diabetes complications.

- ✔ Reducing your risk of a heart attack. This isn't proven, but some evidence suggests that, independent of their effect on glucose control, TZDs may help protect against heart attacks and strokes.

- ✔ Improving fertility. TZDs have been found to increase a woman's fertility if she has polycystic ovary syndrome.

- ✔ Helping preserve your pancreas's ability to make insulin. This isn't as yet fully proven.

- ✔ Preventing (or delaying the onset of) diabetes if you have pre-diabetes. (Pre-diabetes is a condition where your blood glucose levels are increased compared with normal, but not to a level where diabetes is diagnosed. Having pre-diabetes puts you at high risk of eventually developing diabetes.) TZDs are more effective than acarbose or metformin at doing this.

TZDs are unique among OHAs in that their blood glucose–lowering ability may not show up right away; indeed, it can take up to two months before their full benefit is seen. Bottom line: don't be discouraged if, after taking a TZD for two or three weeks, you haven't seen your blood glucose levels go down — it may just take a bit longer for you to see the benefit.

How TZDs might harm you

Possible side-effects from taking TZDs include:

- ✔ Weight gain. Unfortunately, this is a common problem with TZD therapy. (Some of the weight gain may be due to fluid retention.)
- ✔ *Peripheral edema* (ankle swelling).
- ✔ Congestive heart failure. Infrequently, TZDs cause fluid buildup in the lungs due to heart failure; this serious side-effect will make you feel short of breath, especially when you're lying down or if you're exerting yourself. This is more likely to occur if you have pre-existing heart damage (from, say, a previous heart attack).
- ✔ Anemia. TZDs sometime cause very mild anemia. This isn't serious.
- ✔ Fractures. There is some evidence that TZDs increase a woman's risk of arm, hand, and ankle fractures. This is unproven.

When you should not take a TZD

People with the following conditions shouldn't take a TZD:

- ✔ Poor heart function.
- ✔ Serious liver disease.

The safety of TZDs in pregnancy and breastfeeding is unknown. If you're pregnant or breastfeeding, we recommend you discuss it with your physician before taking this medicine.

Precautions to follow if you're taking a TZD

Follow these precautions if you're taking a TZD:

- ✔ If you develop shortness of breath, seek prompt medical attention.
- ✔ Because TZDs may increase some women's fertility (see earlier in this section), if you're a woman of child-bearing age and are not wanting to get pregnant, you need to take appropriate birth control measures.

How to take a TZD

Pioglitazone is usually started in a dose of 15 mg to 30 mg once daily. Rosiglitazone is usually started in a dose of 4 mg once daily. After a few weeks the dose may be increased, under your doctor's supervision, based on your response. You can take TZDs with or without food.

 ## Repaglinide

GlucoNorm

Repaglinide is a helpful drug to control blood glucose levels but in general isn't considered a "first line" drug; rather, doctors typically prescribe it to replace glyburide if glyburide isn't serving your needs sufficiently well.

 Repaglinide stimulates the pancreas to produce more insulin. Insulin, in turn, helps your body move glucose from your blood into your muscle cells where it can be used as fuel or, if in excess supply, into your fat cells where it can be used as storage in the form of fat.

How repaglinide can help you

By lowering your blood glucose levels, repaglinide will reduce your risk of developing diabetes complications. Compared with other OHAs, repaglinide is particularly effective at reducing after-meal blood glucose levels.

How repaglinide might harm you

Repaglinide tends to be tolerated very well and, apart from hypo-glycemia and mild weight gain, side-effects seldom occur.

Repaglinide shouldn't be taken if you have type 1 diabetes.

 The safety of repaglinide in pregnancy and breastfeeding is unknown. If you're pregnant or breastfeeding, we recommend you discuss it with your physician before taking this medicine.

Precautions to follow if you're taking repaglinide

If you have severe liver or kidney disease, you're more at risk of developing hypoglycemia while taking repaglinide. In these circum-stances, keep an especially close eye on your blood glucose levels and be sure to notify your physician if you're getting readings under 4 mmol/L.

How to take repaglinide

Repaglinide is usually started in a dose of 1 mg taken 15 to 30 min-utes before meals. The dose is then gradually increased, under your doctor's supervision, based on your response. The usual maintenance dose is 2 mg to 4 mg per meal. If you skip a meal (not that we're advocating this, of course), skip your dose.

Avoid consuming grapefruit or grapefruit juice because it can affect the level of repaglinide in your blood.

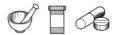

Phosphodiesterase Type 5 (PDE5) Inhibitors

The introduction of PDE5 inhibitors such as sildenafil (Viagra) not only revolutionized the treatment of erectile dysfunction, but also helped to lift the unfortunate stigma that erectile dysfunction (ED) had lived under for too, too long. Table 6-48 lists the PDE5 inhibitors available in Canada.

As we discuss in Chapter 5, sildenafil, the first of the PDE5 inhibitors available in Canada, now shares the limelight with two other members of this drug family, each with slightly different properties, but in most ways being very similar. We discuss sildenafil in more detail below.

The different PDE5 inhibitors work based on the same underlying principles. Increased levels of an enzyme called cGMP allow for blood to flow into the penis, which results in an erection. Phosphodiesterase type 5 (PDE5) is an enzyme that reduces the level of cGMP and therefore reduces the ability to have an erection. PDE5 inhibitors block the action of PDE5. Less PDE5, more cGMP; more cGMP, more blood into the penis; more blood into the penis, more firmness to the organ. Et voila, an erection (and potentially something else) is born.

Table 6-48	PDE5 Inhibitors
Generic Name	*Trade Name(s)*
Sildenafil	Revatio, Viagra
Tadalafil	Cialis
Vardenafil	Levitra

Sildenafil

Revatio, Viagra

Sildenafil has truly been a revolutionary drug, and both the drug and the advertising and hype around it have helped to bring a hitherto often hidden and distressing topic out into the open. Clearly, if you have erectile dysfunction you're not alone: in Canada in 2005 more than 850,000 prescriptions were written for sildenafil!

How sildenafil can help you

Sildenafil can help you in the following ways:

- Obtaining an erection.

- Improving *pulmonary artery hypertension.* (This is a rare disease in which there is increased blood pressure confined to certain arteries in the chest.)

- Treating Raynaud's phenomenon.

How sildenafil might harm you

Possible side-effects from taking sildenafil include:

- Headache, flushing, indigestion. These are the most common side-effects. They aren't serious.

- Altered vision including blurring or abnormal colour discrimination. This seldom occurs.

- *Priapism.* This is a persistent, painful erection (typically lasting several hours or more). It must be treated urgently; otherwise it can lead to permanent erectile dysfunction.

People with the following conditions shouldn't take sildenafil:

- Using nitrate medication. Combined use of nitrates (regardless of the route they're being used: oral, under the tongue, on the skin, etc.) and sildenafil can cause a sudden and potentially dangerous drop in your blood pressure.

- Women. (Sildenafil isn't currently recommended for use by women; however, there are ongoing studies looking at whether this drug might be of value for women with sexual dysfunction or other conditions noted above: see "How sildenafil can help you.")

Precautions to follow if you're taking sildenafil

There are many causes of erectile dysfunction, a number of which require different treatment than sildenafil. Examples include testosterone deficiency or high prolactin hormone levels. Before sildenafil is prescribed for you, your doctor needs to determine whether you might have one of these other causes.

If you're new to the use of the drug and have not had recent intercourse, it's possible that you may have underlying heart disease that has not caused symptoms because you've been inactive. Renewed sexual activity may bring out heart symptoms such as chest discomfort or breathing difficulty. Therefore, keep an eye out for the development of these symptoms and, if they develop, discontinue use of sildenafil until you've been assessed by your doctor.

How to take sildenafil

The usual dose is 50 mg. This is preferably taken about one hour before sexual activity, but may be taken anywhere from one-half to four hours beforehand. Depending on how you respond to the medicine and how you tolerate it, your doctor may recommend in the future you take doses as low as 25 mg or as high as 100 mg. It's recommended that you not exceed one dose per day.

Ingesting a high-fat meal at the time of taking your sildenafil will interfere with its absorption into your body.

Avoid consuming grapefruit or grapefruit juice because it can affect the level of sildenafil in your blood. Don't want to give up grapefruit and not too keen on giving up sex either? Well, you have a tough choice to make, then, because grapefruit and grapefruit juice should not be taken with tadalafil or vardenafil either. Hmm, wonder if grapefruit sales are going down...

Sildenafil requires sexual stimulation in order to work.

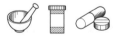

Proton Pump Inhibitors (PPIs)

Proton pump inhibitors: Sounds like something the Klingons would use to sabotage Scotty's engines on the Enterprise. Well, at least here on Earth, proton pump inhibitors (or PPIs) are not used for acts of subterfuge, but rather are used to treat acid-related diseases of the esophagus, stomach, and duodenum.

Parietal cells, found in the lining of the stomach, produce acid with the help of an enzyme called *H-K-ATPase,* which, thankfully has a much more pronounceable name: *proton pump.* Proton pump inhibitors *inhibit* the action of this pump (hence, these drugs are called *proton pump inhibitors*) and as a result less acid is released into the stomach.

PPIs available in Canada are listed in Table 6-49. The various PPIs are very similar in terms of how they work, their side-effects, and so forth.

Table 6-49	Proton Pump Inhibitors
Generic Name	*Trade Name(s)*
Esomeprazole	Nexium, Nexium 1-2-3 A*
Lansoprazole	Hp-PAC*, Prevacid, Prevacid Fas Tab
Omeprazole	Apo-Omeprazole, Losec Capsules, Losec 1-2-3 A*, Losec 1-2-3 M*, Losec MUPS, Losec Tablets
Pantoprazole	Pantoloc
Rabeprazole	Pariet

* This medicine is a combination of different drugs. Refer to the drug label to determine what they are.

 Pantoprazole

Pantoloc

Pantoloc is a highly effective and very well tolerated drug. It's also very commonly used with millions of prescriptions dispensed every year in Canada.

How pantoprazole can help you

By reducing stomach acidity, pantoprazole may help improve the following conditions:

- ✔ Stomach and duodenal ulcers.

- ✔ Gastritis.

- ✔ Gastro-esophageal reflux disease (GERD) including *reflux esophagitis* (inflammation of the esophagus due to acid).

- ✔ Pantoprazole may also be used to prevent ulcers if you're prone to them and are taking potentially ulcer-causing drugs like NSAIDs.

How pantoprazole might harm you

The great majority of people taking this medicine don't experience side-effects. Possible side-effects from pantoprazole include:

- ✔ Headache, nausea, diarrhea. These occur in only a small number of people.

- ✔ Increased risk of hip fracture. This isn't yet proven. (A study that looked at all PPIs together — not just pantoprazole alone — suggested that you're more likely to have a hip fracture if you're over the age of 50 and have taken a PPI for more than one year.)

- ✔ Vitamin B12 deficiency. This is unlikely to occur unless you have been taking pantoprazole for three years or more.

The safety of pantoprazole in pregnancy and breastfeeding is unknown. If you're pregnant or breastfeeding, we recommend you discuss it with your physician before taking this medicine.

Precautions to follow if you're taking pantoprazole

Follow these precautions if you're taking pantoprazole:

- ✔ If you're taking pantoprazole for a stomach ulcer, improvement of your ulcer symptoms does not exclude the (small) possibility that your ulcer is cancerous. For this reason it's important you follow-up with your doctor even if you're feeling better.

- ✔ If you have taken pantoprazole for several years you need to have your vitamin B12 level checked.

How to take pantoprazole

To treat active ulcers or esophagitis, a dose of 40 mg per day is generally used. When taken for prevention, a dose of 20 mg per day is generally used. A tablet should be taken in the morning, with or without food, and should be swallowed whole.

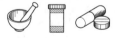

Retinoids

Retinoids are medicines used in the treatment of acne and are available in both oral and topical forms. As we discuss in Chapter 5, when prescription drug therapy is required, a *topical* retinoid is typically a first-line medicine. *Oral* retinoids, on the other hand, are generally reserved for those situations where other medications have not worked sufficiently well. Topical retinoids are very similar to one another. In this section we look in detail at the particularly commonly used topical drug tretinoin. Table 6-50 lists the retinoids available in Canada.

Oral retinoids (and possibly topical retinoids as well) can damage the fetus of a pregnant woman and therefore **must not** be taken if you're pregnant or if you're sexually active and not using sufficient contraception. If you're being considered for retinoid therapy, your doctor needs to discuss these issues in detail with you before you start taking the medicine.

Table 6-50	Retinoids
Generic Name	*Trade Name(s)*
Acitretin	Soriatane
Adapalene	Differin
Isotretinoin	Accutaine Roche, Clarus
Tazarotene	Tazorac Cream, Tazorac Gel
Tretinoin	Rejuva-A, Renova, Retin-A, Retin-A Micro, Retisol-A, Solangé, Stieva-A, Stievamycin Preparations*, Vesanoid, Vitamin A Acid

 Tretinoin

Rejuva-A, Renova, Retin-A, Retin-A Micro, Retisol-A, Solangé, Stieva-A, Stievamycin Preparations*, Vesanoid, Vitamin A Acid

Tretinoin is a topical medication similar in nature to vitamin A.

Tretinoin helps in the treatment of acne by opening skin pores (which decreases the number of pimples being formed) and causing peeling of the skin (which helps the body rid itself of existing pimples). Tretinoin helps sun-damaged skin by changing the skin's water content, the thickness of certain layers of skin, and increasing blood supply to deeper levels of the skin.

How tretinoin can help you

Tretinoin can help you by improving acne and sun-damaged skin (features of this include fine wrinkles, increased pigmentation, and roughness of the skin).

How tretinoin might harm you

Possible side-effects from tretinoin include:

- ✔ Skin redness, flaking, and peeling. If being used to treat acne, these are not truly side-effects as these changes are part of the way the medicine leads to improvement in your acne. (However, see the precautions below.)

- ✔ Skin irritation with mild burning or stinging discomfort.

- ✔ Change in skin pigmentation of the area being treated. This is reversible.

Although the safety of tretinoin in pregnancy and breastfeeding are unknown, because of safety concerns (see above) use of this medicine in these circumstances is usually *not* recommended. If you're pregnant or breastfeeding, we recommend you discuss it in detail with your physician before taking this medicine.

Precautions to follow if you're taking tretinoin

Follow these precautions if you're taking tretinoin:

- ✔ If your skin becomes severely inflamed with marked redness, swelling, and crusting, stop using the tretinoin and contact your physician.

- ✔ Because the drug isn't proven to be safe when taken during pregnancy and because oral forms of this drug are dangerous to take during pregnancy, effective birth control measures are recommended for sexually active women of child-bearing age who are taking tretinoin.

- ✔ Because areas of skin being treated are at increased risk of damage from UV rays, try to avoid exposing these areas to sun, and cover the affected areas with sunscreen and protective clothing when necessary.

How to take tretinoin

This discussion looks specifically at the use of tretinoin to treat acne; however, much of this applies to treating sun-damaged skin also. We recommend in either case you speak to your pharmacist to get specific directions for your particular circumstance.

Tretinoin is taken once daily, preferably at bedtime. Before applying the medicine, wash the skin being treated then gently pat it dry. Wait 20 to 30 minutes, then apply the medicine using a gauze swab or clean fingers. Use the least amount of medicine that will cover the affected area. We discuss general principles regarding the use of topical medicines in Chapter 4.

Additional important things to know about taking tretinoin are

✔ Increased skin irritation can occur from overuse of tretinoin, use of sun lamps or harsh abrasives, or having products such as shampoos, medicated soaps, or waxing aids come into contact with areas of skin that are being treated.

✔ Avoid getting the medicine in your eyes, nose, or mouth.

✔ Tretinoin shouldn't be applied to areas of skin that are severely inflamed or have open sores.

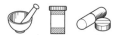

Selective Estrogen Receptor Modulators (SERMs)

This small family of drugs has only two members currently available in Canada. Selective estrogen receptor modulators (SERMs) are sometimes called "designer" estrogens. They have some of the good features of estrogen and generally fewer of the bad. We list the two SERMs available in Canada in Table 6-51. Although these two drugs work in similar ways, they're generally used for different purposes, as we describe in detail below.

Estrogen, the main "female hormone," attaches to estrogen receptors on various cells and influences these cells to perform a variety of functions. SERMs compete with estrogen for these receptors (and generally win), so that these receptors become occupied by the SERM instead of estrogen. The SERM then, depending on where in the body the cells are located, either influences the cells as estrogen would or, alternatively, prevents the cells from being influenced. This selective action of SERMs provides some of the benefits of estrogen therapy without some of the drawbacks.

Table 6-51	Selective Estrogen Receptor Modulators
Generic Name	*Trade Name(s)*
Raloxifene	Evista
Tamoxifen	Apo-Tamox, Gen-Tamoxifen, Nolvadex- D, Novo-Tamoxifen, Tamofen

Raloxifene

Evista

Raloxifene is used for prevention and treatment of osteoporosis in post-menopausal women. It's sometimes referred to as a "bone plus" drug as its effects are not limited just to bone.

How raloxifene can help you

Raloxifene can help you in the following ways:

- ✔ Decreasing the risk of developing some types of breast cancer if you're at high risk for this disease.

- ✔ Preventing or improving osteoporosis. This will decrease your risk of certain types of fractures.

- ✔ Raloxifene will also improve your cholesterol; however, we don't yet know if this particular way of improving cholesterol will reduce the risk of heart disease.

How raloxifene might harm you

Possible side-effects from taking raloxifene include:

- ✔ Hot flushes. These are quite common and often a nuisance, but are not dangerous and tend to improve as the drug is continued. They're most likely to occur in recently post-menopausal women who are naturally getting hot flushes.

- ✔ Leg cramps. These are quite common, and may be unpleasant, but they aren't dangerous.

- ✔ Blood clots in the legs (*phlebitis*), lungs (*pulmonary embolism*), and brain (*stroke*). These are serious, but, fortunately, very infrequent complications.

Raloxifene will not cause you to have menstrual bleeding nor will it increase your risk of cancer of the uterus.

People with the following conditions shouldn't take raloxifene:

- ✔ Men of any age.

- ✔ Women who are of child-bearing age; women who are pregnant or breastfeeding.

- ✔ Previous blood clot.

- ✔ Severe liver disease.

Precautions to follow if you're taking raloxifene

Follow these precautions if you're taking raloxifene:

- ✔ If you get a swollen leg, calf pain, chest pain, or shortness of breath, promptly see your doctor to make sure you do not have a blood clot.

- ✔ If you're going to be having major surgery, stop taking raloxifene at least 72 hours beforehand and restart it only after you're once again up and about. This will reduce your risk of developing a blood clot.

How to take raloxifene

Raloxifene is taken once daily in a dose of 60 mg and may be taken with or without food.

 ## Tamoxifen

Apo-Tamox, Gen-Tamoxifen, Nolvadex- D, Novo-Tamoxifen, Tamofen

Tamoxifen is used primarily in the prevention and treatment of breast cancer, but does have other potential roles as we look at next.

How tamoxifen can help you

Tamoxifen can help you in the following ways:

- ✔ Decreasing the risk of developing some types of breast cancer if you're at high risk for this disease.

- ✔ Decreasing the risk of reoccurrence of some types of breast cancer.

- ✔ Improving fertility if you're a woman of child-bearing age. It does this by helping you to ovulate.

- ✔ Improving some other, uncommon conditions including *gynecomastia* (breast enlargement in males), retroperitoneal fibrosis, and desmoid tumors.

- ✔ Tamoxifen will also improve your cholesterol; however, we don't yet know if this particular way of improving cholesterol will reduce the risk of heart disease.

How tamoxifen might harm you

Possible side-effects from taking tamoxifen include:

- ✔ Nausea.

- ✔ Hot flushes. These are quite common and often a nuisance, but are not dangerous.

- Increased blood pressure.
- *Peripheral edema* (ankle swelling).
- Mood changes including depression.
- Sexual dysfunction.
- "Tamoxifen flare." This is the development of bone pain and skin rash just after starting tamoxifen therapy. Although it may make you appropriately concerned, it's not serious and usually settles within four weeks.
- Vaginal discharge.
- Blood clots in the legs (*phlebitis*), lungs (*pulmonary embolism*), and brain (*stroke*). These are serious, but, fortunately, uncommon complications.
- Cancer of the uterus. This is a serious, but, fortunately, very infrequent complication.

People with the following conditions shouldn't take tamoxifen:

- Previous blood clot.
- Women who are pregnant or breastfeeding.

Precautions to follow if you're taking tamoxifen

Follow these precautions if you're taking tamoxifen:

- If you get a swollen leg, calf pain, chest pain, or shortness of breath, promptly see your doctor to make sure you do not have a blood clot.
- If you're going to be having major surgery, stop taking tamoxifen at least 72 hours beforehand and restart it only after you're once again up and about. This will reduce your risk of developing a blood clot.

How to take tamoxifen

Tamoxifen is taken in a dose of 20 mg to 40 mg (either taken as a single dose or divided into two equal doses) and may be taken with or without food.

Avoid consuming grapefruit or grapefruit juice because it can affect the level of tamoxifen in your blood.

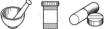

Serotonin (5 HT) Receptor Agonists

Serotonin receptor agonists (or *triptans*) are relative newcomers in the treatment of migraine headache disorders, but have quickly assumed a pre-eminent role in the treatment of this troubling ailment. The serotonin receptor agonists available in Canada are listed in Table 6-52. These drugs are very similar in how they work, how they can help you, and so forth. In this section we look in detail at the particularly commonly used drug sumatriptan.

Table 6-52	Serotonin Receptor Agonists
Generic Name	*Trade Name(s)*
Almotriptan	Axert
Eletriptan	Relpax
Naratriptan	Amerge
Rizatriptan	Maxalt, Maxalt RPD
Sumatriptan	CO Sumatriptan, Gen-Sumatriptan, Imitrex DF Tablets, Imitrex Injection/Autoinjector, Imitrex Nasal Spray, Novo-Sumatriptan, PMS-Sumatriptan, ratio-Sumatriptan, Sandoz Sumatriptan
Zolmitriptan	Zomig, Zomig Nasal Spray, Zomig Rapimelt

 Sumatriptan

CO Sumatriptan, Gen-Sumatriptan, Imitrex DF Tablets, Imitrex Injection/Autoinjector, Imitrex Nasal Spray, Novo-Sumatriptan, PMS-Sumatriptan, ratio-Sumatriptan, Sandoz Sumatriptan

 Multiple theories exist as to what causes migraine headaches and how this form of therapy may work. One suggestion is that excess levels of a naturally occurring chemical messenger (*neurotransmitter*) called *serotonin* stimulate certain pain centres in the brain as well as causing blood vessels in the head to widen (*vasodilate*). Sumatriptan may work by dampening the action of these neurotransmitters on these pain centres and by causing the blood vessels to narrow (*vasoconstrict*). As a result, a migraine headache is eased.

How sumatriptan can help you

Sumatriptan can help you by easing a migraine headache.

This drug is used to treat a migraine *after* it has begun. It's *not* used to prevent a migraine from starting in the first place.

How sumatriptan might harm you

Possible side-effects from taking sumatriptan include:

- Drowsiness.
- Feeling warm.
- (With the nasal spray): nausea, vomiting, bad taste in the mouth.
- Heart attack, stroke, high blood pressure. Fortunately these rarely occur.
- Abdominal pain, diarrhea. These, too, seldom occur.

When you shouldn't use sumatriptan

People with the following conditions shouldn't take sumatriptan:

- Pregnancy, breastfeeding.
- Circulatory diseases such as coronary artery disease, peripheral vascular disease, cerebrovascular disease, Raynaud's phenomenon. We discuss these conditions in Chapter 5.
- Heart rhythm or heart valve disorders.
- Inadequately controlled high blood pressure.
- Severe liver disease.
- Use of ergot-containing medication (for example, Cafergot) within 24 hours or drugs called MAO inhibitors within two weeks.
- Any of the following types of (unusual) migraine: basilar migraines, ophthalmoplegic migraines, hemiplegic migraines.

Precautions to follow if you're taking sumatriptan

Follow these precautions if you're taking sumatriptan:

- Your risk of having circulatory disease (see above) needs to be regularly reviewed by your doctor; if the risk is significant, you may need to discontinue the drug.
- If, after taking a dose, you develop chest discomfort, discontinue using the drug until your doctor has first excluded heart disease.

✔ This drug may make you drowsy, which would make it unsafe for you to perform activities — like driving — that require you to be alert and focused.

✔ Because alcohol may worsen drowsiness, it may be unwise to consume it. We recommend you check with your doctor to find out whether drinking (small amounts of) alcohol would be okay.

How to take sumatriptan

The three ways you can take sumatriptan are

✔ **Nasal spray:** The nasal spray comes in a single-dose container of either 5 mg or 20 mg of sumatriptan. Place the nozzle into a nostril and then push the top and bottom ends of the container toward each other. This will make the medicine spray out of the container into your nose, where it will be absorbed. (Unlike decongestant nose sprays, sumatriptan is *not* given into both nostrils.) It tends to taste awful (as Heather knows all too well!) but it does work quickly, with significant improvement typically occurring within 15 minutes (as Heather also thankfully knows well). If the first dose doesn't work, a second dose can be administered two hours after the first; however, no more than 40 mg should be taken in a 24-hour period.

✔ **Injection:** The medicine is supplied as a pre-filled syringe containing 6 mg of sumatriptan. It's best to inject into the thigh or the upper arm. Significant improvement is expected within 10 to 15 minutes. If you don't get relief from your first injection, taking a second dose is unlikely to help you. (Be sure to use the supplied container to dispose of your used syringe and needle.)

✔ **Oral medicine** (tablets): The tablets come in 25-, 50-, and 100-mg strengths, with the 50-mg dose being the most commonly used. The tablet should be taken with water and swallowed whole. Significant improvement should begin within about 30 minutes. If the first dose is ineffective, a second dose can be taken two hours later; however, no more than 200 mg should be taken in a 24-hour period.

If you get nausea with your migraines, giving sumatriptan by injection or nasal spray is preferred to oral medicine.

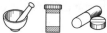

Skeletal Muscle Relaxants

Skeletal muscle relaxants are used, as the name suggests, to relax skeletal muscles. Skeletal muscles are those muscles that move our bodies (and therefore include the muscles in the back, chest, arms, legs, etc.). (Smooth muscles are located internally; for example in the blood vessels, the bladder, and the bowel.) Some skeletal muscle relaxant drugs (methocarbamol and orphenadrine) are available over-the-counter. The skeletal muscle relaxants that are prescription drugs are listed in Table 6-53.

Table 6-53	Skeletal Muscle Relaxants
Generic Name	*Trade Name(s)*
Baclofen	Apo-Baclofen, Gen-Baclofen, Liorisal Oral, Nu-Baclo, PMS-Baclofen, ratio-Baclofen
Cyclobenzaprine	Apo-Cyclobenzaprine, Gen-Cyclobenzaprine, Novo-Cyclobenzaprine, Nu-Cyclobenzaprine, PMS-Cyclobenzaprine, ratio-Cyclobenzaprine

 ## Cyclobenzaprine

Apo-Cyclobenzaprine, Gen-Cyclobenzaprine, Novo-Cyclobenzaprine, Nu-Cyclobenzaprine, PMS-Cyclobenzaprine, ratio-Cyclobenzaprine

Cyclobenzaprine can reduce skeletal muscle pains; however, its role is to complement (not replace) other helpful therapies including plain analgesics (such as acetaminophen) and, when necessary, nonsteroidal anti-inflammatory drugs (NSAIDs) and physiotherapy.

 Cyclobenzaprine does not work directly on the muscles, but rather acts on the brain, where it inhibits the activity of specific nerves; this, in turn, causes skeletal muscles to relax.

How cyclobenzaprine can help you

Cyclobenzaprine can help you by reducing tension, spasm, and discomfort in your skeletal muscles, whether arising from overuse or fibromyalgia. (We have more evidence supporting its benefit in the former than the latter.)

How cyclobenzaprine might harm you

Possible side-effects from taking cyclobenzaprine include:

✔ Drowsiness, fatigue, dizziness, difficulty concentrating and thinking.

✔ Dry mouth, nausea, diarrhea, constipation.

✔ Difficulty emptying the bladder.

✔ Worsening of glaucoma.

✔ Muscle weakness.

✔ Abnormal heart rhythm.

✔ Abnormal liver tests.

Side-effects are much more likely to occur if you're elderly. If you're elderly and can manage without this medicine, you're best to do so.

People with the following conditions shouldn't take cyclobenzaprine:

✔ Liver disease.

✔ Certain heart problems including recent heart attack, heart rhythm disorders and other problems with the heart's electrical system, congestive heart failure.

✔ Hyperthyroidism (unless under control with appropriate therapy).

✔ You shouldn't take cyclobenzaprine if you have taken a drug from the monoamine oxidase (MAO) inhibitor family within the past 14 days, nor should you start taking an MAO inhibitor within 14 days of stopping cyclobenzaprine.

The safety of cyclobenzaprine in pregnancy and breastfeeding is unknown. If you're pregnant or breastfeeding, we recommend you discuss it with your physician before taking this medicine.

Precautions to follow if you're taking cyclobenzaprine

Follow these precautions if you're taking cyclobenzaprine:

✔ Cyclobenzaprine is for short-term use (up to three weeks).

✔ This drug may make you drowsy, which would make it unsafe for you to perform activities — like driving — that require you to be alert and focused.

✔ Because alcohol may worsen drowsiness, it may be unwise to consume it. We recommend you check with your doctor to find out whether drinking (small amounts of) alcohol would be okay.

How to take cyclobenzaprine

The usual dose is 5 to 10 mg taken three times daily. Cyclobenzaprine can be taken with or without food.

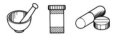

Statins

Statin therapy has been a true panacea when it comes to improving cholesterol levels and reducing the risk of heart disease. Indeed, prior to their introduction, we had a terribly limited number of tools in our cholesterol-fighting arsenal, and what we did have usually worked poorly. There were a mind-boggling 20 million prescriptions filled for statin therapy in Canada in 2005, and atorvastatin, the best-selling prescription drug in the country, accounted for more than half of those.

"Statin" is the very welcome short form for HMG-CoA reductase inhibitors (and even that is the thankfully short form for the even longer term: hydroxymethylglutaryl-coenzyme A reductase inhibitor. Oh my!). Statins available in Canada are listed in Table 6-54.

Table 6-54	Statins
Generic Name	**Trade Name(s)**
Atorvastatin	Caduet*, Lipitor
Fluvastatin	Lescol, Lescol XL
Lovastatin	Advicor*, Apo-Lovastatin, CO Lovastatin, Gen-Lovastatin, Mevacor, Novo-Lovastatin, Nu-Lovastatin, PMS-Lovastatin, RAN-Lovastatin, ratio-Lovastatin, Sandoz Lovastatin
Pravastatin	Apo-Pravastatin, CO Pravastatin, Novo-Pravastatin, Nu-Pravastatin, PMS-Pravastatin, Pravachol, ratio-Pravachol, Sandoz Pravastatin
Rosuvastatin	Crestor
Simvastatin	Apo-Simvastatin, CO Simvastatin, Gen-Simvastatin, Novo-Simvastatin, PMS-Simvastatin, ratio-Simvastatin, Sandoz Simvastatin, Taro-Simvastatin, Zocor

* This medicine is a combination of different drugs. Refer to the drug label to determine what they are.

Because statins are very similar in terms of how they work, how they can help you, their side-effects, and so forth, we discuss them together.

Statins all work well and are generally very well tolerated. We expect that over the next few years there will be increasing numbers of drugs combined with statins, seeing as many people with high cholesterol also need to take other medications (for example, drugs for high blood pressure).

 Most of the cholesterol in our bodies is manufactured within the liver. This process requires the help of an enzyme called HMG-CoA reductase. Statins block (*inhibit*) the action of this enzyme, and as a result the liver produces less cholesterol.

How statins can help you

Statins can help you in the following ways:

- Improving your cholesterol.

- Improving your triglycerides (a type of fat). Of the various statins, atorvastatin and rosuvastatin are particularly effective at doing this.

- Reducing your risk of a heart attack. This benefit is primarily but not exclusively caused by the improvement in cholesterol, because for unclear reasons the risk of a heart attack goes down *even before* the cholesterol levels improve.

- Reducing your risk of another stroke if you have previously had one.

How statins might harm you

Possible side-effects from statin therapy include:

- Muscle aching (most commonly of the arms and legs). This quickly goes away after discontinuing the drug.

- Muscle damage (*rhabdomyolysis*). Fortunately, this occurs only rarely. (See the precaution below.)

- Abnormal liver tests. These are typically mild. Only infrequently does significant liver injury develop.

- Headache, nausea, vomiting, diarrhea, abdominal pain, skin rash. These are not serious, occur in only a small minority of people, and go away quickly upon stopping the drug.

People with the following conditions shouldn't take a statin:

✔ Allergies to *any* statin.

✔ Liver disease or unexplained elevation (beyond three times normal) of certain liver enzyme (*transaminase*) levels on a blood test.

✔ Pregnancy or breastfeeding.

Precautions to follow if you're taking a statin

Follow these precautions if you're taking a statin:

✔ Your doctor should check your liver function prior to and then periodically after you start the medicine.

✔ Minimize or avoid alcohol altogether.

✔ If you develop muscle pains see your doctor promptly.

Many people taking a statin develop a slight (and often transient) elevation of an enzyme called CPK (or CK). This is detected on a blood test and is done to check for muscle injury. A minimal elevation of the CPK, particularly in the absence of muscle discomfort, is usually of no importance and does *not,* in and of itself, require the drug to be discontinued. If, however, your CPK level is more than ten times normal, your statin *should be immediately stopped.*

How to take a statin

These are points to be aware of when taking a statin:

✔ Fluvastatin, lovastatin, pravastatin, and simvastatin should be taken in the evening; atorvastatin and rosuvastatin can be taken any time of day.

✔ As it can take up to four weeks before the full effect of a statin on your blood cholesterol levels is seen, it's usually inappropriate to have your dose changed sooner than that.

✔ The starting dose of a statin, depending on which one you have been prescribed, will vary from 10 mg to 40 mg per day. Your doctor may need to prescribe lower than usual doses if you have kidney failure.

✔ Statins may be taken with or without food (except for lovastatin, which should be taken with food).

✔ Avoid consuming grapefruit or grapefruit juice because it can affect the level of a statin in your blood.

Stimulants

Stimulants are also known as *CNS stimulants* because they increase the activity of certain nerves within the brain. (CNS stands for *central nervous system*.) Stimulants available in Canada are listed in Table 6-55. As we discuss in Chapter 5, dextroamphetamine and methylphenidate are used principally in the treatment of attention-deficit/hyperactivity disorder (ADHD). Because it works quickly and because, if side-effects develop, they wear off quickly (as the medicine is short-acting), methylphenidate is typically the preferred stimulant to treat ADHD. As such, we discuss it in detail below. (Modafanil is a stimulant that is sometimes used to improve alertness in people with certain sleep disorders such as sleep apnea.)

Table 6-55	Stimulants
Generic Name	**Trade Name(s)**
Dextroamphetamine	Dexedrine
Methylphenidate	Apo-Methylphenidate, Apo-Methylphenidate SR, Biphentin, Concerta, PMS-Methylphenidate, Ritalin, Ritalin SR
Modafinil	Alertec

Methylphenidate

Apo-Methylphenidate, Apo-Methylphenidate SR, Biphentin, Concerta, PMS-Methylphenidate, Ritalin, Ritalin SR

Methylphenidate is used in the treatment of attention-deficit/hyperactivity disorder (ADHD) and narcolepsy. It's also sometimes used to treat depression. In this section we look at the use of this drug to treat ADHD; however, general principles regarding this drug apply to all these circumstances.

The precise way in which methylphenidate improves symptoms of ADHD is not known, however it appears to be related to this drug's ability to increase levels of *dopamine* and *norepinephrine* (these are chemical messengers or *neurotransmitters*) in the brain.

How methylphenidate can help you

Methylphenidate may help ADHD by decreasing restlessness and improving attention.

How methylphenidate might harm you

Possible side-effects from taking methylphenidate include:

- ✔ Nervousness, insomnia, decreased appetite, nausea, vomiting, abdominal pain. These are the most common side-effects and are most likely to occur shortly after starting the medicine. These typically go away as the medicine is continued; if necessary, your doctor can reduce the dose to help ease these symptoms.

- ✔ Increased blood pressure and heart rate.

- ✔ Inability for children to have appropriate growth and weight gain with long-term use of this medicine. This is not proven.

- ✔ Increased risk of seizures (especially if you have a known seizure disorder).

- ✔ Dizziness.

- ✔ Worsening of behaviour disturbance and thinking disorders, mood change including sadness, overly variable emotions.

- ✔ Rash, joint pains, scalp hair loss.

- ✔ Abnormal liver tests or blood counts. These rarely occur.

People with the following conditions shouldn't take methylphenidate:

- ✔ Anxiety disorders.

- ✔ Hyperthyroidism.

- ✔ Heart or other cardiovascular disease including insufficiently controlled hypertension.

- ✔ Glaucoma.

- ✔ *Motor tics* (these are sudden, repetitive, rapid movements).

- ✔ Tourette's syndrome or a family history of this.

- ✔ You shouldn't take methylphenidate if you have taken a drug from the monoamine oxidase (MAO) inhibitor family within the past 14 days, nor should you start taking an MAO inhibitor within 14 days of stopping methylphenidate.

The safety of methylphenidate in pregnancy and breastfeeding is unknown. If you're pregnant or breastfeeding, we recommend you discuss it with your physician before taking this medicine.

Precautions to follow if you're taking methylphenidate

Follow these precautions if you're taking methylphenidate:

- ✔ Your blood pressure should be monitored regularly.

- ✔ If a child is not growing and gaining appropriate weight, the medicine should be discontinued.

- ✔ If you experience a seizure while taking this medicine, the drug should be discontinued.

- ✔ Because this drug may make you dizzy, it could make it unsafe for you to perform activities such as driving.

- ✔ Alcohol should be avoided.

- ✔ Blood tests (to check your blood counts as well as your liver function) should be performed periodically.

- ✔ The drug should *not* be stopped without first consulting your doctor.

How to take methylphenidate

Methylphenidate should be started in the lowest possible dose and increased slowly, under your doctor's supervision, based on your response. Your dose and how you take the medicine depends on the particular form of the drug you're prescribed.

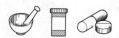

Testosterone

Androgens are defined as "male hormones," but despite this appellation, "male" hormones are actually present in both men *and* women; it's just that in men they're present in much higher amounts. The androgen most familiar to people — and the only one that is available as a medicine — is *testosterone*. Oral and topical testosterone supplements available in Canada are listed in Table 6-56.

Table 6-56	Testosterone
Generic Name	**Trade Names**
Testosterone	Andriol, Androderm, AndroGel, Delatestryl, Depo-Testosterone

R Testosterone

Andriol, Androderm, AndroGel, Delatestryl, Depo-Testosterone

Testosterone attaches to *androgen receptors* in cells and stimulates these cells to make proteins responsible for a number of normal processes such as making muscle, making hair, and, ahem, making hay. If you lack sufficient androgen, you may develop muscle weakness, hair loss (most notably in the armpits and genital areas), and sexual dysfunction, in which case taking testosterone can improve the situation.

How testosterone can help you

If you're lacking sufficient testosterone in your body, taking testosterone supplements can help you by

- ✔ Stimulating the growth of bone, muscle, and body hair.

- ✔ Restoring male fertility.

- ✔ Improving libido and, for men, improving erectile function.

How testosterone might harm you

Possible side-effects from testosterone include:

- ✔ Acne.

- ✔ Irritation of the skin at the site of a testosterone patch.

- ✔ *Peripheral edema* (ankle swelling).

- ✔ A high level of cholesterol and/or hemoglobin in your body. (Hemoglobin is the substance in the blood that carries oxygen.)

- ✔ For men, breast swelling (*gynecomastia*) and erectile dysfunction. (Although in some men testosterone helps erectile dysfunction, it can sometimes make things worse, not better.)

- ✔ For women, abnormal hair growth, a change in the voice, and enlargement of the clitoris.

Testosterone is much more likely to harm you if you're taking it inappropriately (for example, if you're not lacking this hormone but are taking it for bodybuilding purposes).

People with the following conditions shouldn't take testosterone:

- ✔ Breast or prostate cancer, if you're a man.

- ✔ Serious heart, kidney, or liver disease.

✔ A high calcium level in your blood.

✔ Pregnancy or breastfeeding.

Precautions to follow if you're taking testosterone

Follow these precautions if you're taking testosterone:

✔ Avoid having your partner come in contact with your topical application of testosterone. (Depending on the type of topical application you're using, there is the risk that if your partner is in contact with it, the testosterone could get into her system and lead to excess levels of this hormone in her body.)

✔ Have periodic blood tests to check your testosterone level as well as your hemoglobin and cholesterol levels.

How to take testosterone

Important points about taking topical testosterone include:

✔ Apply topical testosterone in patch form (Androderm) once daily, in the late evening, immediately after opening the package. Apply it to a clean, dry area of skin on the abdomen, back, upper arms, or thighs.

✔ Apply topical testosterone in gel form (AndroGel) once daily, in the morning, to a clean, dry area of skin on the shoulders, upper arms, or abdomen.

The package inserts for topical testosterone products give *very* detailed descriptions of how to take these medications. We recommend you read the insert very carefully.

Topical testosterone should *not* be applied to the scrotum or penis, as doing so may result in transfer of the medicine to your partner during sexual contact.

Oral testosterone (in the form of Andriol) is usually started in a dose of 60 to 80 mg taken two times per day, and the dose is then adjusted by your doctor after a few weeks. Andriol should be swallowed whole (that is, not chewed, crushed, and so on) and taken with food.

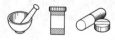

Thyroid Hormones

As we discuss in Chapter 5, if your thyroid gland is unable to make enough thyroid hormone (that is, you have *hypothyroidism*), you take thyroid hormone supplements to make up for this deficiency. Although there are three different types of thyroid hormone medicine, more than 99 percent of the time (99.4 percent, to be precise!) it's L-thyroxine (also known as levothyroxine or T4) that is used. Liothyronine (T3) is, with rare exception, used only as short-term therapy during certain phases of thyroid cancer treatment. Desiccated thyroid is almost never used. Thyroid hormones available in Canada are listed in Table 6-57.

Table 6-57	Thyroid Hormones
Generic Name	*Trade Name(s)*
L-thyroxine (T4)	Eltroxin, Euthyrox, Synthroid
Liothyronine (T3)	Cytomel
Desiccated Thyroid	Thyroid Hormone

 L-thyroxine

Eltroxin, Euthyrox, Synthroid

L-thyroxine is the main thyroid hormone made in the body.

 Thyroid hormones control the rate at which a number of normal body processes (bowel habits, periods, metabolism, and so on) take place. Thyroid hormone supplements, taken in usual doses, perform exactly the same functions.

How L-thyroxine can help you

L-thyroxine can help you in the following ways:

- ✔ Preventing/reversing symptoms of hypothyroidism if you have an underfunctioning thyroid.

- ✔ Shrinking a *goiter* (thyroid swelling).

- ✔ If you have previously had thyroid cancer, making it less likely that you will have a recurrence of thyroid cancer. It's also used to shrink metastases if you have thyroid cancer that has spread to other parts of the body.

How L-thyroxine might harm you

If taken in the correct dose, side-effects aren't expected to occur. The one exception to this is the occasional circumstance where mild and temporary hair loss develops (it's unclear whether this is actually caused by the medication).

People with the following conditions shouldn't take L-thyroxine:

✔ *Hyperthyroidism* (thyroid overfunctioning).

✔ Untreated *adrenal insufficiency* (underfunctioning of the adrenal glands).

L-thyroxine may be safely taken if you're pregnant or breastfeeding.

Precautions to follow if you're taking L-thyroxine

Follow these precautions if you're taking L-thyroxine:

✔ If, shortly after starting L-thyroxine or having the dose increased, you develop chest pains or palpitations, seek prompt medical attention.

✔ If you have diabetes and are being newly treated for hypothyroidism, your blood glucose levels may rise. For this reason, check your blood glucose levels more often during the first few weeks after starting treatment or having your dose increased. If your blood glucose levels rise, contact your physician.

✔ Taking both L-thyroxine together with liothyronine (T3) offers no proven advantage (and presents some disadvantages) over taking L-thyroxine alone.

✔ Thyroid hormone requirements may increase during pregnancy. If you're pregnant, have regular blood work done to determine this.

✔ Because the amount of thyroid hormone absorbed into your body can vary depending on the manufacturer of a thyroid supplement (even if the strength of the thyroid pill is the same), it's best to stick with the same brand of L-thyroxine. It doesn't matter which brand, so long as you're consistent. (You may need to discuss this with your pharmacist, as he may change suppliers from time to time and need to order your medicine in for you.)

Occasionally, doses as high as 0.25 mg per day are required. As this is not common, the location of that crucial decimal may be missed and the dose mistakenly interpreted as a similar-looking .025 mg per day. This may *look* similar on paper, but it's a *ten-fold difference* in strength. For this reason, if you're prescribed either

0.25 mg per day or 0.025 mg per day, we recommend you double-check your thyroid prescription with the pharmacist before you leave the drugstore.

How to take L-thyroxine

For a very simple medicine, there are a whole bunch of things to know about taking L-thyroxine:

- ✔ L-thyroxine is taken once daily, with water and on an empty stomach at least 30 minutes before eating.

- ✔ L-thyroxine shouldn't be taken within four hours (before or after) of taking calcium or iron supplements, or antacids that contain aluminum or magnesium.

- ✔ If you're elderly or have heart disease you should be started on a very low dose (such as 0.025 mg per day) and the dose should slowly be increased (typically no more frequently than every four weeks or so). The one exception occurs when you have suddenly become hypothyroid (such as after thyroid surgery), in which case you can be started on full doses right away.

- ✔ To know if you're on the correct dose, have your thyroid status checked on a blood test done, in general, about four to eight weeks after starting the medicine or having your dose adjusted. Most people require between 0.075 and 0.175 mg of L-thyroxine per day (the more you weigh, the higher the dose you will generally need).

- ✔ Your dose should be adjusted based on your blood test results, not on your symptoms. Adjusting the dose based on symptoms is likely to lead to (potentially dangerous) under- or overdosing.

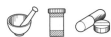

Tricyclic Antidepressants (TCAs)

Many different classes of medicine are used to treat depression. (See "Antidepressants" earlier in this chapter.) Among these are tricyclic antidepressants — however, as this class of medicine has broader uses (as we discuss below), it's typically classified on its own. Despite their name, tricyclic antidepressants (TCAs) are often used for conditions other than depression. (The term *tricyclic* refers to the presence of three carbon "rings" within its chemical structure.) Table 6-58 lists the TCAs available in Canada. In this section we look in detail at the particularly commonly used TCA, amitriptyline.

Table 6-58	Tricyclic Antidepressants
Generic Name	*Trade Name(s)*
Amitriptyline	Apo-Amitriptyline, Novo-Triptyn
Clomipramine	Anafranil, Apo-Clomipramine, CO Clomipramine, Gen-Clomipramine
Desipramine	Apo-Desipramine, Norpramin, Nu-Desipramine, PMS-Desipramine, ratio-Desipramine
Doxepin	Apo-Doxepin, Novo-Doxepin, Sinequan
Imipramine	Apo-Imipramine, Novo-Pramine, Tofranil
Maprotiline±	Novo-Maprotiline
Nortriptyline	Apo-Nortriptyline, Aventyl, Gen-Nortriptyline, Novo-Nortriptyline, Nu-nortriptyline, ratio-Nortriptyline
Trimipramine	Apo-Trimip, Nu-Trimipramine

± *Maprotiline is, technically speaking, a tetracyclic antidepressant. However, as it shares much in common with tricyclic antidepressants, it's customarily grouped with them.*

 Amitriptyline

Apo-Amitriptyline, Novo-Triptyn

Amitriptyline, discovered almost 70 years ago, retains a key role in the treatment of several ailments. Thank goodness there's no mandatory retirement age for (good) drugs!

 Nerve cells communicate with one another by sending out chemical signals called *neurotransmitters*. Amitriptyline works by increasing the amount of these messengers, specifically ones called *serotonin* and *norepinephrine*. Serotonin and norepinephrine then influence the way certain other cells behave.

How amitriptyline can help you

Amitriptyline can help you in the following ways:

- ✔ Improving depression.

- ✔ Reducing pain from certain forms of nerve injury, such as *diabetic peripheral neuropathy*. (We discuss neuropathy in Chapter 5.)

- ✔ Other, less proven uses are many and include the treatment of bed wetting (*nocturnal enuresis*), insomnia, fibromyalgia, irritable bowel syndrome, and the prevention of migraine headaches.

How amitriptyline might harm you

Possible side-effects from amitriptyline include:

- ✔ Dry mouth, blurred vision, constipation. These are the most common side-effects.
- ✔ Drowsiness.
- ✔ Faintness (especially upon first arising from a bed or from a chair).
- ✔ Weight gain.
- ✔ Reduced white blood cell count. (See below.)

You may find some relief from a dry mouth by taking sips of water or by sucking on hard candy or chewing sugarless gum. Also, having a persistent dry mouth can increase your risk of cavities, so be sure to look after your teeth well and have regular dental care.

People with the following conditions shouldn't take amitriptyline:

- ✔ Recent heart attack.
- ✔ Congestive heart failure.
- ✔ You shouldn't take amitriptyline if you have taken a drug from the monoamine oxidase (MAO) inhibitor family within the past 14 days, nor should you start taking an MAO inhibitor within 14 days of stopping amitriptyline. There are rare exceptions to this.

The safety of amitriptyline in pregnancy and breastfeeding is unknown. If you're pregnant or breastfeeding, we recommend you discuss it with your physician before taking this medicine.

Precautions to follow if you're taking amitriptyline

Follow these precautions if you're taking amitriptyline:

- ✔ If you have heart disease, your doctor should perform periodic electrocardiograms (EKGs).
- ✔ Because there is the (remote) possibility that amitriptyline will lower your white blood cell count and therefore put you at risk of an infection, contact your doctor if you develop a fever, bad sore throat, yellow or greenish phlegm, or other symptoms suggesting you have an infection. (Your doctor should then order a blood test to check your white blood cell count.)
- ✔ Some people find their urine turns blue or green. This isn't serious and, ahem, will not make you prone to telling off-colour jokes.
- ✔ The medicine should — whenever possible — not be stopped suddenly.

✔ This drug may make you drowsy, which would make it unsafe for you to perform activities — like driving — that require you to be alert and focused.

✔ Because alcohol may worsen drowsiness, it may be unwise to consume it. We recommend you check with your doctor to find out whether drinking (small amounts of) alcohol would be okay.

✔ There is some evidence that taking antidepressants — particularly in the early stages of treatment — can lead to thoughts of suicide. If you have such thoughts, seek urgent medical care.

Because amitriptyline can make you prone to heart rhythm problems during surgery, if you will be having an operation we recommend you ask your doctor whether you should discontinue the medication in advance of the surgery.

How to take amitriptyline

Amitriptyline is typically started in a low dose, with the dose then gradually increased, under your doctor's supervision, based on your response. The usual starting dose varies depending on the condition being treated:

✔ Depression: 25 mg three times per day.

✔ Neuropathy and fibromyalgia: 10 to 25 mg at bedtime.

✔ Migraine prevention: 10 mg at bedtime.

Amitriptyline may be taken with or without food.

Avoid consuming grapefruit or grapefruit juice because it can affect the level of amitriptyline in your blood.

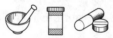

Xanthine Oxidase Inhibitor

Allopurinol is the only member of the xanthine oxidase class of drugs approved for use in Canada. Table 6-59 lists the trade names for this drug.

Table 6-59	Xanthine Oxidase Inhibitor
Generic Name	**Trade Names**
Allopurinol	Apo-Allopurinol, Novo-Purol, Zyloprim

℞ *Allopurinol*

Apo-Allopurinol, Novo-Purol, Zyloprim

 During the normal process of breaking down proteins, our bodies produce a substance called xanthine. With the help of an enzyme called xanthine oxidase, xanthine is then broken down to a molecule called uric acid. Excess uric acid levels can lead to gout and, sometimes, kidney disease. Allopurinol works by inhibiting the activity of xanthine oxidase; this results in lower levels of uric acid and, thus, a lower likelihood of developing these complications.

How allopurinol can help you

Allopurinol can help you in the following ways:

- ✔ Preventing attacks of gout.

- ✔ Reducing your risk of developing uric acid kidney stones and *uric acid nephropathy*. (Uric acid nephropathy is a condition in which uric acid is deposited in the kidney and damages it. If severe, this can lead to kidney failure.)

- ✔ Shrinking *tophi*. Tophi are large, sometimes disfiguring, deposits of uric acid that may form in various parts of the body — especially the earlobes and the fingers.

How allopurinol might harm you

Most people taking allopurinol don't experience any side-effects. Possible side-effects from taking allopurinol include:

- ✔ Rash. This is typically very mild, but on rare occasion can be severe.

- ✔ Nausea, vomiting, diarrhea.

- ✔ Abnormal liver tests, liver inflammation.

- ✔ Low blood counts.

- ✔ Drowsiness.

 Allopurinol should *not* be started during an attack of gout. (Taking allopurinol during an attack can make the misery of an attack even worse.) As we discuss in Chapter 5, allopurinol should be started only after an attack has completely settled.

 The safety of allopurinol in pregnancy and breastfeeding is unknown. If you're pregnant or breastfeeding, we recommend you discuss it with your physician before taking this medicine.

Precautions to follow if you're taking allopurinol

Follow these precautions if you're taking allopurinol:

- ✔ Allopurinol should be discontinued at the first sign of a skin rash. Otherwise, allopurinol should not be stopped unless you speak to your physician first.

- ✔ Blood tests (to check your blood counts as well as your liver and kidney function) should be performed prior to, and then periodically after, starting the medicine. This is particularly important if you have liver or kidney disease.

- ✔ If you're taking allopurinol and then develop an attack of gout, *don't stop* the drug (this can make the attack worse).

- ✔ Stay well hydrated.

- ✔ This drug may make you drowsy, which would make it unsafe for you to perform activities — like driving — that require you to be alert and focused.

- ✔ Because alcohol may worsen drowsiness and because it may decrease the effectiveness of allopurinol, it may be unwise to consume it. We recommend you check with your doctor to find out whether drinking (small amounts of) alcohol would be okay.

How to take allopurinol

The key points about taking allopurinol to prevent gout include:

- ✔ The dose of allopurinol ranges from 100 mg all the way up to 800 mg per day. If you're taking more than 300 mg your dose should be divided up and taken two to three times per day.

- ✔ In the early stages of treatment, allopurinol can trigger an attack of gout. To reduce this risk:

  - • Allopurinol is generally started in a low dose, with the dose then progressively increased, under your doctor's supervision, based on your uric acid level on a blood test.

  - • Colchicine or a nonsteroidal anti-inflammatory drug (NSAID) is recommended during the first three to six months of therapy.

- ✔ Allopurinol can be taken with or without food, but if it's upsetting your stomach, taking it with food is a good idea.

Part IV
Common Concerns

The 5th Wave   By Rich Tennant

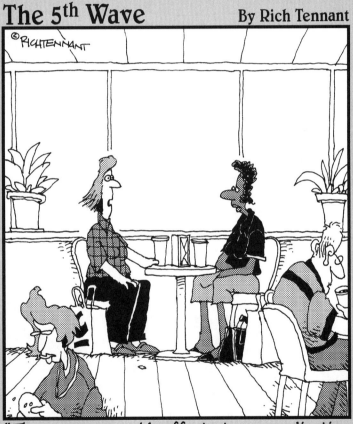

"There are some side-effects to my medication, like headaches, nausea, and weight gain. Not unlike the holidays at my in-laws."

In this part . . .

We look at special situations regarding prescription drug therapy — such as side effects and drug interactions, taking medications while you're pregnant, and dealing with emergencies — and offer suggestions and recommendations to help you contend with them.

Chapter 7

Side-Effects and Drug Interactions

In This Chapter

▶ Understanding what side-effects are and recognizing their various forms

▶ Discovering how to avoid side-effects from your medications

▶ Knowing what to do if you experience a side-effect

▶ Recognizing and avoiding possible drug interactions

*A*s physicians, we're thrilled to have so many medications available to help our patients feel better, be healthier, and, often, live longer. Yet at the same time, we're saddened and frustrated that the medications we use have the potential to cause harm. Fortunately, drugs are much more likely to do good than bad. Indeed, most people taking most drugs experience no side-effects at all. Nonetheless, that's not much consolation to the poor person who starts taking amoxicillin only to wake up the next day looking like a two-legged leopard.

In this chapter we look at why side-effects occur and what you can do to help avoid them. We also explore how prescription drugs can interact with other drugs, foods, herbs, and other "natural" products, and how you can reduce this risk.

Understanding Side-Effects

Although we use the term *side-effect* throughout this book, the official term for what we're talking about is an "adverse reaction" or an "adverse effect." Not that we're averse to these terms, but because both doctors and patients typically call side-effects, well, side-effects, we've opted to stick with this usage.

A side-effect is an unintended consequence, or result, from taking a medicine. Although, quite appropriately, people typically think of side-effects as being bad (such as developing a skin rash from taking an antibiotic), on occasion they can be good (for example, in someone who's taking tamsulosin to treat prostatism and finds the "side-effect" of lowering blood pressure has helped his hypertension).

In this chapter we focus our discussion on side-effects of a negative nature, because the negatives are both more common and, almost always, more likely to raise concerns.

Many different types of side-effects exist. Sometimes people react to the actual medicine in a product, sometimes to a non-medicinal ingredient. Sometimes a drug is perfect for the treatment of one of your health problems, but makes another one of your ailments worse. Sometimes a dose is simply too strong, and sometimes even the smallest dose causes a problem. We look at these and other important types of side-effects in this section. Following that, we look at what you can do in the event you have a side-effect (see "What to do if you experience a side-effect" later in this chapter).

Allergic reactions

Contrary to what is often thought, allergic reactions make up only a small percentage of side-effects that people experience from their medications. Also, allergic reactions are very specific types of side-effects as we discover in this section.

Mary Jackson was a 30-year-old homemaker who was seldom sick. On this occasion, however, she had come down with a wretched sore throat and felt miserable. She saw her doctor, who found she had a throat infection due to a streptococcus germ ("strep throat") and gave her a prescription for penicillin (a drug she had taken uneventfully a couple of years before). As soon as she got home from the drugstore, her pill bottle in hand, she took a dose. Shortly thereafter, Mary realized she was scratching her abdomen. She looked down and saw red welts (hives). She then noticed her lips felt puffy, and soon she started to wheeze. Alarmed, Mary called 911. Upon their arrival, the paramedics immediately administered epinephrine (adrenaline) and whisked her to hospital. By the time she got to the emergency department her symptoms had eased, and with further treatment in the ER she remained well. Mary had experienced an allergic reaction to penicillin.

Most drug allergies are related to antibodies. As in Mary's case in the preceding anecdote, antibodies may be formed to a drug the first time you take it, but typically don't cause problems until you take the drug again at some future time.

These are the most common symptoms of a drug allergy:

- ✔ Skin rash, often in the form of hives (typically, itchy red bumps)
- ✔ Itchiness of the skin and/or eyes
- ✔ Wheezing
- ✔ Swelling of the lips and/or tongue

If you develop these symptoms after taking a medicine, seek medical attention — urgently, if you have either of the last two symptoms on the list.

If it's confirmed you had an allergic reaction to the drug, do not take the medicine again. It's wise to obtain a piece of medical identification (typically in the form of a bracelet or necklace) stating you have an allergy to the drug. (Such jewellery is available through MedicAlert — www.medicalert.ca — and is also commonly available in pharmacies and jewellery shops.)

If you've had an allergic reaction to one type of penicillin, you are at increased risk of allergic reaction to other types of penicillin (and cephalosporins). It's called *cross-sensitivity,* and it applies to certain other drug families as well. (To find out which oral antibiotics are relatives of penicillin, refer to Table 6-10.)

To lower your risk of an allergic reaction to a drug, before you're prescribed/dispensed a medicine be sure to tell your physician and pharmacist the drugs to which you've reacted in the past so that they can avoid giving you the same or a related drug in the future.

 Most side-effects are not due to allergies, so to avoid confusion and to make sure you're not excluded from future use of potentially helpful drugs, when speaking to health care professionals it's best to say you are *intolerant of* (rather than *allergic to*) a drug unless you're certain you had an allergic reaction. We discuss drug intolerance in more detail later in this section.

Dose-related side-effects

A dose-related side-effect is a side-effect that occurs because the amount of medicine you are taking is too strong for your needs.

 Rhoda Diamond was a charming 75-year-old woman who had successfully contended with diabetes for five years. Her glucose levels, however, had recently climbed, and her doctor added a low dose of glyburide (a medicine used to reduce blood glucose levels) to her existing drug therapy. Rhoda's blood glucose levels improved but were still above target, so her doctor asked her to increase the dose. Two days later her doting husband, an early riser, realized Rhoda had overslept. He went in to awaken her only to find her wandering around the bedroom — she was confused, pale, and sweaty. He tested her blood glucose and found it was extremely low. He helped her drink some juice, and within a few minutes Rhoda was back to her normal self. Rhoda had experienced a dose-related side-effect.

Dose-related side-effects can occur for a number of reasons. One is if you're overly responsive to usual doses of a drug (as was the case with Rhoda's experience in the preceding anecdote). Another is having excessive amounts of a drug in your body, which can occur for several reasons including:

- ✔ **Being unable to properly eliminate a drug from the body.** For example, if you're taking a drug that exits the body through the kidneys, but you have kidney failure so are unable to rid your body of the medicine. See Chapter 2 for more on this process.

- ✔ **Consuming other drugs, herbs, or "natural products" that cause your prescription drug to accumulate in higher levels in the body.** (See "Drug–complementary and alternative medicine interactions" later in this chapter.)

- ✔ **Being prescribed too high a dose.**

- ✔ **Intentionally ingesting too much (that is, overdosing).**

Another less common form of dose-related side-effect is related to a cumulative effect of the drug on your body. In this situation, it takes many doses over an extended period of time before a side-effect shows itself — an example is eye damage occurring after months or years of amiodarone therapy. The great majority of drugs do not cause cumulative toxicity.

Side-effects from your drug acting where you'd rather it didn't

As wonderful as prescription drugs can be, they are often not all that bright and don't know to work on one place in the body and not another.

Marshall Weston, a 30-year-old aspiring corporate executive, had mild asthma readily controlled with the occasional dose of salbutamol. When Marshall developed rapid weight loss and palpitations he knew something was amiss. He saw his doctor and was quickly diagnosed as having hyperthyroidism (thyroid overactivity). Marshall's doctor prescribed anti-thyroid medication and, because he knew it takes a couple of weeks to have much benefit, he also prescribed propranolol (a type of beta blocker) to try to quickly ease Marshall's palpitations. A couple of days later Marshall noticed his heart pounding had settled, but he had become increasingly breathless and wheezy with his worst asthma in years. He saw his doctor and was told to immediately discontinue the propranolol. His asthma resolved soon thereafter.

Why did this happen to Marshall? His medicine acted not only where it helped him (the beta receptors in his heart), but also where it hurt him (the beta receptors in his lungs). Propranolol has never met a beta receptor it didn't like. To propranolol, the beta receptors in your lungs look similar to the beta receptors in your heart, so it affects both. As a result, it can help one problem (easing palpitations, for example) and worsen another (triggering asthma).

Before your doctor prescribes a drug, she customarily checks to see whether it may interfere with any other health issues you have. If she thinks it may, she either will not prescribe the drug, or will alert you to things to watch for. Nonetheless, if your doctor doesn't specifically bring this issue up, it cannot hurt — and it may be a big help — for you to ask your doctor if the prescription you are being given might adversely affect other ailments you have.

Some side-effects are very predictable and are not due to an unrelated health condition. For example, if you're taking a medicine (such as oxybutynin) to treat overactive bladder, the drug acts not only on acetylcholine receptors in the bladder, but also on similar receptors elsewhere in the body. The result can be, for example, a bothersome dry mouth. The drug simply doesn't know that you want it to go to one place in your body and not another. In cases like this, you may have to decide whether the side-effects you're experiencing are bothersome enough to outweigh the benefits of the medicine you're taking. (In the case of oxybutynin you can take some measures to lessen dry mouth; we discuss these in Chapter 6.)

Kate didn't mind taking antibiotics to clear up her chest infection. In fact, if they were going to help her get better quickly she was all for it: she had an overseas trip coming up and didn't want anything getting in the way. After starting her treatment she was thrilled to find she was feeling better. However, her joy quickly turned to dismay when she developed a vaginal discharge. She saw her doctor, who diagnosed a vaginal yeast infection. She was given a different antibiotic, and soon thereafter bade both her infection and Canada "au revoir."

Kate's antibiotic had killed off not only the bacteria infecting her chest, but also the protective, necessary bacteria that live in the vagina — as a result, she'd developed a vaginal yeast infection. You've heard the old expression "Give someone a hammer and everything looks like a nail"? Well, give a body an antibiotic and sometimes every germ looks like dinner. We all have essential bacteria in our bodies. These are present mostly in our bowels (we excrete *billions* of bacteria each day in our stool), but are also found in our mouths, on our skin, and, in women, in the vagina. These protective bacteria live in a fine balance. If the balance is disturbed — as happened to Kate — some germs may run roughshod over the others, resulting in an infection.

Idiosyncratic reactions

Idiosyncratic reactions to a drug are those side-effects that are unpredictable and not related to the drug's mechanism of action. They typically occur for no obvious reason.

Harriet Brooks, a 45-year-old homemaker and mother of two, came down with fever, chills, back pain, and foul-smelling urine. She promptly saw her doctor, who diagnosed her with a bladder infection and gave her a prescription for sulfamethoxazole-trimethoprim. A few days later she noticed lots of tiny red spots on her skin, and bleeding gums when she brushed her teeth. Harriet went to see her doctor, who sent her for a blood test and found she had a very low platelet count (platelets are cells in the blood that prevent bleeding). She stopped the drug, and soon thereafter her platelet count was back to normal. Harriet had experienced an *idiosyncratic reaction* to her sulfamethoxazole-trimethoprim.

Idiosyncratic drug reactions can at times be very dangerous. They may include bone marrow damage, hepatitis, lung inflammation, and heart damage — to name but a few. Fortunately, serious idiosyncratic reactions are uncommon. In Chapter 6 we point out important idiosyncratic reactions that may occur from certain prescription medicines.

As with other possible side-effects, if while taking a prescription drug you develop new symptoms you cannot readily explain it's best to contact your doctor to make sure you're not experiencing a reaction to your medicine.

Drug intolerance

Being intolerant of a drug is a non-specific reaction — basically, a drug "just doesn't agree with you."

Norman, Roger, Craig, and David were sitting in the doctor's office, patiently (well, sort of patiently) waiting while reading the most current magazines in the office — you know, the *Time* magazine that talks about the forthcoming Seoul Olympics, and the *Maclean's*

looking at whether Trudeau will be re-elected. By coincidence, they all had the same ailment (a throat infection), were all the same age, were all in excellent health, and had no other symptoms. Dr. Jones prescribed the same antibiotic for each of them. Two days later they were all back to see the doctor, and they were not a happy lot. Norman had nausea. Roger had the runs. Craig had cramps. David had dizziness. Dr. Jones had them each discontinue their antibiotic, and their symptoms quickly settled. Though their symptoms differed, what Norman, Roger, Craig and David had in common was that they were all intolerant of their medication.

Typically, an intolerance to a medicine relates to known and predictable properties of a drug. For example, an antibiotic called erythromycin commonly causes nausea, a simple intolerance. An intolerance differs from an allergy (which is related to the immune system and typically causes specific symptoms such as a skin rash) and differs from the unpredictable nature of idiosyncratic reactions. Drug intolerance is very common, is typically not serious, and goes away quickly (sometimes, however, only after the drug is stopped).

Side-effects from non-medicinal ingredients

That little pill you're about to swallow (or enema you're about to insert, or inhaler you're about to puff...) contains a heck of a lot more than just the medicine you see on the prescription label. Non-medicinal ingredients may include preservatives, colouring agents, lubricants, buffers, fillers, flavours, and more. Sometimes, people experience side-effects due to these other ingredients.

Consider the following three examples of side-effects from non-medicinal ingredients:

- ✔ Mohammed developed abdominal cramps a few weeks after starting Trasicor. His celiac disease had flared because the pills contained gluten.

- ✔ Juan started passing inordinate amounts of flatus and developed loose stools after starting to take Capoten and Gen-Indapamide. His lactose intolerance had acted up because the pills contained lactose.

- ✔ Suchitra was gasping for air moments after taking her first capsule of Prometrium. Fortunately, her EpiPen was handy: she injected herself and was able to regain her breath. Suchitra had a severe peanut allergy and hadn't realized the capsule contained peanut oil.

If you have a history of allergies, sensitivities, or other types of reactions, before you start taking a newly prescribed medicine be sure to find out from your pharmacist what is in your medicine apart from the actual drug. If the medicine contains something to which you are known to adversely react, speak to your pharmacist or your doctor about what different medicine you can take in its place.

In Chapter 2 we discuss non-medicinal ingredients in more detail.

How to Avoid Side-Effects

As we discuss in the preceding section, medicines can cause many different types of side-effects. Indeed, it's a wonder and a blessing most people experience none! Although it's impossible to guarantee that you won't experience a side-effect, you can improve the odds. We look at how to do this next.

Questions to ask your doctor before you leave the office

 To minimize the risk of side-effects from your new prescription drug, before you leave your doctor's office be sure to ask your doctor whether your medicine:

- ✔ **May unfavourably affect any other health problems you have.** This one's especially important if you're seeing an unfamiliar doctor, such as in an emergency department or walk-in clinic, or even meeting a specialist for the first time — he may not have your previous medical records to review.

- ✔ **May interact with other drugs (prescription and non-prescription) you're taking.** We discuss drug interactions later in this chapter.

- ✔ **Is safe to take during pregnancy or breastfeeding.** (Assuming there's a possibility either of these situations apply to you.)

- ✔ **Is related to drugs that gave you side-effects in the past.**

Depending on your doctor's answers to these questions, you may need to have your medicine changed to something else. (For more questions to ask your doctor about your medication, see Chapter 3.)

Questions to ask your pharmacist before you leave the pharmacy

To minimize the risk of side-effects from your new prescription drug, before you leave your pharmacy be sure to ask your pharmacist whether your medicine:

- ✔ **Should be taken with or without food** (or if it doesn't matter).

- ✔ **Requires you to avoid certain foods** (such as grapefruit or grapefruit juice), salt substitutes, or alcohol.

- ✔ **May contain other ingredients to which you might react.** (This applies only if you have other health issues, such as celiac disease, a peanut allergy, and so on, as we discuss earlier in this chapter.)

- ✔ **May interact with other drugs you're taking** (prescription and non-prescription). We discuss drug interactions later in this chapter. (We know we already suggested you ask your doctor this question, but it's so important we suggest you ask *both* of them.)

- ✔ **Requires you avoid sun exposure.** (Some drugs cause a skin rash if you're out in the sun, a condition called *photosensitivity.*)

- ✔ **Requires you to gargle and/or rinse your mouth after a dose** (as is the case with some inhalers).

For more questions to ask your pharmacist about your medication, see Chapter 3.

Questions to ask yourself before you take your new medicine

To minimize the risk of side-effects from your new prescription drug, before you take your first dose be sure to ask yourself the following questions:

- ✔ **Am I clear on the instructions my doctor and pharmacist gave me, and were all my questions answered?** (For more, see the lists above and in Chapter 3.)

- ✔ **Do I understand the prescription label's instructions?**

- ✔ **Do I understand the warning labels the pharmacist affixed to the container?**

If the answer is no to any of these three questions, we recommend you seek clarification from your doctor or pharmacist as soon as possible. (Next time, take this book with you and look over the questions here and in Chapter 3 *before* you leave the doctor's office or the pharmacy.) Getting things clarified *while you're still there* saves time and avoids the risk you won't be able to get in touch with your health care providers later in the day. Also, be sure to complete the Cheat Sheet at the front of this book for each prescription drug you are taking.

What to Do If You Experience a Side-Effect

If you think you're experiencing a side-effect from a prescription drug, we recommend the following action:

- ✔ **Quickly assess whether the situation is urgent.** If, for example, you take a dose of your new medicine and moments later you become wheezy, your lips and tongue swell, and you're short of breath, call 911 immediately — you're likely having a very serious allergic reaction. Conversely, if you've taken a medicine for a couple of days and develop a bit of nausea — well, this isn't urgent. All degrees of reactions need to be considered on an individual basis.

- ✔ **Notify the appropriate member of your health care team.** For non-urgent situations (ones not requiring immediate attention), contact the most appropriate member of your health care team at your earliest opportunity to let them know what has happened and to find out whether you should continue taking the drug or stop. Generally, the most appropriate person to contact is the physician who prescribed your medicine. If she's not available, call your family physician (of course, it may have been your family physician who prescribed the drug). If he's not available and you have any reason to think your symptoms can't wait until you can reach him, call your provincial/territorial urgent health care line (if one exists) or your pharmacist.

  (Ideally, when you first get a prescription, you discuss with your doctor right then and there what to do in the event you later run into side-effects.)

- ✔ **Report the event to Health Canada.** If you've consulted with your doctor or pharmacist and the consensus is you've experienced a side-effect to a prescription drug, it's wise to notify Health Canada (particularly if it is serious). Overseeing bodies such as Health Canada can effectively monitor the safety of medicines only by keeping records that are as thorough as possible. Health Canada can be reached either on the Web (www.hc-sc.gc.ca) or by phone (1-866-234-2345).

Understanding Drug Interactions

A *drug interaction* is the process wherein a drug interacts with another drug — or some other, non-medicinal substance — resulting in an enhanced or a reduced effect (or some other unrelated effect). For example, let's say that like many people you are on a common iron supplement (such as ferrous sulfate) to treat anemia, and you take a commonly used antacid (such as Maalox) to treat heartburn. These are two fine and effective drugs. Yet, in fact, if you take them at the same time, the Maalox blocks a significant amount of the iron from getting into your system (so the iron pill you just took is less likely to help you). This is a common example of a drug interaction (which, in this case, is causing a reduced effect of a medicine).

To reduce your chances of experiencing a drug interaction we recommend you ask your doctor whether a new drug might interact with any other drug you're taking (prescription or non-prescription) *before* you start the new drug. Also ask your pharmacist. (We're aware it's redundant, but we're talking about your safety here!)

You can also look up drug interactions yourself on the Web. Two excellent Web sites for this purpose are `www.drugdigest.org` and `www.epocrates.com`.

Although a drug interaction can occur if you take certain medicines too close together, most drug interactions in fact occur regardless whether you take the medicines at the same moment or not. It's the fact you're taking the products at all, not the specific times at which you are ingesting them, that's important.

Drug–drug interactions

Many drugs can have their actions altered if you're also taking other drugs. Although on occasion this is helpful, the majority of the time it's not. Drugs can interact with other drugs by

- **Reducing the absorption of a prescription drug.** The iron/antacid example in the preceding section illustrates this point. Drugs that can reduce absorption of other drugs include antacids, cholestyramine, calcium, and iron. You won't derive the benefit from it you're supposed to if you don't absorb your medicine sufficiently well.

- **Increasing the potency or amount of the prescription drug in your blood.** An example is the antibiotic *sulfamethoxazole/ trimethoprim,* which can increase the potency of *methotrexate.*

- **Increasing the risk of side-effects.**

Because of the potential for drug–drug interactions, your doctor may need to avoid prescribing certain combinations of medicines. In other cases, she may need to prescribe a smaller or larger dose of a drug.

Sometimes, drugs known to interact can still be used together and in their usual doses, but more frequent blood-test monitoring may be required.

In the case of drugs (such as antacids) that interfere with the absorption of prescription medicines, generally you can deal with this by taking the prescription drug at least two hours before or after taking the antacid (if this applies to a drug you've been pre-scribed, your physician and/or pharmacist should let you know about this precaution).

Drug–food interactions

Foods you eat can interact with your prescription drug(s) by

- ✔ **Reducing absorption of your medicine.** To ensure proper absorption of your prescription drug from your gut into your body, many drugs are taken on an empty stomach. (On the other side of the coin, some medicines need to be taken on an empty stomach for the opposite reason: food unduly *increases* their absorption.) We discuss this issue in more detail in Chapter 4.

- ✔ **Reducing metabolism of your medicine.** Grapefruit is proba-bly the best known example of a food that can alter the way the body handles a medicine, potentially leading to danger-ously high levels of the drug in your blood. We discuss this issue in more detail in Chapter 4.

- ✔ **Causing inconsistent action of your medicine.** One notable example is the inconsistent action of warfarin (a potent "blood thinner") if you're getting overly variable quantities of vitamin K in your diet. As we discuss in more detail in Chapter 6, if you're taking warfarin it's important to be consistent in the amount of vitamin K you consume.

Drug–alcohol interactions

Alcohol and a large number of drugs don't, ahem, mix well together. Possible drug–alcohol interactions are

✔ **Excess sedation** (that is, making you overly sleepy).

✔ **Disulfiram reactions.** Disulfiram (Antabuse) is a drug used in the treatment of alcoholism. It works by making you feel ill if you consume alcohol. Symptoms include nausea, vomiting, headaches, and flushing.

✔ **High blood pressure.** This can occur if you're taking a monoamine oxidase (MAO) inhibitor and consume alcohol.

✔ **Hypoglycemia (low blood glucose).** This is likely to be a problem only if your diabetes is treated with drugs — such as glyburide or insulin — that may cause low blood glucose.

Depending on the drug in question, limited consumption (rather than complete elimination) of alcohol may be sufficient to avoid alcohol–drug interactions. Check with your pharmacist to find out if your medication can interact with alcohol and, if so, how much — if any — alcohol you may safely consume.

Drug–complementary and alternative medicine interactions

As we discuss in Chapter 2, *complementary and alternative medicines* (CAMs) include certain herbs, vitamins (often in high dose), minerals, amino acids, and dietary supplements typically given outside the scope of mainstream medical practice. In the same way that many of these products can lead to side-effects when taken in isolation, so too can they interact with prescription drugs. For this reason, if you are taking a CAM, be sure to let your doctor and your pharmacist know this before you start taking a new prescription medicine.

Certain CAMs can interact with your prescription drug(s), causing

✔ **Reduced potency of the prescription medicine.** For example, Coenzyme Q10 may decrease the potency of warfarin, leading to dangerous blood clotting.

✔ **Increased potency of the prescription medicine.** Again using warfarin as an example — which we do because it's such a commonly used and potentially dangerous drug — garlic can increase the potency of warfarin, potentially leading to dangerous bleeding.

✔ **Altering the amount of the prescription medicine in the blood.** For example, if you take digoxin, St. John's wort can cause the level of digoxin to fall, which could result in a deterioration in your heart condition.

Because St John's wort can dangerously interact with so many drugs, in some places in the world it's available only by prescription. We strongly recommend that you not take St. John's wort and prescription medicine together unless you, your doctor, and your pharmacist have first determined that your prescription drug(s) do not interact with this product.

Drug–sunshine interactions

Sunshine gets such a bad rap these days, what with skin cancers and all, we hate to add to the guilt many of us feel (us included) when we throw caution to the wind and venture out on a sunny day "without adequate sun protection," but...

Yup, there's a but here. A number of drugs can make you prone to a rash upon sun exposure (called a *photosensitive skin rash*). Examples include amiodarone, ciprofloxacin, and tetracycline, and dozens more exist. (If you're prescribed a drug with this effect, your pharmacist typically informs you of this precaution when dispensing the drug to you.)

If you're taking a drug that can cause a rash, you need to — you guessed it — use appropriate sun protection.

Chapter 8

Prescription Drugs for Moms-to-Be, Kids, and Seniors

● ●

In This Chapter

▶ Taking prescription drugs if you are pregnant or breastfeeding

▶ Helping your child take a medicine

▶ Avoiding accidental drug overdose in children

▶ Monitoring your child's use of stimulant medication to treat ADHD

▶ Keeping seniors organized and safe with their prescription medicines

● ●

Safety is always a priority with prescription drug therapy, especially for pregnant or breastfeeding women, the elderly, and households with young children. In this chapter we look at these special situations. We also look at how you can help your child take oral medicines and what you can monitor if you have a child with attention-deficit hyperactivity disorder (ADHD) being treated with stimulant medications like methylphenidate (Ritalin).

Drug Safety for Women Who Are Pregnant or Breastfeeding

No situation demands greater caution than the use of prescription drugs during pregnancy. Complicating matters is the general lack of proof a medicine is completely safe for the fetus of a pregnant woman. Indeed, the precise risks to a fetus are unknown for more than 90 percent of prescription drugs. A medicine may appear safe based on tests involving pregnant laboratory animals, but no guarantee exists the drug is equally safe when taken by a pregnant woman. Similarly, the safety (to the infant) of taking prescription drugs during breastfeeding is often not fully known.

If you take prescription medicines and are contemplating pregnancy, we cannot recommend strongly enough that you discuss with your doctor what is to be done regarding your drug therapy — in particular, if (and when) you should discontinue your prescriptions — *before* attempting to conceive. (We say this in the interests of being cautious; reassuringly, very few drugs are proven to be unequivocally dangerous if taken during pregnancy.)

Looking at whether a drug is safe when pregnant or breastfeeding

Because limited information exists on the safety of most medicines when taken during pregnancy and breastfeeding, the best policy is to avoid prescription drugs in these situations whenever possible. Nonetheless, sometimes you simply cannot. Here are some examples of when you may need to take a prescription medicine:

- A chronic illness (such as asthma or diabetes)

- Certain types of complications from pregnancy, such as high blood pressure

- An ailment — say, for example, pneumonia — unrelated to pregnancy or breastfeeding but requiring immediate treatment

How a prescription medicine may harm a fetus

A pregnant woman and her fetus each have their own blood circulation, but the placenta allows many substances to travel from mother to fetus — and it often doesn't discriminate between those that are good (such as nutrients) and those that are bad (such as alcohol).

Adverse ways prescription drugs may affect a fetus include the following:

- **Abnormal organ development leading to birth defects.** Because the fetus's organs form early during pregnancy, it's the stage of greatest risk. Perhaps the most notorious example is the formation of abnormal limbs in the offspring of many women who took a drug called thalidomide.

- **Abnormal but reversible organ function.** One example is the goiter (thyroid swelling) a fetus may develop when a pregnant woman takes an anti-thyroid medicine, such as propylthiouracil. (The goiter goes away after birth.)

✓ **Miscarriage.**

✓ **Premature labour.**

✓ **Damage to the placenta leading to insufficient passage of nutrients into the fetus's circulation.** This, in turn, can cause the fetus (and, subsequently, the newborn) to be too small.

How a prescription medicine may harm a breastfeeding infant

Many prescription medicines taken by a breastfeeding woman do not cause problems for the infant. Others, however, can. For example, minocycline can lead to discoloured teeth in the infant if taken by a breastfeeding woman for more than 10 days. Another example is the lethargy that can occur in the breastfeeding infant of a woman taking diazepam.

Whether a drug is likely to harm a breastfeeding infant depends on a number of factors, including:

✓ **The particular drug being taken.**

✓ **How much of the drug accumulates in the baby's system.** This in turn depends on several things, including:

  • How much of the drug enters the mother's breast milk.

  • How much (if any) of the drug present in the mother's breast milk gets absorbed into the baby's system.

  • How much breast milk the infant consumes. (This varies depending on whether the baby is also consuming other foods and liquids.)

  • How quickly the infant eliminates the drug from its body.

 If you wish to continue breastfeeding but have been prescribed a medicine that makes doing so unsafe, consider pumping and discarding your breast milk for the duration of your drug therapy. In many cases, pumping can maintain your ability to produce milk so that when you've completed your prescription you can resume breastfeeding. Check with your doctor to find out how long you should wait following the last dose of your medicine to safely resume breastfeeding.

How the safety of drugs taken during pregnancy and breastfeeding is classified

The main resource doctors use when looking up information on drug safety is a book called the *Compendium of Pharmaceuticals and Specialties* (CPS). However, Canada does not have a formalized classification system for measuring drug safety during pregnancy and breastfeeding. The CPS summarizes the safety data, but does not assign it specific rankings.

FDA drug classification during pregnancy

This table shows the classification system used by the United States Food and Drug Administration (FDA). The majority of drugs tend to fall into Category C, which basically comes down to, "We don't know whether it's safe or not, so we have to use our best judgment."

Category	Description
A	Adequate, well-controlled studies in pregnant women have not shown an increased risk of fetal abnormalities.
B	Animal studies have revealed no evidence of harm to the fetus; however, no adequate and well-controlled studies in pregnant women exist.
	or
	Animal studies have shown an adverse effect, but adequate and well-controlled studies in pregnant women have failed to demonstrate a risk to the fetus.
C	Animal studies have shown an adverse effect and no adequate and well-controlled studies in pregnant women exist.
	or
	No animal studies have been conducted and no adequate and well-controlled studies in pregnant women exist.
D	Studies, adequate well-controlled or observational, in pregnant women have demonstrated a risk to the fetus. However, the benefits of therapy may outweigh the potential risk.
X	Studies, adequate well-controlled or observational, in animals or pregnant women have demonstrated positive evidence of fetal abnormalities. The use of the product is contraindicated* in women who are or may become pregnant.

* Contraindicated, in this context, means a drug should not be used

The United States does have a classification system for drug use during pregnancy. However, because of the paucity of available data on prescription drug use in this context, its value is somewhat limited. Because you may come across it in your travels (both literally and figuratively), we present it in the sidebar "FDA drug classification during pregnancy" in this section.

You can look up your drug's FDA classification at www. epocrates.com.

What to do if you're taking a prescription drug and then find out you're pregnant

If you've been taking a prescription drug and then discover you're pregnant, your mind may immediately fill with worry that the medicine has harmed your fetus. So let us reassure you that very brief exposure to most prescription drugs isn't likely to have damaged your fetus.

If you're taking a prescription medicine and then find out you're pregnant, it's essential to seek urgent consultation with your doctor so together you can make a prompt decision regarding whether the drug should be discontinued. You and your doctor will need to consider several factors including why you're taking it in the first place, its risk to the fetus (which depends on the specific properties of the drug and on your stage of pregnancy), and the other therapies available (both prescription and non-prescription).

Until you speak with your doctor, don't stop taking your medicine unless you're certain it's safe to do so. Suddenly discontinuing a prescription drug may have its own risks (for example, suddenly discontinuing an anticonvulsant puts you at increased risk of seizures, as we discuss in Chapter 6).

An excellent resource on prescription drug therapy in the setting of pregnancy and breastfeeding is the site run by the Motherisk Clinic of the Hospital for Sick Children in Toronto (on the Web at www.motherisk.org).

Drug Safety for Children

In all likelihood, your child will be the recipient of a few prescriptions during her childhood (think earaches, sore throats, certain skin rashes . . .). Be prepared by being versed in some of the finer points of safely and effectively administering medications to children. We discuss these in this section.

Generally, a child's dose is based on body weight — the greater the weight, the larger the dose. Nonetheless, when it comes to drug dosages, children aren't just little adults. For instance, some drugs are metabolized in children more slowly than in adults, so a proportionately smaller dose is needed. Conversely, some drugs are metabolized in children more quickly than in adults, so a proportionately larger dose is required.

Children also differ from adults when it comes to drug side-effects. Depending on the medicine in question, youngsters can be more or even uniquely susceptible to certain side-effects (such as impaired bone growth from long-term oral corticosteroid therapy, which may result in a failure to achieve full adult height), or they may experience side-effects opposite to what an adult might experience (such as the agitation some children develop after taking certain antihistamines that more typically cause sedation in adults). Every time you're handed a prescription for your child, speak to your physician and pharmacist about what side-effects the child may experience (so that you know what to keep an eye out for), and find out what to do if a side-effect does occur. And if you have children in your household ensure that you store all medications safely — theirs and yours.

Consider the following ways to help your child stay safe around prescription drugs:

- ✓ **Store prescription medicines safely.** The best place to store your medicines is in a locked cabinet. (We discuss additional storage issues in Chapter 4.)

- ✓ **Keep your medicines in child-resistant containers.** (This may not always be possible; for example, if you have severe arthritis making it impossible for you to open this type of container.)

- ✓ **Don't take your medicine in front of your child; she may try to mimic you at some other time.**

- ✓ **Never refer to medicine as candy or a treat.** Although this may be a tempting way to coax your child to take a prescribed medicine (we remember being tempted ourselves), doing so may encourage the child to take medicines inappropriately if, for example, they came across an open pill bottle or found errant pills on the floor.

Special issues regarding your child's use of stimulant medicines to treat Attention-Deficit/Hyperactivity Disorder (ADHD)

As we discuss in Chapter 5, ADHD is a disease, typically diagnosed in childhood, characterized by difficulty paying attention, being overly active and acting impulsively. In this section we look at what you can watch for if your child is taking stimulant medication to treat this condition. (Stimulant drugs are the most commonly used form of medication to treat ADHD. In Chapter 6 we look in detail at methylphenidate, a specific form of stimulant drug.)

ANECDOTE

A parent's worst nightmare: The open pill bottle

Keeping medicines safely out of a child's reach is of paramount importance.

Heather well remembers a time when she was 7 years of age and visiting a friend's house. She and her friend, Jill Harris, had just come in from playing, and at Heather's insistence had gone upstairs to see Jill's little brother. They found him sitting happily on his parents' bed, heartily snacking away on some cherished treat, his cheeks chipmunk-size, saliva dripping down his chin.

As they moved closer they found a half-empty bottle of ASA on the bed and a few pills in his hand. With alarm in her voice, Jill called for her mother. In a flash, Mrs. Harris ran into the room from the adjoining bathroom. Instantly sizing up the situation she immediately called an ambulance, which arrived in short order. As the ambulance pulled away, Heather, Jill and Mrs. Harris jumped into a car and followed the ambulance to the hospital.

As they waited in the ER, Heather remembers Mrs. Harris pacing, beside herself with worry. After what seemed like an interminable wait, the doctor emerged from the examining room. "I was just gone for a moment," Mrs. Harris immediately said to the doctor. "I just went to the bathroom. He was fine. I..." The doctor looked at her reassuringly and said, "Your son is doing just fine. You got him here soon enough." Mrs. Harris sobbed with relief then, composing herself once again, said to the doctor, "I had no idea there was an open pill bottle lying around. It'll never happen again; that's for sure." And, Jill recently told Heather, it never did.

ASK YOUR DOCTOR

When the doctor hands you the prescription for a stimulant medication, discuss the specific goals of treatment for your child with the doctor and how you'll know they are being achieved. Also, as we discuss below, you can help your doctor by monitoring your child. Be sure to ask your doctor what you are to do with your observations.

Things you can monitor include the following:

- ✔ Improvement in positive traits such as attentiveness

- ✔ Reduction in negative traits such as impulsive behaviour

- ✔ Your child's mood

- ✔ Your child's growth and weight

- ✔ The development of drug side-effects such as nervousness, decreased appetite, insomnia, nausea, vomiting, and abdominal pain (We discuss these and other side-effects in more detail in Chapter 6.)

How to help your child swallow a medicine

Getting a child to swallow a necessary (but not very palatable) medication can be as difficult as persuading them to eat those delectable Brussels sprouts on their plate. (Here we help you with the former and, as for the latter we simply wish you the best of luck!) Although, as we discuss below, you can be flexible with your child regarding some things, your child must take the dose. If your child is to benefit from their medicine, there's simply no other choice.

Depending on your child's age, the specific medicine in question, and whether the medicine is in pill or liquid form, you can try some of the following to help your child swallow a dose:

- **Use a helpful tool such as a specially designed dropper or syringe.** (Your pharmacist can help you select the best one for your child's needs.)

- **Have your child create a special "medicine cup" that he can decorate** (with stickers, for example).

- **Camouflage the bad taste by mixing the medicine in with a pleasant, fruity drink.** You can also mix it in with a good-tasting food such as chocolate pudding. (Before you do this, let your child know what you're up to; otherwise she may not trust her food again.)

- **Have your child take the medicine with a straw.** The medicine will go further back in the mouth, where the taste may not be as evident. Also, the act of using a straw may distract your child from the stuff being swallowed.

- **Praise your child liberally for having taken a dose.** You might also consider rewarding her with a sticker or other memento. (Our kids called this "a bribe.")

- **For an infant, gently but firmly keep her lips together as you insert the liquid medicine with a dropper into her mouth. Keep her lips together until she's swallowed the medicine.**

Ask your child's doctor (or your pharmacist) which of the preceding tips would be appropriate for your particular child and the specific drug being taken. Also, be sure to ask the doctor for her own favourite tips; you can be sure she has a whole bunch.

Drug Safety for Seniors

As people get older, most of us require increasing numbers of pre-scription drugs. And with each new prescription comes one more thing to know — actually, *many* more things, because drugs can be so complicated! In this section we look at drug-related issues that seniors often need to contend with, and provide some tips to help seniors ensure that their prescription drugs work safely and effectively.

Considering special risks for seniors

Although for some seniors taking prescription drugs is not much — or even any — different from taking medicines in earlier stages of life, many people in their later years have additional health issues influencing which drugs are prescribed in what doses, and what needs to be done to make sure they're taken properly. For example, seniors are at increased risk of having

✔ **Reduced kidney function.** You may need to avoid drugs that are eliminated from the body through the kidneys, or to use the drugs in lower doses.

✔ **Liver damage.** You may need to avoid drugs that are elimi-nated from the body through the liver, or to use the drugs in lower doses.

✔ **Arthritis or muscle weakness.** You're not very likely to have a good response to your fancy-shmancy new medication if you can't even take a dose because opening the pill bottle's "childproof" top requires Herculean brawn. (We'd rent out our teenage boys to help you, but we need them at home to open jars for us!)

✔ **Increased sensitivity to medicines.** You may experience side-effects from levels of a drug in the bloodstream that might be fine in a younger person.

✔ **Memory or other thinking problems.** If you experience this common predicament, consider enlisting help from your family members or friends, pharmacist, and doctor.

Time to clean house

Seniors are at increased risk of getting their medicines muddled, so unnecessary, outdated, or unused medications must not be kept around the home.

Marcia Greenbaum was a frail, retired, 80-year-old widow contending with a variety of health concerns including some recent problems with her memory. Fiercely independent, she had refused her daughter's overtures to move into a supervised living situation and remained at home on her own. Her daughter, Rebecca, called her at least twice a day to make sure all was well.

One day, to Rebecca's alarm, Mrs. Greenbaum sounded confused and groggy over the phone. Rebecca rushed over, to find her mother slumped in a chair. She had been incontinent and she was dazed and disoriented. Food was scattered over the kitchen floor, and on the counter were open containers of lorazepam, oxazepam, acetaminophen with codeine, and hydroxyzine (an antihistamine). Some of the prescriptions had been issued years before.

Mrs. Greenbaum was rushed to the hospital, where a diagnosis of (unintentional) drug overdose was made. She improved over the next couple of days and was ready for discharge. In the meantime, Rebecca stopped by her mother's house and collected every medicine bottle on the premises, filling a grocery bag to overflowing. On their way home from the hospital the two women stopped by their drugstore. There, they sat down with the pharmacist as he discarded dozens of old, unused, and expired medicines and then carefully organized Mrs. Greenbaum's current prescriptions into a blister pack dispenser (we discuss these below), which separates each dose for each day for an entire week. Every week thereafter Rebecca stopped by the pharmacy to get a new, filled, dispenser. No pill bottle or other type of medicine container was again to grace the Greenbaum residence, and no further dosing misadventures took place.

Helpful ways for seniors to stay organized with their prescription medicines

Sadly, stories of older adults being rushed to the emergency room for accidental drug overdose aren't rare; faulty memory may cause a senior to take a daily drug twice in one morning or an entire array of drugs when they were only supposed to take one or two. When a senior lives alone with no one to watch or help remember when to take medicines, the risk increases.

Whether you're past a certain age or not, it never hurts to start forming good drug organizing habits that will serve you even better as you get older. To help stay organized with your prescription drugs, follow these tips:

✔ **Never keep unnecessary prescription medication around your house.** This includes old, unused, or partially used prescriptions.

✔ **Always keep your prescription medicines in their original containers or a special dispenser.** You may decide — or your loved ones or health care providers may suggest — that you'd have an easier time keeping track of your drugs if they were organized in a *7-day pill organizer,* a special dispenser with separate compartments for medicines you take at certain times of the day for an entire week. (See Figures 8-1 and 8-2 for illustrations of the two most common types of such containers: blister packs and dosettes.) These containers typically have a week's worth of medicines divided into the appropriate number of small, labelled chambers.

Dosettes have little opening doors, so anyone can fill the dispenser. Blister packs, on the other hand, have sealed compartments and can be filled only by a pharmacist. Each method has pros and cons. A dosette provides greater flexibility — you can fill it yourself, and it's reusable (that is, you can refill it each week). A blister pack provides an extra margin of safety because only the pharmacist can fill it (and he can affix a prescription label to the back of the blister pack at the same time). We recommend you discuss these issues with your pharmacist to ensure that you make the best choice for your particular circumstances.

✔ **Ask your doctor to prescribe medicines requiring the least frequent dosing.** Also ask your doctor if some of your prescribed drugs are available in a format combining two different medicines. (Note that combined medicines may not be covered by some drug plans that do cover both drugs when taken separately.)

✔ **Be as routine as possible in the way you take your prescription medicines.** For instance, keep all your medicines in the same place, and take them at consistent times.

Every time you see the doctor, bring *all* your medicines (in their original containers or, if you're using a 7-day pill organizer, bring it *and* a list of your drugs). Your doctor will check to ensure that you still need them and that you're taking them properly. Also, arrange with your pharmacist to periodically sit down with her to have your medicines reviewed. (Whenever possible make a point of using the same pharmacist, so that she can get to know you and your needs. In Chapter 3 we discuss, in detail, the roles of the pharmacist.)

Even if you know with certainty what medicine you're taking based on its colour, shape, and size, your doctor will surely hesitate to make treatment decisions based on this information, because dozens of different drugs may look virtually identical. We strongly recommend that you *not* rely on your memory as your guide when you recount to your doctor or pharmacist what medicines you're taking. Even the best memory is not as reliable as having your pills in their *labelled containers* sitting in front of you when you see your health care provider. (Incidentally, we give this same advice to people of any age.)

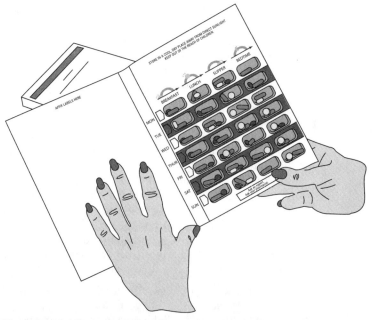

Figure 8-1: A *blister pack* 7-day pill organizer.

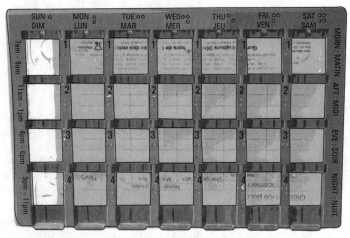

Figure 8-2: A *dosette* 7-day pill organizer.

Watching out for special side-effects in seniors

Anybody, regardless of age, can experience side-effects from medications. If a drug commonly causes nausea in a teenager, then taking it is likely also going to make you feel nauseated if you're the grandparent of the teenager. Nonetheless, certain side-effects are more likely to occur when you're of a more advanced age. Here are some of the more common side-effects — and recommendations on how to deal with them:

- ✔ **Sleepiness, fatigue, and altered thinking:** Many medicines can cause these side-effects, including benzodiazepines (typically used to treat anxiety and sleep disorders), narcotic analgesics, and beta blockers. (We discuss these medicines in Chapter 6.)

  If you're experiencing these side-effects, let your doctor know. Sometimes, simply reducing the dose can help. Other times, the drug may need to be discontinued. Your doctor can discuss with you which of these choices is best. Also, alcohol tends to makes these symptoms worse, so avoiding alcohol may help.

- ✔ **Dry mouth, constipation, difficulty passing urine:** These are examples of *anticholinergic* side-effects and can be caused by many different drugs — including, unsurprisingly, by *anticholinergics.* You may find some relief from your dry mouth by taking frequent sips of water, sucking on hard candy, or chewing sugarless gum. (Because having a persistent dry mouth can increase your risk of cavities, be sure to look after your teeth well and have regular dental care.) You can help avoid constipation by consuming a fibre-rich diet and, if necessary, taking an over-the-counter stool softener such as docusate.

- ✔ **Faintness upon standing:** Certain medications used to treat high blood pressure and other conditions can cause an excess drop in blood pressure upon standing. It's especially likely to occur soon after you start the medicine. If you're prescribed a medicine with this potential side-effect, your doctor should initially prescribe the lowest possible effective dose. Also, we recommend that you

  - Take your first dose at bedtime (unless your doctor advises you otherwise).

  - Stand for a moment before walking away from your chair or bed to make sure that you do not feel faint. If you do feel faint, sit (or, if necessary, lie) back down.

✓ **Dehydration (from diuretics):** Most diuretics (such as hydrochlorothiazide, for example) cause only a modest increase in the amount of urine you produce and dehydration is unlikely to occur. Some diuretics (such as metolazone or, sometimes, furosemide), however, can cause a profound increase in urine and can put you at risk of dehydration. You can monitor your fluid status by weighing yourself daily. If you are losing weight too rapidly (as determined by your doctor), this may indicate excess fluid is being lost from your body. Be sure to ask your doctor how much weight loss (if any) is expected and at what point to contact her if weight loss occurs.

If you're experiencing side-effects from your medication, in most cases you will need to talk to your doctor before you stop taking it. In Chapter 7 ("What to Do If You Experience a Side-Effect") we provide detailed advice on this topic. Also, we recommend that you complete the Cheat Sheet at the front of this book, where you can write in what your doctor advises you to do in the event you experience a side-effect. (In Chapter 6 we look at a variety of specific medications and point out side-effects seniors need to be especially vigilant for.)

Chapter 9

Dealing with Emergencies and Hospitalizations

● ●

In This Chapter

▶ Determining whether to seek emergency treatment

▶ Knowing how to handle an overdose

▶ Considering your options if you accidentally run out of medicine

▶ Understanding the essentials about prescription drugs given in a hospital

● ●

*P*rescription medicines are wonderful tools in our quest for good health, but they have very real dangers, too. Few dangers are as great as taking an overdose of medicine. In this chapter we look at this important issue. (In Chapter 7, we discuss the other great hazard of prescription drug therapy: serious side-effects and what to do about them.) Also in this chapter, we look at some important issues surrounding prescription drug therapy you might receive in a hospital setting.

Can It Wait? Deciding When You Require Emergency Medical Attention

Here is the most straightforward piece of advice that we can give in the entirety of this book: If you ever think something might be an emergency, treat it as an emergency. Better to do that and find out it wasn't an emergency after all than to assume everything's fine only to find out things weren't fine at all.

ANECDOTE

Simply too, too much

Sometimes, a person takes too much of a medication to intentionally harm oneself; other times, taking a drug overdose is unintentional. In either case, it can create life-threatening consequences...

Rosalie had suffered from migraine headaches for years, and to her great dismay the attacks had become increasingly frequent and increasingly severe. And now, into the umpteenth hour of her worst migraine ever, she was feeling wretched. She called in sick to work, went to the medicine cabinet, and took a couple of generic ASA. That didn't help, so an hour later she took a couple more. Still not feeling better, she returned to her bathroom and pulled out a bottle of Extra-Strength Bufferin. Four of those later, still not feeling better, she dragged herself out of bed and took a few Aspirin. Not improved, she took some Norgesic then some Novasen, but these, too, were to no avail. She found some old Fiorinal and Percodan. Those didn't help either. Pill after pill went down in Rosalie's desperate efforts to gain relief from her agony.

Later that day Rosalie's husband, Peter, arrived home and, to his horror, found Rosalie disoriented, confused, and breathing rapidly. He immediately called 911, and soon thereafter Rosalie was whisked to the hospital. About an hour later the doctor came to the waiting room and told Peter Rosalie had overdosed on ASA. "How could that be?" Peter asked in astonishment. "She'd never do that!" "Peter," the doctor replied, "it was an accident. She didn't intentionally overdose, she was just trying to feel better and didn't realize the different products she was taking all contained the same medicine: ASA."

Rosalie was admitted to the Intensive Care Unit and, fortunately, was soon much better. Later, she was started on propranolol as preventive therapy for her migraines and, though not completely free of further attacks, they occurred far less often.

What are prescription drug emergencies? Some examples include:

- ✔ **Known or suspected drug overdose.** (We talk about this in the next section.)
- ✔ **Severe allergic reaction.** Symptoms suggesting this include swollen lips and tongue, wheezing, and shortness of breath.
- ✔ **Anything more than trivial quantities of bleeding if you are on an anticoagulant** ("blood thinner") such as warfarin.
- ✔ **Palpitations and faintness if you are on an anti-arrhythmic.**

Some situations require medical attention but are not emergencies. Some examples include:

- ✔ Minor gastrointestinal side-effects from a drug, such as having mild nausea or a few abdominal cramps after taking an antibiotic such as erythromycin.

✔ Longstanding side-effects, such as having a persisting cough from taking an ACE inhibitor.

✔ Fatigue that develops shortly after starting a medicine, such as a beta blocker.

Dealing with an Overdose

A drug overdose occurs when you take more than the recommended or prescribed amount of a medicine. Although technically this includes accidentally taking even a single extra dose, doing so is very rarely a danger. Of greater concern — and what we're referring to here — is taking a substantially greater quantity of a medicine than is prescribed.

If you ever take an overdose, or are assisting someone who has (or you think *may* have), call for help — even if the person feels and looks completely well. If he or she is fully alert, oriented, and appears reasonably well, then it's appropriate to first call your regional poison control centre (see the numbers in the nearby sidebar "Poison Control Centre phone numbers"). In all other cases, it's best to call 911 (or, if you're in an area that doesn't have 911 service, whatever emergency number is applicable to your locale).

While you wait for emergency personnel to arrive, you can do the following things to help a person who has overdosed:

✔ If necessary, perform cardiopulmonary resuscitation (CPR). The details of how to do this are beyond the scope of this book — however, in all cases, if the person isn't breathing properly check to see whether he's choking on something.

You can find out more about CPR through the Canadian Red Cross (www.redcross.ca/firstaid) and St. John Ambulance Canada (www.sja.ca).

✔ If the person is not alert and no evidence of possible spinal cord injury is present, roll him onto his side so that if he vomits he won't choke. (Because improperly moving a person with a spinal cord injury can worsen the damage, if there's *any* question about whether the individual has a spinal cord injury, *never* move him — just wait for the paramedics to arrive.)

✔ Do *not* try to get the person to vomit unless instructed to do so by emergency personnel.

✔ If the person has diabetes, is alert, and may have low blood glucose (from, for example, having taken an overdose of a drug such as glyburide or insulin), help them swallow a sugar-containing product such as juice.

✔ After the individual you're assisting has been suitably looked after, check the person, the room they were found in, the bed-room, the bathroom, the kitchen, the medicine cabinet, and all other possible locations for medicine bottles or other drug containers (whether empty or not). Collect these and give them to the emergency personnel — doing so could provide invaluable information to assist with the person's treatment in the emergency department.

Poison Control Centre phone numbers

Poison control centre phone numbers for the different regions of Canada are listed here. And remember, phone numbers can change, but 911 will always be 911. If any emergency contact number you're trying to use changes and no alternate number is provided when you call, just dial 911.

British Columbia:

  Lower Mainland: 604-682-5050

  Remainder of BC: 1-800-567-8911

Alberta: 1-800-332-1414

Saskatchewan: 1-800-667-4545 or 1-800-363-7474

Manitoba: 204-787-2591

Ontario: 1-800-268-9017 or 1-800-267-1373

Quebec: 1-800-463-5060

New Brunswick: 506-857-5555 or 506-648-6222

Nova Scotia: 902-428-8161

PEI: 1-800-565-8161

Newfoundland and Labrador: 709-722-1110

Yukon: 403-667-8726

Northwest Territories: 867-669-4100

Nunavut: 867-979-7350

If, at your leisure (that is, *not* during an emergency), you want to find out more about the Canadian Association of Poison Control Centres, you can find it on the Web at www.capcc.ca.

What to Do If You Run Out of Your Prescription Medicine

People regularly run out of things they need. Sometimes it's as benign as no milk for Sunday morning pancakes because you have three teenagers who routinely think nothing of finishing off a few litres of your finest skim to wash down four dozen chocolate-chip cookies. And sometimes you're sure you have enough gas to make it to the next station but, well, you don't. (Ian very clearly remembers picking up his first new car and running out of gas on the way home from the dealership!)

In the case of prescription drugs, unexpectedly finding out that you have no medicine left can surely be anxiety-provoking. So, right off, let us reassure you it's very seldom indeed that missing a dose or two of a prescription medicine presents a threat to your health. Also, don't feel sheepish about the oversight — this situation happens to lots of people.

 Having said that, surely you want to avoid the situation in the first place, so be sure to regularly check the amount of medicine you have left, pick up refills as necessary, and contact your physician if you need a new prescription because you have no refills left. (Oh, and remember to check your fuel gauge before you whiz by that gas station!)

In Chapter 4 we look at what to do when you're travelling and have forgotten your prescription medicine back home. If, however, you're in your own neck of the woods, have run out of your medication, have no refills left, and your doctor isn't available, you can try the following (in order):

1. Speak to your pharmacist. Most pharmacists are able to provide you with a few doses to tide you over until you can reach your doctor. Or, if not, they can at least tell you whether your medication refill can or can't wait.

2. If Step 1 didn't help, phone your provincial/territorial urgent health care line (if one operates where you're located). Let them know what medicine you're missing, and it's likely they'll be able to tell you whether it's something that can or can't wait.

3. If Steps 1 and 2 didn't help, visit a walk-in-clinic. Let them know what medicine you're in need of. If at all possible, show them your empty prescription container to confirm the details of your medicine. In most cases, they'll be able to give you a new prescription. (The most notable exception is when you're looking for drugs that could be sold on the street — narcotics, for example.)

4. If Steps 1, 2, *and* 3 didn't help, visit the local hospital emergency department. This, of course, is not the ideal use of such a facility, but if you're stuck, you're stuck. Again, if at all possible show them your empty prescription container.

If you end up having to go the emergency department in search of a prescription refill, don't be surprised if the reception you get is on the frosty side. Most emergency department personnel are not overly thrilled about dealing with these sorts of issues. But at least they'll almost certainly be able to help you — and hey, it's not going to happen again.

Your Prescription Drugs and Hospitalizations

So, you have your prescription drugs all sorted out. You know which ones you take at breakfast and which ones you take at supper. You know the red and white capsule is to help your blood pressure, and the white round pill is to help your diabetes. You know you need to take the pink pill with food, and the blue one on an empty stomach. But wait — all of a sudden you've ended up in hospital with some new health problem, and you're being given all sorts of different pills and at different times than you're accustomed to.

Should you be concerned? Should you ask the nurse and doctor about this or simply rely on their expertise? And what if you have questions about your new drugs but, because of illness, you're unable to ask them? What then? We look at these and other related issues in this section.

Your prescription drugs and the emergency department

If, whenever you walk into an emergency department you are seen immediately and are on your way home five minutes later, this section doesn't apply to you. If you are one of the remaining 99.99999 percent of Canadians, please read on...

Having one's careful routine for taking prescription drugs forcibly interrupted can be very disconcerting as Melissa Jennings, a meticulous 72-year-old woman, discovered. Apart from troublesome high blood pressure, her health had always been excellent — at least it had been until earlier that day, when she developed chest pains landing her in the emergency department. Mrs. Jennings was interviewed first by the nurse and then by the doctor, and she provided both of them with the details about her medications. After examining Mrs. Jennings, the emergency department physician, Dr. Raphael, said, "It's not yet clear what the cause of your pain is, but it doesn't appear likely to be serious. We'll run some tests and I'll be back in an hour or two." As the doctor made her way to the door, Mrs. Jennings looked at her watch and, with concern, called out to the doctor. "Doctor, wait. I missed my hydrochlorothiazide dose from this morning." "Not to worry, Mrs. Jennings," Dr. Raphael reassured her as she left the room. Returning a couple of hours later, Dr. Raphael advised her patient the tests were excellent, her pain was likely due to some muscular strain, and she could go home. Mrs. Jennings was thrilled with the good news, but perplexed about the casual approach to her prescription medicine.

Mrs. Jennings was understandably surprised that the precise timing with which she customarily took her medicine was treated so nonchalantly when she was in the emergency department. She (wisely) knew it's best to take prescription medicines exactly as prescribed — however, what she hadn't been made aware of was that when you're being closely monitored in an emergency department and the health care staff know what drugs you're taking, it's highly unlikely any harm will come to you if you delay a dose of your usual medicines or, for many medicines, miss a dose altogether. Several reasons exist, including:

- ✔ Hardly any medicine absolutely, positively, must be taken without fail at a specific time each and every day. And if you are taking such a drug, the staff almost always recognize this fact and give you the required medicine.

- ✔ If you have a potentially serious problem, in all likelihood while you're in the emergency department you'll be very closely supervised — so, for example, if your blood pressure rises, or your heart rate goes up, you'll quickly be attended to.

- ✔ Perhaps most important of all, if you're being evaluated for a possibly serious condition (such as a heart attack, stroke, kidney failure, or severe infection), it's often best *not* to take your usual drugs because you may be either medically unstable or at risk of becoming medically unstable. In these cases the health care team may give you special medications to deal with your immediate situation, and these can conflict with your usual drugs.

This information applies only to situations where you have made the emergency room staff aware of your medications and you're being closely monitored. It's entirely different from the situation where — alas — you've been asked to wait (and wait and wait and wait...) in the appropriately named "waiting room." In this circumstance, we suggest you speak with the emergency room staff, make them aware of the prescription drugs you're taking, and ask them specifically whether, while you wait, you should or should not take these medications.

Everyone is fallible, and blind faith in health care providers is not a great idea. So there's no harm — and potentially much good — in doing just as Mrs. Jennings did in the preceding anecdote and reminding the emergency department staff that you've missed a dose of your medicine or that one is due. They may simply reassure you that it's not a problem, or they may be pleased to have a reminder to give you your medicine.

Your prescription drugs and the inpatient wards

One of the most common concerns we hear from our patients who have recently been in hospital is that, while they were hospitalized, they felt they had lost control over their drug therapy. The following anecdotes illustrate some typical examples of this.

- ✔ Jonathan normally takes a white circular tablet called metoprolol. The nurse comes in and hands him a light red coloured capsule and tells him it's the same medicine. He wonders whether she's right.

- ✔ Alphonse has taken lorazepam daily for many months. He's been in hospital for several days now and has become agitated and has developed nightmares. He points out to the medical staff that he hasn't received his lorazepam since he was admitted.

- ✔ Emma takes oral contraceptives. She was admitted to hospital two days earlier and hasn't taken a dose since. She is uncertain whether she hasn't been given a dose because she's not supposed to be taking them or because she's supposed to be taking her own supply.

- ✔ Priya brought all her medications with her when she went to the hospital so she could show them to the staff. Now, four days later and ready to be discharged, she asks the ward clerk to give her medicines back. The drugs cannot be located. Priya wonders whether she did the right thing by bringing them with her.

Here are things you can do to help avoid confusion, mistakes, or just plain hassles surrounding your drug therapy when you've been hospitalized:

- ✔ Do bring *all* your prescription and non-prescription drugs (not just a list) with you whenever you go to the hospital. When the nurse or doctor is looking at the medicine containers you brought with you, be sure to let them know if you're taking your medicines in a way that differs from what the prescription labels say.

- ✔ After the nurse and doctor have looked at them and written down the necessary information, ask them whether you should keep any with you in your room to administer yourself during your stay in hospital (as might be the case if, for example, you are to continue your oral contraceptives). Send your other medicines home with a relative or friend.

- ✔ Keep a list of your usual prescription drugs (preferably by generic name) and their doses in your hospital room in case you need to refer to it.

- ✔ If you've previously been advised not to suddenly discontinue a drug (such as lorazepam in the anecdote above) and you don't see it among the medicines you're being given, ask the doctor if he is substituting an equivalent (not necessarily identical) type of drug. If not, let him know you were previously advised not to suddenly stop the drug. (He may be unaware of this, or, much more likely, there may be an important medical reason leading him to not continue it.)

- ✔ If you're given an unfamiliar-looking drug, ask what its generic name is. (We talk about generic drugs in Chapter 2.) It's not unusual for a drug to have the same name as a drug you normally take but to look very different. Some drugs have many different manufacturers, each using its own particular manufacturing process. (Of course, if you have any doubt, ask the nurse to double-check what the drug is.)

- ✔ When the nurse double-checks your name before giving you your medication, don't consider it a perfunctory measure. Listen to what he or she says, and make sure it is indeed your name. Even better, show your arm band to the nurse.

- ✔ If you're too unwell to ask questions about your medications, ask a loved one or trusted friend to do so on your behalf. Appointing only *one* individual to serve this role will help avoid misunderstandings (both for the hospital staff and for you). Ideally, you would make this arrangement before you ever have occasion to be hospitalized. (If you are hospitalized unexpectedly you may be too ill to do this at that time.)

✔ If you're being given a medication at a different time from when you normally take your drug, double-check with the nurse that the difference is not significant.

✔ If you have diabetes and are accustomed to managing your condition with insulin, let your doctor and nurse know if you want to stay involved in managing your insulin dosing and administration during your stay in hospital. (Assuming, of course, you're well enough to do so.) It's especially important when you're using an insulin pump device, because the hospital staff may not be all that familiar with one.

Your prescription drugs when you're discharged from hospital

We'd love to be able to insert the sound of a drum roll here, because this is crunch time. Indeed, seldom do we see more confusion — and potential danger — regarding prescription drugs than when someone is newly discharged from hospital.

When you arrive home you'll almost certainly have the following two things in your possession:

✔ New prescriptions to be filled at the pharmacy.

✔ Your old medicines.

If you're like many people, you may be unclear as to what you're to do with your old drugs, and in particular whether your new prescriptions replace your old drugs or are to be taken in addition to your old drugs. We now look at how to avoid this confusion.

Things to do before you leave the hospital

It's customary for the doctor to come by your room at the time of discharge (or shortly prior) to review with you the medicines you're to take at home. Whenever possible try to find out when the doctor will be coming by, so you can arrange to have a family member or trusted friend in attendance (you know what they say about two sets of ears, eh?).

When you speak with the doctor, make sure you are clear whether the prescriptions she hands you are to *replace* your old drugs or are to be taken in *addition* to your old drugs. If they are to replace *some* of them, be sure you're clear on which ones. Ask the doctor to write it out for you.

Things to do immediately after you leave the hospital

 We recommend that as soon as possible after discharge from hospital you take *all* of your old medicines *and* your new prescriptions to your pharmacist. Ask the pharmacist to do the following three things:

✔ Discard those of your old medicines you are not to take.

✔ Give you back the old medicines that your doctor wants you to continue.

✔ Fill the prescriptions for new medicines you're in need of.

When your doctor discharged you from hospital you were probably given detailed instructions to enable you and your pharmacist to readily carry out the above tasks. If your doctor did not provide instructions, or if they are unclear, your pharmacist can call your doctor to clarify.

 Because it is so terribly important to make sure there's no confusion regarding your drugs when you're sent home from hospital — imagine you've had a heart attack and a few days later are sent home only to then have lifesaving medications omitted! We must do everything possible to avoid this — we'll risk redundancy and reiterate the following two points:

✔ Do not leave hospital unless you are 100 percent certain what drugs your doctor wants you to take after discharge.

✔ Do not leave the pharmacy unless you are 100 percent certain what drugs your pharmacist has dispensed to you and you are equally certain they match the instructions the doctor previously gave you.

Okay, crunch time's over — please insert imaginary sound of cymbals clashing triumphantly here!

Chapter 10

Coping with the Costs of Prescription Drugs

- -

In This Chapter

▶ Working with your doctor to cut costs

▶ Discovering how your pharmacist can help you rein in costs

▶ Keeping up with government programs that can save you money

▶ Considering extras your private insurer can offer

▶ Accessing programs offered by the pharmaceutical companies themselves

▶ Looking into buying prescription drugs over the Internet

- -

Doesn't it seem like every day you read a story in the newspaper talking about the prohibitive cost of some new "breakthrough" medication? Indeed, some new drugs may cost upward of $2,000 to $3,000 *per month!* Although that's a rarity, it remains the case the monthly cost for many newer prescription drugs is often more than $100. And if you're taking several medications, you can be looking at thousands upon thousands of dollars in drug costs each and every year. In this chapter, we look at possible ways you can save on the cost of your prescription drugs.

How Your Doctor Can Help You Save Money

 Your doctor may be able to help you save some of your hard-earned cash. Consider asking your doctor the following questions:

> ✔ "If there are several different and equally good types of drugs to choose from, can you prescribe the least expensive one?"

✔ If you're being started on a drug that's new to you: "Can you prescribe only a small supply so if I react poorly and have to stop the drug I won't have spent money on medicine I won't be using?" (A downside is that if you end up staying on the drug you'll have to pay another dispensing fee to the pharmacist — sooner rather than later.)

✔ If you're being prescribed a refill for a drug you've taken uneventfully for a while and will continue to be on indefinitely: "Can you prescribe several months' supply so I won't have to pay as many dispensing fees to the pharmacist?"

✔ "Do you have drug samples I could have?" (Some doctors keep samples in their offices, some don't.)

✔ "If the drug comes in different doses that are all priced the same, can I get a higher dose and split it?" (Some medicines are priced the same regardless of the strength of the dose, so if you need, for example, a 20-mg dose you'd save money by obtaining 40-mg-strength doses and taking only half at a time. Note, however, that not all doses can be split, as we discuss in Chapter 4.)

✔ If you have a drug plan that covers over-the-counter drugs, but only when they're prescribed: "Can I have a prescription for this medicine?" (This accounts for why ASA — an over-the-counter product — has more prescriptions written for it than just about any other medicine in the country.) Bear in mind, however, that getting a prescription for a drug such as ASA that's available relatively inexpensively without a prescription does, naturally enough, increase overall health care costs, though not to the individual.

Some doctors charge a fee to patients if they're requested to authorize a prescription by phone or fax. If your doctor has this policy be sure to keep tabs on how many refills you have left (you can find the information on the drug container, as we discuss in Chapter 3), and if you're running out remember to ask your doctor for a new prescription at the time of your appointment.

Pharmacists often know more than physicians about the costs of drugs, especially when it comes to, say, the feasibility of pill split-ting to save money. So, if your doctor isn't sure about some of these issues bring them up with your pharmacist, who can then contact your doctor with suggestions.

How Your Pharmacist Can Help You Save Money

Your pharmacist may be able to help you save some money. Consider asking your pharmacist the following questions:

✔ "Is the prescription I've been given for a product that's also available over-the-counter?" Over-the-counter products typically are less expensive than prescription drugs — they also don't require a dispensing fee. So, if you don't have a drug plan, you could purchase such a product less expensively by buying it without the prescription. (ASA is an example of an over-the-counter drug you may be given a prescription for, most typically if you're being discharged from hospital after having had a heart problem or stroke.)

✔ "Do you accept seniors' cards (or drug benefits cards)?" Most pharmacies gladly do so.

Why do prescription drugs cost so much?

A year's supply of many newly developed prescription drugs may run you over $1,000. Is this appropriate? Well, it's a highly contentious issue with much debate (and worse) over whether these costs are excessive. Some of the factors in determining the price you pay for that new prescription medicine include:

✔ **The pharmaceutical company's costs for research and development, marketing, and administration.** (Thousands of molecules — that is, potential future drugs — are studied for every one eventually making it to market.)

✔ **The pharmaceutical company's profits.**

✔ **The pharmacy's fees.** (These fees include their costs for overhead — including what it costs them to maintain an inventory of medicine in their pharmacy — and a fee for their time and expertise in properly dispensing the medicine.)

Pharmaceutical companies estimate their costs to get a new drug to market at about US$800 million and indicate they have only a limited time to recoup these costs before their patent expires and generic versions of the drug come on the market. Others contest these figures. It's a heated debate, to say the least.

The Government of Canada, through the Patented Medicine Prices Review Board, is involved in determining the price of prescription drugs. You can read more about the Board and about how prices are set at www.pmprb-cepmb.gc.ca.

One way pharmacists help save you money is automatic. By government mandate, they must substitute less expensive, generic versions of drugs for more expensive branded versions. For example, if your doctor writes a prescription for Zocor (a trade name version of simvastatin), your pharmacist automatically substitutes a less expensive generic version (such as Apo-Simvastatin, CO Simvastatin, and so on). The one exception to this automatic substitution policy occurs when your doctor writes "no substitution" on the prescription. We discuss this issue further in Chapter 2.

 The fees pharmacists charge can vary a fair bit, so you might consider shopping around to find the best price. Bear in mind, however, that factors other than just cost are important when deciding on the right pharmacist for you. We discuss the many important roles of the pharmacist in Chapter 3.

How the Government Can Help You

Different levels of government may be able to assist with your prescription drug costs; how they do this depends on your particular circumstances.

Typically, your *provincial/territorial government* can provide financial assistance for prescription drug costs if you

- ✔ Are a senior.
- ✔ Are receiving social assistance.
- ✔ Have a disease resulting in disproportionately higher drug costs (this is highly variable).
- ✔ Belong to a household where drug costs exceed a certain percentage of household income.

You can find out more regarding your provincial/territorial government drug coverage policies at the Health Canada Web site: www.hc-sc.gc.ca.

The *federal government* also provides financial assistance to cover the cost of prescription drugs for certain people, including those who are

- ✔ First Nations or Inuit.
- ✔ A current member or veteran of the Canadian Forces.
- ✔ A member of the RCMP.

The federal government allows deductions from your income tax for a number of "qualifying medical expenses," including a portion of your prescription drug costs. (Although the deductions may not cover the full amount of your medical expenses, every little bit helps.) You can find out more at www.cra-arc.gc.ca/tax.

How Your Private Health Insurer Can Help You

If you have private health insurance, your insurer likely covers some portion of the costs of your prescription medicines. Which medicines they cover, what percentage of the cost they cover, and whether they have a total annual or lifelong cumulative ceiling for the amount they cover depends on your particular insurer and policy.

How the Pharmaceutical Industry Can Help You

Some brand-name drug manufacturers have policies to help people obtain certain medicines. If you have neither private coverage nor the financial means to afford a product, ask your doctor and/or pharmacist whether they're aware of such a "compassionate care program" (also known as a "patient assistance program") that might assist you. However, because programs are highly variable, you likely need to contact the company directly to find out availability and details. Be aware that, depending on the nature of the particular program, the company may ask you to provide evidence (such as an income tax return) to demonstrate your financial need.

 You can find out the name and phone number of the drug company that manufactures your medicine by asking your pharmacist.

Buying Prescription Drugs over the Internet

If you're like us, you're routinely inundated with spam email messages offering to sell you "low-cost prescription drugs." You probably reflexively hit the "delete" button — but at the same time wonder whether at least some Internet purveyors of prescription drugs are reputable.

Verified Internet Pharmacy Practice Sites

To help you know whether you're dealing with a reputable Internet pharmacy, the National Association of Pharmacy Regulatory Authorities established the Canadian Verified Internet Pharmacy Practice Sites (VIPPS) program (www.napra.org/docs/0/586/716.asp). It's designed to work — at least in theory — so that if you go to an Internet pharmacy Web site and it displays a VIPPS seal, you're assured this pharmacy has been found to meet a certain minimum standard including "meaningful consultation between patients and pharmacists." In practice, no pharmacy has yet signed up with the VIPPS program.

The Internet is still a "Wild West" in many ways, none moreso than in the plethora of online pharmacy Web sites. Many of these sites are of dubious character, and some are downright fraudulent. If you decide to buy your prescription drugs through the Internet it's essential that, as a lawyer would say, you do your "due diligence." The old adage "buyer beware" has never been more true.

The National Association of Pharmacy Regulatory Authorities (NAPRA; www.napra.org), a Canadian organization that oversees Canadian pharmacies, is working to bring some order to this chaos with the VIPPS program (Verified Internet Pharmacy Practice Sites), but the project has not been successful to date. Another organization you may come across in your Internet travels is the Canadian International Pharmacy Association (www.ciparx.ca), whose logo adorns the sites of a number of Internet pharmacies and whose stated aim is to "advocate for patients' rights to afford-able medications." It is, however, an association of bodies with a special interest, not a dispassionate, regulatory body. Accordingly, consider this when evaluating Internet sites carrying its seal.

So, then, is it a good idea to buy your prescription drugs from an Internet pharmacy? We do have some concerns — the most deeply felt is our belief that pharmacists are not automatons simply handing over pill bottles. We consider pharmacists invaluable resources, there to help you take your medicines safely and effec-tively, and we're concerned this type of help won't be routinely available when you buy your drugs over the Internet.

For more information on Canadian Internet pharmacies, we suggest you visit the NAPRA Web site (www.napra.org).

Part V
The Part of Tens

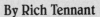

The 5th Wave   By Rich Tennant

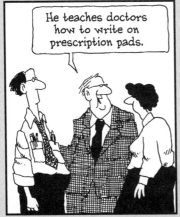

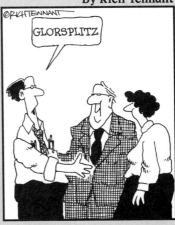

In this part . . .

*W*e get to pretend we're David Letterman and offer our own Top Ten Lists. From a look at the best-selling prescription drugs in Canada to our dream of a Multipill, this part is packed with interesting facts, hopes for the future, and miscellaneous observations.

Chapter 11

Ten Changes We Hope to See in the World of Prescription Drug Therapy

In This Chapter

▶ Managing the costs of prescription drugs

▶ Remembering to take your medicines

▶ Replacing a fistful of drugs with a Multipill

*T*he longer we're in practice, the more evident it becomes to us there's lots of room for improvement in the world of prescription drug therapy. Given a sufficiently sturdy soap box we could probably list hundreds of suggestions, but because this is a "Part of Tens" we'll confine ourselves to our top ten. These are certainly arguable, and we ask for your forgiveness and indulgence if we've omitted those you might have included.

So, without further ado, here (in no particular order) are our top ten dreams we hope to see fulfilled in the world of prescription drug therapy.

A Catastrophic Drug Plan

Though we're not by any stretch of the imagination politicians or economists, as physicians who routinely see patients who can't afford needed drugs and medical supplies we can say with some authority a problem does exist — and it needs fixing. Some people have chronic illnesses like diabetes or debilitating forms of inflammatory arthritis requiring thousands upon thousands of dollars to manage and simply do not earn enough to pay for these expenditures while putting food on the table and a roof over their heads. They're either not covered by — or, at the very least, not sufficiently covered by — existing drug plans or programs. Often, these patients tell us they can't afford to fill a specific, new prescription or that they've stopped taking some or even all of their drugs for financial reasons. So, for people in this position we'd love to see a catastrophic drug plan to provide the monies to help pay for their drugs and medical supplies.

Drugs That Say What They Are

Medicines commonly have the manufacturer's name or logo or abbreviation imprinted on their surface, and they may have some numbers to give clues as to their strength, but what they don't routinely have is anything to tell us what the drug actually *is*. It's a lot more important to you and to your doctor to know what medicine you're taking than whose assembly line it came from. We extend kudos to companies that imprint the name of the drug on their products, and suggest the others follow suit!

More Skepticism about New Drugs

Here's a phenomenon we've never been enamored with: Why is it when a new drug hits the market it's often widely used even if it offers no major advantage over older (and often cheaper) drugs boasting a long track record of safety and effectiveness?

Of course, if a new drug is truly a breakthrough product and can treat conditions that had no particularly good therapy beforehand, then we're all for trying it. But if all it has to offer is yet another variation on an old theme (what we in the medical business call a "me too" drug), or is a novel drug but without sufficiently proven value or safety, we'd rather be cautious, give it some time, and see whether the new drug on the block truly is a good choice.

Better Package Inserts and Information Sheets

As we discuss in Chapter 3, some drugs are accompanied by package inserts or information sheets, some are not. Some of these are detailed, some are vague. Some list dozens of potential side-effects, some just a few. Sometimes they tell you if you should take your medicine with food, sometimes they leave you guessing.

In the interests of drug safety, we believe that order must be made of this chaos and that package inserts or information sheets not only should be made mandatory, but also should be consistent in their layout and the types and amounts of information that they provide.

More Quality Time with Your Pharmacist

Waiting in line to pick up your prescription isn't quality time! Finding out more about the drugs you're taking is.

Pharmacists have many years of education and are experts when it comes to prescription drug therapy. What a shame, then, that so much opportunity for the consumer of prescription drugs (that's you!) to glean information from these experts is wasted. Heck, we learn from them all the time.

Some pharmacists consider counselling patients to be part of the job. And some pharmacists consider it *the most important part* of the job. We'd like to see all pharmacists adopt the latter attitude. In certain places in Canada the powers-that-be are working on this very issue, and either have in place or are developing programs to reimburse pharmacists for time spent performing this teaching.

Better Medical News Reporting

We know some excellent medical reporters who are well trained, do their homework, spend significant time researching their stories, and present a well-balanced and objective summary of a piece of medical news. Regrettably, the stories we see more often are either sensationalistic and overly negative leading to unnecessary fears, or, conversely, little more than wire-service quotes from self-serving news releases presented without context or background information. Is it any wonder, therefore, that so many people have their hopes dashed when they hear about a new "wonder drug" that turns out to be decidedly less than wonderful?

More Certainty about a Drug's Effectiveness and Tolerability

Sayed takes penicillin and in a matter of days his infection is gone. Sam takes penicillin and his infection doesn't budge. Tara takes penicillin and doesn't have a whiff of a side-effect. Tom takes penicillin and spends the next day sick to his stomach. Same drugs, different responses. Is there a way that physicians could better predict who will do well with a drug and who won't?

Medical studies are very helpful at showing the *big* picture, such as the *percentage* of people that a drug will help and the *percentage* of people that a drug will hurt. They can also often reveal the *types* of people who are most likely to benefit from a drug and the *types* of people who are most likely to be harmed by a drug. But that's a far cry from predicting how a *specific* person will respond to a *specific* drug. People are simply too complex, and medical science simply not yet advanced enough to provide that level of precision. Medical science is making progress, but still has a ways to go.

Smarter Technology

In our experience, most people have *some* familiarity with the drugs they're taking and may know the names or the doses of their medicines, but it's certainly the rare person who knows *all* the relevant details about his or her drugs.

To help out, we've created the Cheat Sheet located at the front of this book, which allows you to record this key information. We recognize that not everyone will take advantage of this tool — and besides, what if your Cheat Sheet is at home while you're on a stretcher in the Emergency Department in Whistler, B.C., because you twisted your ankle while heli-skiing to celebrate your 80th birthday? Wouldn't it be great if the emergency room nurse or doctor could simply borrow your keychain dongle (such as a USB memory drive or other highly portable electronic storage device), plug it into the ER computer, and immediately see a list of all your drug information (and other medical information too, if you so choose)? This so-called smart technology is available, it just hasn't made it to routine use in the health care setting as yet.

Easier Ways to Know When It's Time to Take Your Medicine

Although doctors have thousands of prescription drugs in our medical arsenal, even the best of pharmaceutical weaponry is of little value in the fight against diseases if the ammunition is never used. Put another way, if your pill never leaves the pill bottle, it's not going to help you.

It can be so darn hard to remember to take a medicine, especially if you're taking a whole bunch at different times — particularly mid-day. Pharmacists can offer helpful tools such as 7-day pill organizers (which we discuss in Chapter 8), but these can be cumbersome if you need to take medicines when you're away from home. You can purchase pill bottles with an alarm in the cap, but they're not cheap. You could set an alarm on your watch or your cell phone (or your PDA or other electronic tool), but that can be a hassle. You could have a workmate or friend or family member call to remind you. You could even tie a string around your finger!

So with these and so many other reminder systems available, surely no one ever forgets to take a dose of their medicine, right? Oh, if only it were so. The truth is most people *do* miss doses (we've even done it ourselves!). What's needed is a better way of alerting us when it's time to take a medicine. (Have a special trick you use to remember to take your medicine? We'd love to hear it. Our email address is noted at the end of this chapter.)

Multipills

Many people are on more than one medication. And the more drugs to take, the less convenient it is. So why not combine one's different medicines, size permitting, into one big "Multipill"? The idea isn't novel; in 2003 Drs. Wald and Law suggested a "Polypill" consisting of a statin, three different blood pressure medicines, folic acid, and ASA be given to everyone 55 years of age and older and also to everyone with cardiovascular disease.

What we'd love to see, however, is a Multipill custom-designed for each individual containing just *your* prescribed medicines. The science is already partly there — various combinations of *two* drugs are available (for example, metformin and rosiglitazone, and ACE inhibitors and diuretics). So let's go the whole nine yards and pack three, four, five or more drugs into a pill. As long as the pills were kept to a manageable size, it'd be a heckuva lot easier to take (and to remember to take) than the customary fistful of medicines so many people now contend with.

(P.S. We're not holding our breath on this one: overcoming the obstacles to achieve a Multipill unique to each person's requirements would be similar in difficulty to climbing Mount Everest. In a blizzard. In a bathing suit! Of the many obstacles to creating a Multipill, we'll point out just one: You may be on drugs — like calcium and L-thyroxine — that must be taken at separate times.)

And a Final Fantasy...

More idealistic, perhaps, than anything else we wish for in this chapter, our two ultimate dreams regarding prescription drug therapy are:

- ✔ Affordable drugs that always work well and never cause side-effects.
- ✔ A population so healthy we can misplace our prescription pad and not give it a second thought — it wasn't being used anyway!

Have a "top ten" wish of your own? Feel free to share it with us at drugs@ianblumer.com.

Chapter 12

Ten Not-So-Trivial Facts about Prescription Drugs

In This Chapter

▶ Discovering what Canadians spend on prescription medicines

▶ Finding out what drugs are most commonly used in Canada

▶ Tallying up the number of pharmacists and pharmacies in this country

*E*ver wonder how much Canadians spend on prescription drugs? Or what are the most commonly used prescription medicines north of the 49th? And why is it your dose of a medicine may have changed, but the size of the pill you're taking has stayed the same? Well, if these questions have ever crossed your mind — or even if they haven't! — you've turned to the right chapter. Here, we present Heather and Ian's ten favourite not-so-trivial facts about prescription drugs.

How Many New Prescription Drugs Are Approved Each Year in Canada?

Each year, the Government of Canada (through Health Canada) is asked to approve more than 4,000 requests from pharmaceutical manufacturers regarding prescription drugs. Four thousand! Alas, the overwhelming majority of these requests are for decidedly unexciting and non-novel things such as a new name for an old drug, new "indications" (approval to market an already existing drug to treat a condition for which the drug had not been previously officially approved), new doses, and so on.

Only about 80 "new" drugs are submitted for approval each year, and of these only a small number are for truly new types of medicines. The rest often consist of what doctors call "me too" drugs, meaning medications that technically are new, but in fact represent no great therapeutic advance. They're really just one more addition to an already plentiful drug family.

How Much Do Canadians Spend on Prescription Drugs?

It's estimated that in 2005 Canadians spent a whopping $20 billion on prescription drugs. How much money is that? Well, for $20 billion you could build 20 Confederation Bridges. Or, if you prefer, forget the bridges — more than one seems a bit redundant anyhow — and go out and buy 40,000 shiny, new Rolls-Royce automobiles. (Though, to be perfectly honest, we think that sounds kind of indulgent and wonder whether you might be happy enough with just a dozen or so.)

And what did Canadians get for our hard-earned $20 billion? We got 400 million prescriptions. Which means the average Canadian spent $600 and got 12 prescriptions. The biggest spenders on prescription drugs: people living in Ontario. The smallest spenders on prescription drugs: people living in Nunavut.

How Expensive Is It to Run a Drug Study?

Elsewhere in this book we talk about the surprisingly small number of people participating in drug studies before a prescription medicine comes to market. One reason is, no doubt, the huge cost of doing this type of research. Indeed, it's estimated that the company running a drug trial spends $5,000 per subject (depending on the nature of the study)! Performing large, multinational drug studies can cost well over $100 million.

This money goes toward the considerable task of organizing the study (including establishing the protocol to be followed and having it reviewed by the appropriate regulatory bodies), creating, completing, and storing study documents, paying research staff, providing the study medication (and, sometimes, a placebo), reimbursing laboratories for processing lab samples, and on and on.

How Often Do People <u>Improperly</u> Take Their Prescription Medicines?

Feeling badly because you forgot a dose of your medicine? Conscience bothering you because you never had that last prescription filled? Well, don't let guilt get the best of you, because you're certainly in good company. Indeed, fewer than half (!) of all people take their prescription medicines exactly as prescribed. Not that we think this is a good thing, mind you (because it's definitely not). Rather, it's just the plain reality of the situation. So thank goodness you're reading this book, because now you will be armed with all manner of tips to help you stay on track with your drugs!

What Are the Best-Selling Prescription Drugs in Canada?

The top ten best-selling drugs (by trade name) in Canada in 2005 — and the number of prescriptions written for these drugs — are listed below. Drumroll, please:

Trade Name	*Number of Prescriptions Written*
Lipitor	11,235,295
Synthroid	9,095,566
Altace	8,175,128
Norvasc	5,503,293
Effexor XR	5,011,190
Asaphen	4,529,704
Tylenol #3	4,473,694
Pantoloc	3,878,328
Ratio-Salbutamol	3,737,814
Apo-Furosemide	3,578,193

As you can see, Lipitor — a cholesterol-reducing statin — is way ahead of even the second most commonly prescribed drug, with more than 11 million prescriptions written in 2005.

What Are the Best-Selling Prescription Drug Classes in Canada?

The top five best-selling *classes* of drug in Canada in 2005 are:

Trade Name	Number of Prescriptions Written
Anti-depressants	25,326,488
Drugs for dyslipidemia (typically, high LDL cholesterol)	21,846,752
Tranquillizers (includes lorazepam, risperidone, oxazepam, quetiapine, olanzapine, and a few others)	20,896,509
Angiotensin converting enzyme (ACE) inhibitors (includes ACE inhibitors in combination with other drugs)	16,661,911
Antibiotics	16,498,625

As the table reveals, the dominant classes of drugs in Canada are those used for mood/psychiatric ailments, cardiovascular disease/cholesterol problems, and infections.

How Often Are Prescription Drugs Used for "Unapproved Indications"?

When a prescription drug is first released, the pharmaceutical company that manufactures it submits a request to the Government of Canada to permit the drug to be marketed as helpful in the treatment of a specific condition (or conditions). When the government grants approval, the drug is said to have an "approved indication" or a "labelled indication" to treat condition A or condition B or whatever.

However, this approval does not restrict the drug for this use. In fact, about 20 percent of the time prescription drugs are used for non-approved (so-called "off-label") purposes. This isn't necessarily a bad thing. Indeed, it's very often a good thing, because it allows doctors to prescribe — and patients to use — drugs in ways experience shows works, even if they're not officially sanctioned. One particularly common example is the use of amitriptyline, a tricyclic antidepressant, to treat pain from nerve damage caused by, for instance, diabetes ("diabetic peripheral neuropathy").

How Many Pharmacists Are Practising in Canada?

As of January 1, 2006, there were about 30,000 licensed pharmacists in Canada. That's about one pharmacist for every 1,100 Canadians. (Twice as many physicians as pharmacists practise in Canada.) Ontario has about 10,000 pharmacists, and on the other end of the spectrum Nunavut has 16. The majority of pharmacists work in community pharmacies; however, a significant number work elsewhere, such as in hospitals.

How Many Pharmacies Are in Canada?

Canada has 8,000 pharmacies, which works out to about one pharmacy per 4,125 Canadians. Based on our informal observations this is considerably smaller than the ratio of donut shops to Canadians, which we estimate at 1:1.

How Much Medicine Is in a Pill?

The pill/tablet/capsule you hold in your hand may contain a surprisingly small amount of active ingredient (that is, the actual medicine), with the bulk comprising non-medicinal ingredients (which we discuss in Chapter 2). A good illustration is L-thyroxine. This medicine comes in strengths from as little as 0.025 mg all the way to as much as 0.30 mg — a more than tenfold difference in strength, yet every single one of these doses comes in a pill of the same size.

Drug Index

● ●

Detailed descriptions of individual drugs are in bold. Drugs marked with an asterisk are combination drugs; refer to the drug label to determine what they are.

3TC, 282. *See also* lamivudine
5 alpha-reductase inhibitors. *See* alpha-reductase inhibitors
5-aminosalicylic acid, 141, **187-188.** *See also* aminosalicylates
5-ASA. *See* 5-aminosalicylic acid
5-fluorouracil, 168
17 beta estradiol, 374, **375-377**

● *A* ●

abacavir, 282
abraclonide, 340
acarbose, 118, 388, **389-390,** 394
Accolate, 370. *See also* zafirlukast
Accupril. *See* quinapril
Accuretic*. *See* hydrochlorothiazide; quinapril
Accutane Roche, 402. *See also* isotretinoin
ACE inhibitors. *See* angiotensin converting enzyme inhibitors
Acebutolol, 290
acetaminophen, 23, 70, 88, 105, 129, 142, 148, 152, 161, 235, 236, 382
acetaminophen with codeine, 70, 158
acetazolamide, 327, 344
acetylsalicylic acid. *See* ASA
acitrecin, 402
Actonel, **296-298.** *See also* risedronate
Actonel Plus Calcium*, **296-298.** *See also* risedronate
Actos, 388, **394-396.** *See also* pioglitazone

Acular, Acular LS, **384-387.** *See also* ketorolac
acyclovir, 114, 134, 158, **288-290**
Adalat XL, 300. *See also* nifedipine
adapalene, 96, 402
adefovir, 133
adrenaline. *See* epinephrine
adrenergic agonist eye drops, 127
adrenergic agonists, 340
Advair Diskus*, 356, 357, **359-360, 363-364.** *See also* fluticasone; salmeterol
Advair Inhalation Aerosol*, 356, 357, **359-360, 363-364.** *See also* fluticasone; salmeterol
Advicor*, **413-415.** *See also* lovastatin
Advil, **384-387.** *See also* ibuprofen
Aerolizer, 80
Agenerase Capsules, 283. *See also* amprenavir
Agenerase Oral Solution, 283. *See also* amprenavir
Aggrenox*, **272-274.** *See also* ASA; dipyridamole
agonists, **174**
Airomir, 356, **357-359.** *See also* salbutamol
Aldactazide 25*, 50*, 327, **330-332, 332-334.** *See also* hydrochlorothiazide; spironolactone
Aldactone, 327, **330-332.** *See also* spironolactone
alendronate, 67, **296-298**
Alertec, 416. *See also* modafinil
Alesse 21*, 28*, 97, 306. **307-309.** *See also*

ethinyl estradiol; levonorgestrel; oral contraceptives
alfuzosin, 155, 178
allopurinol, 128, 145, 426
almotriptan, 408
alpha-adrenergic antagonists. *See* alpha blockers
alpha adrenergic blockers. *See* alpha blockers
alpha blockers, 120, 154, 155, 178-181
alpha glucosidase inhibitor, 388
Alphagan, Alphagan P, 340, **341-342.** *See also* brimonidine
alpha-reductase inhibitors, 108, 155, 182-183
alprazolam, 162, 194
alprostadil, 124
Altace, 487. *See also* ramipril
Alvesco, 357. *See also* ciclesonide
Alzheimer's disease medications, 183-186
amantadine, 149, 153, 267
aminoglycosides, 114, 205, 208-210
Amaryl, 388. *See also* glimepiride
amcinonide, 315
Amcort, 315. *See also* amcinonide
Amerge, 408. *See also* naratriptan
amiloride, 327
aminosalicylates, 186-188
amiodarone, 55, 103, 104, **200-202,** 434, 444
amitriptyline, **424-426,** 489
amlodipine, 300, **301-302**
amoxicillin, 23, 70, 113, 121, 122, 158, 161, 164, 166, 207, **219-220,** 431
amoxicillin-clavulanate, 158

ampicillin, 67, 207
amprenavir, 283
anabolic steroids, 134, 313
Anafranil, 424. *See also*
  clomipramine
analgesics, 63, 105, 123,
  125, 128, 129, 142, 144,
  148, 152, 235, 236, 274,
  382, 411
analogs, 174
Anandron, 225. *See also*
  nilutamide
Anaprox, Anaprox DS,
  385-387. *See also*
  naproxen
anastrozole, **225-226**
Andriol, 418, **419-420.** *See*
  also testosterone
AndroDerm, 418, **419-420.**
  See also testosterone
AndroGel, 418, **419-420.** *See*
  also testosterone
angiotensin converting
  enzyme inhibitors, 38,
  102, 113, 130, 131, 137,
  143, 147, 160, 189-191,
  331, 461, 488
angiotensin receptor
  antagonists. *See*
  angiotensin receptor
  blockers
angiotensin receptor
  blockers, 130, 131, 137,
  143, 144, 192-194, 331
Ansaid, 384, **385-387.** *See*
  also flurbiprofen
Antabuse, 98, 443. *See also*
  disulfiram
antacids, 68, 423, 441, 442
antagonists, 174
anti-androgens, 111, 225,
  229, 330
anti-anxiety drugs, 194-199
anti-arrhythmics, 199-203,
  460
antibiotics, 51, 96, 114, 121,
  126, 128, 141, 154, 158,
  161, 164, 204-224, 435,
  437, 488
anticancer drugs, 224-229
anticholinergic inhalers,
  107, 112
anticholinergics, 139, 150,
  153, 229-232, 267, 457
anticoagulants, 104, 110,
  160, 232-237, 460
anticonvulsants, 123, 152,
  237-249, 449

antidepressants, 72,
  249-257, 488
antidiabetic agents (oral).
  See hypoglycemic
  agents (oral)
anti-epileptic drugs. *See*
  anticonvulsants
anti-estrogens. *See*
  aromatase inhibitors
antifungal agents, 108
antihistamines, 99, 121,
  150, 158, 261-264, 350,
  450
antihyperglycemic agents.
  See hypoglycemic
  agents (oral)
anti-hypertensives, 144
anti-inflammatories, 274
antimycobacterials. *See*
  antituberculosis drugs
antiplatelet agents, 274
antipsychotics, 109
antiretroviral drugs, 135
anti-thyroid agents, 138
antiviral agents, 114, 136,
  142, 158
anxiolytics. *See* anti-anxiety
  drugs
Apo-Acebutolol, 290. *See*
  also acebutolol
Apo-Acetazolamide, 327.
  See also acetazolamide
Apo-Acyclovir, **288-290.** *See*
  also acyclovir
Apo-Alendronate, **296-299**
Apo-Allopurinol, 426,
  427-428. *See also*
  allopurinol
Apo-Alpraz, Apo-Alpraz
  TS,194. *See also*
  alprazolam
Apo-Amiloride, 327. *See*
  also amiloride
Apo-Amilzide*, 327. *See*
  also amiloride;
  hydrochlorothiazide
Apo-Amiodarone, **200-202.**
  See also amiodarone
Apo-Amitriptyline, **424-426.**
  See also amitriptyline
Apo-Amoxi, Apo-Amoxi
  Clav*, 207, **219-220.** *See*
  also amoxicillin
Apo-Atenidone*, 290,
  291-293, 327. *See also*
  atenolol; chlorthalidone
Apo-Atenol, 290, **291-293.**
  See also atenolol

Apo-Azathioprine, **351-353.**
  See also azathioprine
Apo-Baclofen, 411. *See also*
  baclofen
Apo-Beclomethasone, 313.
  See also
  beclomethasone
Apo-Benztropine, 267. *See*
  also benztropine
Apo-Bisoprolol, 290. *See*
  also bisoprolol
Apo-Brimonidine, 340,
  341-342. *See also*
  brimonidine
Apo-Bromazepam, 194. *See*
  also bromazepam
Apo-Bromocriptine, 267,
  335-337. *See also*
  bromocriptine
Apo-Butorphanol, 377. *See*
  also butorphanol
Apo-Capto, **189-191.** *See*
  also captopril
Apo-Carbamazepine, 237,
  238-240. *See also*
  carbamazepine
Apo-Carvedilol, 291. *See*
  also carvedilol
Apo-Cefaclor, 206. *See also*
  cefaclor
Apo-Cefuroxime, 206. *See*
  also cefuroxime
Apo-Cephalex, 206,
  210-211. *See also*
  cephalexin
Apo-Chlorax*, 194. *See also*
  chlordiazepoxide
Apo-Chlordiazepoxide, 194.
  See also
  chlordiazepoxide
Apo-Chlorpropamide, 388.
  See also
  chlorpropamide
Apo-Chlorthalidone, 327.
  See also chlorthalidone
Apo-Ciproflox, 206,
  212-213. *See also*
  ciprofloxacin
Apo-Citalopram, 250,
  253-254. *See also*
  citalopram
Apo-Clindamycin, 206,
  214-215. *See also*
  clindamycin
Apo-Clobazam, 194, 237.
  See also clobazam
Apo-Clomipramine, 424.
  See also clomipramine

Apo-Clonazepam, 195, 237, **240-242.** *See also* clonazepam

Apo-Clonidine, 176. *See also* clonidine

Apo-Clorazepate, 195. *See also* clorazepate

Apo-Cloxi, 207. *See also* cloxacillin

Apo-Clozapine, **277.** *See also* clozapine

Apo-Cromolyn, 357. *See also* sodium cromoglycate

Apo-Cyclobenzaprine, **411-413.** *See also* cyclobenzaprine

Apo-Desipramine, 424. *See also* desipramine

Apo-Dexamethasone, 314. *See also* dexamethasone

Apo-Diazepam, 195. *See also* diazepam

Apo-Diclo, Apo-Diclo Rapide, Apo-Diclo SR, 384, **385-387.** *See also* diclofenac

Apo-Diflusinal, 384, **385-387.** *See also* diflusinal

Apo-Diltiaz, Apo-Diltiaz CD, Apo-Diltiaz SR, 300, **302-304.** *See also* diltiazem

Apo-Dipyridamole, 272. *See also* dipyridamole

Apo-Divalproex, 237, **242-243.** *See also* divalproex

Apo-Domperidone, 337, **338-339.** *See also* domperidone

Apo-Doxazosin, 178, **179-180.** *See also* doxazosin

Apo-Doxepin, 424. *See also* doxepin

Apo-Doxy, Apo-Doxy Tabs, 208. *See also* doxycyclines

Apo-Erythro Base, Apo-Erythro EC, Apo-Erythro-ES, Epo-Erythro-S, 207. *See also* erythromycin

Apo-Etodolac, 384, **385-387.** *See also* etodolac

Apo-Fenofibrate, 347, **348-349.** *See also* fenofibrate

Apo-Feno-Micro, Apo-Feno-Super, 347, **348-349.** *See also* fenofibrate

Apo-Flavoxate, 230. *See also* flavoxate

Apo-Floctafenine, 384, **385-387.** *See also* floctafenine

Apo-Fluconazole, Apo-Fluconazole-150, 257, **258-259.** *See also* fluconazole

Apo-Flunisolide, 313, 314. *See also* flunisolide

Apo-Fluoxetine, 250. *See also* fluoxetine

Apo-Fluphenazine, 276. *See also* fluphenazine

Apo-Flurazepam, 195. *See also* flurazepam

Apo-Flurbiprofen, 384, **385-387.** *See also* flurbiprofen

Apo-Flutamide, 225. *See also* flutamide

Apo-Fosinopril, 189, **190-191.** *See also* fosinopril

Apo-Furosemide, 327, **328-330,** 487. *See also* furosemide

Apo-Gabapentin, 238, **243-244.** *See also* gabapentin

Apo-Gemfibrozil, 347. *See also* gemfibrozil

Apo-Gliclazide, 388. *See also* gliclazide

Apo-Glyburide, 388, **390-391.** *See also* glyburide

Apo-Haloperidol, Apo-Haloperidol LA, 276. *See also* haloperidol

Apo-Hydro 327, **332-334.** *See also* hydrochlorothiazide

Apo-Hydroxychloroquine, 351. *See also* hydroxychloroquine

Apo-Hydroxyzine, 261, **263-264.** *See also* hydroxyzine

Apo-Ibuprofen, 384, **385-387.** *See also* ibuprofen

Apo-Imipramine, 424. *See also* imipramine

Apo-Indapamide, 327. *See also* indapamide

Apo-Indomethacin, 384, **385-387.** *See also* indomethacin

Apo-Ipravent, 357, **360-362.** *See also* ipratropium

Apo-ISDN, 381. *See also* Isosorbide Dintrate

Apo-Keto, Apo-Keto-E, Apo-Keto SR, 384, **385-387.** *See also* ketoprofen

Apo-Ketoconazole, 257. *See also* ketoconazole

Apo-Ketorolac, 384, **385-387.** *See also* ketorolac

Apo-Ketotifin, 261. *See also* ketotifin

Apo-Labetalol, 291. *See also* labetalol

Apo-Lamotrigine, 238, **244-246.** *See also* lamotrigine

Apo-Leflunomide, 352. *See also* leflunomide

Apo-Levobunolol, 340. *See also* levobunolol

Apo-Levocarb, Apo-Levocarb CR, 267, **268-270.** *See also* levodopa/carbidopa

Apo-Lithium Carbonate, Apo-Lithium Carbonate SR, 371, **372-373.** *See also* lithium

Apo-Lorazepam, **195-197.** *See also* lorazepam

Apo-Lovastatin, **413-415.** *See also* lovastatin

Apo-Loxapine, 277. *See also* loxapine

Apo-Medroxy, **375-377.** *See also* medroxy-progesterone acetate

Apo-Mefenamic, **385-387.** *See also* mefenamic acid

Apo-Meloxicam, **385-387.** *See also* meloxicam

Apo-Metformin, Apo-Metformin Coated, 388, **392-393.** *See also* hydrochlorothiazide; metformin

Apo-Methazide*, **176-178.** *See also* hydrochloro-thiazide; methyldopa

Apo-Methoprazine, 277. *See also* methotrimeprazine

Apo-Methotrexate, 352, **353-355.** *See also* methotrexate

Apo-Methyldopa, **176-178.** *See also* methyldopa

Apo-Methylphenidate, Apo-Methylphenidate SR, **416-418.** *See also* methylphenidate

Apo-Metoclop, 338. *See also* metoclopramide

Apo-Metoprolol, Apo-Metoprolol (Type L), 290, **291-293.** *See also* metoprolol

Apo-Metronidazole, 207, **217-219.** *See also* metronidazole

Apo-Minocycline, 208. *See also* minocycline

Apo-Moclobemide, 250. *See also* moclobemide

Apo-Nabumetone, **385-387.** *See also* nabumetone

Apo-Nadol, 291. *See also* nadolol

Apo-Napro-Na, Apo-Napro-Na DS, **385-387.** *See also* naproxen

Apo-Naproxen, Apo-Naproxen EC, Apo-Naproxen SR, **385-387.** *See also* naproxen

Apo-Nifed, Apo-Nifed PA, 300. *See also* nifedipine

Apo-Nitrazepam, 195. *See also* nitrazepam

Apo-Norflox, 206. *See also* norfloxacin

Apo-Nortriptylene, 424. *See also* nortriptyline

Apo-Oflox, 206. *See also* ofloxacin

Apo-Omeprazole, 400. *See also* omeprazole

Apo-Oxaprozin, **385-387.** *See also* oxaprozin

Apo-Oxazepam, 195. *See also* oxazepam

Apo-Oxybutynin, **230-232.** *See also* oxybutynin

Apo-Paroxetine, 250. *See also* paroxetine

Apo-Pen VK, 207. *See also* penicillin V

Apo-Perphenazine, 277. *See also* perphenazine

Apo-Pimozide, 277. *See also* pimozide

Apo-Pindol, 291. *See also* pindolol

Apo-Piroxicam, **385-387.** *See also* piroxicam

Apo-Pravastatin, **413-415**

Apo-Prazo, 178. *See also* prazosin

Apo-Prednisone, 314, **317-319.** *See also* prednisone

Apo-Primidone, 238. *See also* primidone

Apo-Prochlorazine, 277. *See also* prochlorperazine

Apo-Propranolol, 291, **293-295.** *See also* propranolol

Apo-Ramipril, 189. *See also* ramipril

Apo-Salvent, Apo-Salvent CFC Free, 356, **357-359.** *See also* salbutamol

Apo-Selegiline, 267. *See also* selegiline

Apo-Sertraline, 250. *See also* sertraline

Apo-Simvastatin, **413-415,** 474. *See also* simvastatin

Apo-Sotalol, 291. *See also* sotalol

Apo-Sulfatrim*, Apo-Sulfatrim DS*, Apo-Sulfatrim Oral Suspension*, Apo-Sulfatrim Pediatric Tablets*, 207, **221-222.** *See also* sulfamethoxazole/trimethoprim*

Apo-Sulin, **385-387.** *See also* sulindac

Apo-Temazepam, 195. *See also* temazepam

Apo-Tenoxicam, **385-387.** *See also* tenoxicam

Apo-Terazosin, 178. *See also* terazosin

Apo-Terbinafine, 257, **259-261.** *See also* terbinafine

Apo-Tetra, 208, **223-224.** *See also* tetracycline

Apo-Tiaprofenic, **385-387.** *See also* tiaprofenic acid

Apo-Ticlopodine, 272. *See also* ticlopidine.

Apo-Timol, 291. *See also* timolol

Apo-Timop, 340, **342-343.** *See also* timolol

Apo-Tolbutamide, 388. *See also* tolbutamide

Apo-Trazadone, Apo-Trazadone D, 251. *See also* trazodone

Apo-Triazide*, 327, **332-334.** *See also* hydrochlorothiazide; triamterene

Apo-Triazo, 195. *See also* triazolam

Apo-Trifluoperazine, 277. *See also* trifluoperazine

Apo-Trihex, 267. *See also* trihexyphenidyl

Apo-Trimebutine, 338. *See also* trimebutine

Apo-Trimip, 424. *See also* trimipramine

Apo-Valproic Acid, 238, **242-243.** *See also* valproic acid

Apo-Verap, Apo-Verap SR, 300. *See also* verapamil

Apo-Warfarin, 232, **233-235.** *See also* warfarin

Apo-Zopiclone, 195, **198-199.** *See also* zopiclone

apraclonidine, 127, 340

Aptivus, 283. *See also* tipranavir

Arava, 352. *See also* leflunomide

ARBs. *See* angiotensin receptor blockers

Aricept, Aricept RDT, **184-185.** *See also* donepezil

Arimidex, **225-226.** *See also* anastrozole

Aristocort C, Aristocort R, 314. *See also* triamcinolone

Aromasin, 225. *See also* exemestane

aromatase inhibitors, 111, 225

Arthrotec*, **384-387.** *See also* diclofenac

ASA, 23, 88, 102, 113, 129, 130, 142, 160, 164, 235, 236, **272-274**, 275, 384, 451, 460, 472, 473, 483. *See also* nonsteroidal anti-inflammatory drugs

Asacol-800, **187-188**. *See also* 5-aminosalicylic acid

Asaphen, Asaphen E.C, **272-274**. *See also* ASA

aspart, 117, 365, **367-369**

Aspirin, 66, 188, **272-274**, 460. *See also* ASA

AT receptor blockers. *See* angiotensin receptor blockers

Atacand, **192-194**. *See also* candesartan

Atacand Plus*, **192-194**, 327, **332-334**. *See also* candesartan; hydrochlorothiazide

Atarax 261, **263-264**. *See also* hydroxyzine

atazanavir, 283

atenolol, 162, 290, **291-293**

Ativan, **195-197**. *See also* lorazepam

atomoxedine, 108, 250

atorvastatin, 146, **413-415**

Atrovent HFA Inhalation Aerosol, Atrovent Inhalation Aerosol, Atrovent Inhalation Solution, 357, **360-362**. *See also* ipratropium

atypical antipsychotics. *See* second-generation antipsychotics

Avalide*, **192-194**, 327, **332-334**. *See also* hydrochlorothiazide; irbesartan

Avandamet*, 37, 388, **392-393**, **394-396**. *See also* metformin; rosiglitazone

Avandaryl*, 388, **394-396**. *See also* glimepiride; rosiglitazone

Avandia, 388, **394-396**. *See also* rosiglitazone

Avapro, **192-194**. *See also* irbesartan

Avelox, 206. *See also* moxifloxacin

Aventyl, 424. *See also* nortriptyline

Avodart, 182. *See also* dutasteride

Axert, 408. *See also* almotriptan

Azatadine, 261

azathioprine, 121, 351, **352-353**

Azilect, 267. *See also* rasagiline

azithromycin, 112, 113, 122, 126, 128, 153, 206, **216-217**. *See also* macrolides

Azopt, 341. *See also* brinzolamide

• *B* •

baclofen, 149, 411

Barriere-HC, 315, **325-326**. *See also* hydrocortisone

Baycol. *See* cerivastatin

beclomethasone, 106, 313, 357

Bellergal Spacetabs*, 238. *See also* phenobarbital

benazepril, **189-191**

BenzaClin*, 206, **214-216**. *See also* clindamycin

Benzamycin*, 207. *See also* erythromycin

benzodiazepines, 102, 103, 162, 194, 195, 256, 457

benztropine, Benztropine Omega, 267

Berotec Inhalation Aerosol, Berotec Inhalation Solution, 356. *See also* fenoterol

beta blockers, 12, 101, 103, 104, 127, 129, 130, 131, 137, 138, 144, 149, 162, 200, 435, 457, 461

beta-1 selective beta blockers, 290

beta-2 agonists, 106, 107, 112, 356

Betaderm, 315. *See also* betamethasone

Betagan, 340. *See also* levobunolol

betahistine, 120, **349-351**

Betaloc, Betaloc Durules, 290, **291-293**. *See also* metoprolol

betamethasone, 314, 315

betaxolol, 340

bethanechol, 149

Betoptic S, 340. *See also* betaxolol

bezafibrate, 347

Bezalip SR, 347. *See also* bezafibrate

Biaxin, Biaxin BID, Biaxin XL, 206. *See also* clarithromycin

bicalutamide, 225, **226-227**

biguanide, 388

bimatoprost, 341

binding resins, 304

biological response modifiers, 105, 147, 156

biologics. *See* biologic response modifiers

Biphentin, **416-417**. *See also* methylphenidate

bisoprolol, 290

bisphosphonates, 151, 296-299

Blephamide*, 207, 314, **317-319**. *See also* prednisolone; sulfacetamide

blockers, 174

blood thinners. *See* anticoagulants

Bonefos, 296. *See also* clodronate

Brevicon*, 306, **307-309**. *See also* ethinyl estradiol; norethindrone

Bricanyl Turbuhaler, 356. *See also* terbutaline

brimonidine, 127, 340, **341-342**

bromazepam, 194

bromocriptine, 136, 140, 267, **335-338**

budesonide, 313, 314, 357

Bufferin, **272-274**, 460. *See also* ASA

bumetanide, 327

bupropion, 116, 159, 251, **255-257**

Burinex, 327. *See also* bumetanide

buserelin, 225

buspirone, 102

butoconazole, 257

butorphanol, 377

• *C* •

cabergoline, 136, 335

Caduet*, 37, 300, **301-302, 413-415.** *See also* atorvastatin; amlodipine
Cafergot, 409
calcipotriol, 156
calcitonin, 151
calcitriol, 144. *See also* vitamin D
calcium, 23, 68, 92, 174, 213, 226, 229, 247, 297, 298, 299, 322, 332, 423, 441, 484
calcium acetate, 144
calcium carbonate, 144
calcium channel blockers, 101, 103, 104, 129, 137, 147, 200
CAMs. *See* complementary and alternative medicines
candesartan, **192-194**
Candistatin, 257. *See also* nystatin
Canesten Topical, Canesten Vaginal, **257.** *See also* clotrimazole
Capex, 315
Capoten, **189-191**, 437. *See also* captopril
captopril, 67, 145, **189-191**
carbachol, 341
carbamazepine, 109, 123, 237, **238-240**
carbidopa, 153
Carbolith, 371, **372-373.** *See also* lithium
carbonic anhydrase inhibitor, 127, 327, 341, 344
cardioselective beta blockers. *See* beta-1 selective beta blockers
Cardizem, Cardizem CD, 300, **302-304.** *See also* diltiazem
Cardura, 178, **179-180.** *See also* doxazosin
carvedilol, 291
Casodex, 225, **226-227.** *See also* bicalutamide
Catapres, 176. *See also* clonidine
Caverject, 124. *See also* alprostadil
cefaclor, **206**
cefprozil, **206**

Ceftin, 206. *See also* cefuroxime
cefuroxime, 113, 158, 206
Cefzil, 206. *See also* cefprozil
Celebrex, **384-387.** *See also* celecoxib
celecoxib, **384-387**
Celexa, 250, **253-254.** *See also* citalopram
Cellcept, 352. *See also* mycophenolate
cephalexin, 206, **210-211**
cephalosporins, 128, 206, 210-211, 220, 433
cerivastatin, 14
CES Tablets, 374, **375-377.** *See also* conjugated estrogens
chlordiazepoxide, 194
chlorpromazine, 276
chlorpropamide, 388
chlorthalidone, 327
cholesterol absorption inhibitor, 304
cholestyramine, 118, 141, 147, 441, 304
cholinergic agonist eye drops, 127
cholinergic agonists, 341
cholinesterase inhibitors, 99, 183, 184
Cialis, 397. *See also* tadalafil
Cicatrin, 205, **208-210.** *See also* neomycin
ciclesonide, 357
ciclopirox, 162, 257
cilazapril, **189-191**
Ciloxan, **206, 212.** *See also* ciprofloxacin
Cipro HC*, 206, **212-213,** 315, **325-326.** *See also* ciprofloxacin; hydrocortisone
Cipro Oral Suspension, Cipro Tablets, Cipro XL, 206, **212-213.** *See also* ciprofloxacin
Ciprodex*, 206, **212-213,** 314, **323.** *See also* ciprofloxacin; dexamethasone
ciprofloxacin, 206, **212-213,** 444
Cirpralex, 250. *See also* escitalopram
cisapride, 14

citalopram, 250, **253-254**
clarithromycin, 113, 153, 161, 164, 206
Clarus, 402. *See also* isotretinoin
Clasteon, 296. *See also* clodronate
clavulanate, 113
Clavulin*, 23, 207, **219-220.** *See also* amoxicillin; clavulanate
Climara Patch, 374, **375-377.** *See also* 17 beta estradiol
clindamycin, 96, 122, 166, 206, 213, **214-216**
Clindasol, 206, **214-216.** *See also* clindamycin
Clinda-T, 206, **214-216.** *See also* clindamycin
Clindets, **206, 214.** *See also* clindamycin
Clindoxyl*, 206, **214-216.** *See also* clindamycin
clioquinol, 257
clobazam, 194, 237
Clobetasol, 315
clobetasone, 315
Clobex Preparations, 315. *See also* clobetasol
clodronate, 296
clomiphene, 21, 140
clomipramine, 151, 424
clonazepam, 156, 195, 237, **240-242**
clonidine, 148, 176
clopidogrel, 102, 113, 130, 160, 272, **274-276**
Clopixol, Clopixol-Acuphase, Clopixol Depot, 277. *See also* zuclopenthixol
clorazepate, 195
Clotrimaderm, 257. *See also* clotrimazole
clotrimazole, 257
cloxacillin, 207
clozapine, 11, 157, **277**
Clozaril, 277. *See also* clozapine
CO Alendronate, **296-299.** *See also* alendronate
CO Atenolol, 290, **291-293.** *See also* atenolol
CO Azithromycin, 206, **216-217.** *See also* azithromycin

CO Bicalutamide, 225, **226-227.** *See also* bicalutamide

CO Ciprofloxacin, 206, **212-213.** *See also* ciprofloxacin

CO Citalopram, 250, **253-254.** *See also* citalopram

CO Clomipramine, 424. *See also* clomipramine

CO Clonazepam, 195, 237, **240-242.** *See also* clonazepam

CO Fluoxetine, 250. *See also* fluoxetine

CO Gabapentin, 238, **243-244.** *See also* gabapentin

CO Glimepiride, 388. *See also* glimepiride

CO Levetiracetam, 238. *See also* levetiracetam

CO Lovastatin, 413, **414-415.** *See also* lovastatin

CO Meloxicam, **385-387.** *See also* meloxicam

CO Metformin Coated, 388, **392-393.** *See also* metformin

CO Norfloxacin, 206. *See also* norfloxacin

CO Paroxetine, 250. *See also* paroxetine

CO Pravastatin, 413, **414-415.** *See also* pravastatin

CO Risperidone, 277, **280-282.** *See also* risperidone

CO Simvastatin, 413, **414-415,** 474. *See also* simvastatin

CO Sotalol, 291. *See also* sotalol

CO Sumatriptan, **408-410.** *See also* sumatriptan

CO Temazepam, 195. *See also* temazepam

CO Terbinafine, 257, **259-261.** *See also* terbinafine

CO Zopiclone, 195, **198-199.** *See also* zopiclone

codeine, 70, 116, 118, 129, 377

Codeine Contin, 377. *See also* codeine

Coenzyme Q10, 443

CO-Etidronate, 296, **298-299.** *See also* etidronate

colchicine, 128, 428

Colestid, 304. *See also* colestipol

colestipol, 304

Combigan*, 340, **341-342, 342-343.** *See also* brimonidine; timolol

Combivent Inhalation Aerosol*, **356, 357.** *See also* ipratropium; salbutamol

Combivent Inhalation Solution*, 356, 357, **357-359, 360-362.** *See also* ipratropium; salbutamol

Combivir*, 282. *See also* lamivudine; zidovudine

CO-Mirtazapine, 251. *See also* mirtazapine

complementary and alternative medicines, 443

COMT inhibitors, 267

Comtan, 267. *See also* entacapone

Concerta, **416-418.** *See also* methylphenidate

conjugated estrogens, 374, **375-377**

contraceptives. *See* Depo-Provera; IUDs; morning-after pill; oral contraceptives; transdermal contraceptive patches; transvaginal contraceptive rings

Cordarone, 55, **200-202.** *See also* amiodarone

Corgard, 291. *See also* nadolol

Cortef, 314. *See also* hydrocortisone

Cortenema, 315. *See also* hydrocortisone

corticosteroids, 97, 105, 106, 107, 112, 113, 120, 121, 128, 132, 141, 149, 150, 156, 158, 167, 213, 312-326, 357, 450

cortisone, 314

Cortisone Acetate, 314. *See also* cortisone

Cortisporin*, 314. *See also* hydrocortisone

Cortisporin ear/eye suspension*, 314. *See also* hydrocortisone

Cortisporin Eye/Ear Suspension Sterile*, 205, **208-210**

Cortisporin Ointment*, 205, **208-210,** 314. *See also* hydrocortisone; neomycin

Cortisporin Otic Solution Sterile*, 205, **208-210.** *See also* neomycin

Cortoderm, 315, **325-326.** *See also* hydrocortisone

Cosopt*, Cosopt Preservative-Free*, 340, 341, **342-343, 344-345.** *See also* dorzolamide; timolol

Coumadin, 68, 232, **233-235.** *See also* warfarin

coumarins, 232

Covera-HS, 300. *See also* verapamil

Coversyl Plus*, 327, 189, **190-191.** *See also* indapamide; perindopril

Cozaar, **192-194.** *See also* losartan

Crestor, 413, **414-415.** *See also* rosuvastatin

Crixivan, 283. *See also* indinavir

Cutivate, 315. *See also* fluticasone

Cyclen*, 306, **307-309.** *See also* ethinyl estradiol; norgestimate

cyclobenzaprine, **411-413**

Cyclocort, 315. *See also* amcinonide

cyclophosphamide, 351

cyclopyrrolone derivative, 195

cyclosporine, 121, 351

Cytomel, 421. *See also* liothyronine (T3)

Cytovene capsules, 288. *See also* ganciclovir

Cytoxan, 351. *See also* cyclophosphamide

• *D* •

Dalacin C, Dalacin C Flavoured Granules, 206, **214-216**. *See also* clindamycin
Dalacin T Topical Solution, 206, **214-216**. *See also* clindamycin
Dalacin Vaginal Cream, 206, **214-216**. *See also* clindamycin
Dalmacol*, 377. *See also* hydrocodone
dalteparin, 233, **235-237**
danazol, 123
darbepoetin, 144
darifenacin, 230
Darvon-N, 378. *See also* propoxyphene
Daypro, **385-387**. *See also* oxaprozin
DDAVP. *See* desmopressin
decongestants, 158
Delatestryl, 418, **419-420**. *See also* testosterone
delavirdine, 283
Demerol, 40. *See also* meperidine
Demulen*, 306, **307-309**. *See also* ethinyl estradiol; ethynodiol diacetate
Depakene, 238, **242-243**. *See also* valproic acid
Depo-Provera, 115, 123, 148, **307-309**, **375-377**. *See also* medroxy-progesterone acetate
Depo-Testosterone, 418, **419-420**. *See also* testosterone
Dermatop, 315. *See also* prednicarbate
Dermovate, 315. *See also* clobetasol
desiccated thyroid, 421
desipramine, 143, 424
desmopressin, 109
Desocort, 315. *See also* desonide
desogestrel, 306
desonide, 315
desoximetasone, 315
Desyrel, 251. *See also* trazodone

Desyrel Dividose, 251. *See also* trazodone
Detemir, 117, 365, **366-369**
Detrol, Detrol LA, 140, 230. *See also* tolterodine
dexamethasone, 97, 150, 314
Dexasone, 314. *See also* dexamethasone
Dexedrine, 416. *See also* dextroamphetamine
dextroamphetamine, 108, 416
Diabeta, 388, **390-391**. *See also* glyburide
Diamicron, Diamicron MR, 388. *See also* gliclazide
Diane-35, 97, 134, 306, **307-309**. *See also* cyproterone acetate; ethinyl estradiol
Diastat, 195, 447. *See also* diazepam
diazepam, 195, 447
Dicetel, 338. *See also* pinaverium
Diclectin*, 150, 261, **262-263**. *See also* doxylamine/pyridoxine
diclofenac, 384, **385-387**
didanosine, 282
Didrocal*, 296, **298-299**. *See also* etidronate
Didronel, 296, **298-299**. *See also* etidronate
diethylpropion, 265
Differin, 402. *See also* adapalene
Diflucan-150, 257, **258-259**. *See also* fluconazole
diflucortolone, 315
diflusinal, 384, **385-387**
digoxin, 103, 104, 132, 200, **202-203**, 443
dihydropyridine, 137, 300
Dilantin, 40. *See also* phenytoin
Dilantin Capsules, Dilantin Infatabs, Dilantin-30 Suspension, Dilantin-125 Suspension, 238, **246-248**. *See also* phenytoin
Dilaudid, 377. *See also* hydromorphone
diltiazem, 103, 104, 144, 300, **302-304**
dimenhydrinate, 120

Dimetane Expectorant-DC*, 377. *See also* hydrocodone
Diovan, **192-194**. *See also* valsartan
Diovan-HCT*, **192-194**, 327, **332-334**. *See also* hydrochlorothiazide; valsartan
Dipentum, 187. *See also* olsalazine
diphenhydramine, 121, 142. *See also* antihistamines
diphenoxylate, 118
Diprolene Glycol, **315**. *See also* betamethasone
Diprosone, 315. *See also* betamethasone
dipyridamole, 160, 272
disease-modifying antirheumatic drugs, 105
Diskus, 80
disulfiram, 98, 443
Ditropan, Ditropan XL, 140, **230-232**. *See also* oxybutynin
diuretics, 120, 122, 143, 144, 334, 372, 458, 484
divalproex, 129, 237, **242-243**
Dixarit, 176. *See also* clonidine
DMARDS. *See* disease-modifying antirheumatic drugs
domperidone, 337, **338-339**
donepezil, 184, **184-185**
dopamine, 153
dopamine agonists, 136, 140, 153, 267
dopamine antagonists, 338
dopamine precursors, 267
dorzolamide, 341, **344-345**
Dostinex, 335. *See also* cabergoline
Dovobet*, 315. *See also* betamethasone
doxazosin, 155, 178, **179-180**, 181
doxepin, 424
Doxycin, 208. *See also* doxycycline
doxycycline, 97, 112, 113, 153, 157, 158, 161, 208
doxylamine/pyridoxine, 150, 261, **262-263**
Dristan, 317
drospirenone, 306, **307-309**

DuoTrav*, 340, 341, **342-343.** *See also* timolol, travoprost
Duovent UDV*, 356, 357, **360-362.** *See also* fenoterol; ipratropium
Duragesic 12, Duragesic 25, Duragesic 50, Duragesic 75, Duragesic 100, 377. *See also* fentanyl
Duralith, 371, **372-373.** *See also* lithium
dutasteride, 182

• *E* •

Ebixa, 184, **185-186.** *See also* memantine
econazole, 257
Ecostatin, 257. *See also* econazole
Edecrin, 327. *See also* ethacrynic acid
EES 200, EES 400, EES 600, 207. *See also* erythromycin
efavirenz, 283
Effexor XR, 250, **251-253,** 487. *See also* venlafaxine
eflornithine, 134
eletriptan, 408
Elidel, 352. *See also* pimecrolimus
Eligard, 225. *See also* leuprolide
Elocom, 315. *See also* mometasone
Eltroxin, **421-423.** *See also* L-thyroxine (T4)
Emadine, 261. *See also* emedastine
emedastine, 261
emergency contraceptive therapy, 307
Emo-Cort, 315, **325-326.** *See also* hydrocortisone
emtricitabine, **282**
Emtriva, 282. *See also* emtricitabine
Enablex, 230. *See also* darifenacin
Enca, 208. *See also* minocycline
Endatadine, 267. *See also* amantadine
Endocet*, **378-380.** *See also* oxycodone
Endodan*, **378-380.** *See also* oxycodone

enfuvirtide, 283
enlalapril, 189, **190-191**
enoxaparin, 233, **235-237**
entacapone, 153, 267
Entocort Capsules, 314. *See also* budenoside
Entocort Enema, 314, **324-325.** *See also* budenoside
epinephrine, 24, 83, 99, 200, 432
EpiPen, 24, 83, 99, 437
EpiPen Jr., 83
Epival, 237, **242-243.** *See also* divalproex
eprosartan, **192-194**
ergotamine, 129
Erybid, 207. *See also* erythromycin
Eryc, 207. *See also* erythromycin
Erysol*, 207. *See also* erythromycin
erythromycin, 96, 97, 112, 114, 126, 157, 207, 437, 460
erythropoietin, 144
escitalopram, 250
esomeprazole, 400
Estalis Patch, **375-377.** *See also* norethindrone acetate; 17 beta estradiol
Estalis Sequi Patch, **375-377.** *See also* norethindrone acetate; beta estradiol
Estrace Tablet, 374, **375-377.** *See also* 17 beta estradiol
Estracomb Patch, **375-377.** *See also* norethindrone acetate; 17 beta estradiol
Estraderm Patch, 374, **375-377.** *See also* 17 beta estradiol
Estradot Patch, 374, **375-377.** *See also* 17 beta estradiol
Estring, 374, **375-377.** *See also* 17 beta estradiol
Estrogel, 374, **375-377.** *See also* 17 beta estradiol
estrogen, 145, 152, 166, 374
estropipate, 374, **375-377**
etezimibe, 304
ethacrynic acid, 327
ethambutol, 163, 285

ethinyl estradiol, 306, 375
ethopropazine, 267
ethosuximide, 237
ethynodiol diacetate, 306
Etibi, 285. *See also* ethambutol
etidronate, 296, **298-299**
etonogestrel, 306
Euflex, 225. *See also* flutamide
Eumovate, 315. *See also* clobetasone
Euthyrox, **421-423.** *See also* L-thyroxine (T4)
Evra, 306, **307-309.** *See also* ethinyl estradiol; norelgestromin
Exelon, 184. *See also* rivastigmine
exemastane, 225
ezetimibe, 146, **304-305**
Ezetrol, **304-305.** *See also* ezetimibe

• *F* •

famciclovir, 114, 134, 158, 288
famotidine, 23
Famvir, 288. *See also* famciclovir
fast-acting insulins, 365. *See also* insulin
felodipine, 300
Fem HRT, **375-377.** *See also* ethinyl estradiol; norethindrone acetate
fenofibrate, 347, **348-349**
fenoterol, 356
fentanyl, 377
ferrous gluconate, 100. *See also* iron
ferrous sulphate, 100, 441. *See also* iron
fibrates, 146, 347-349
finasteride, 108, 134, **182-183**
Fiorinal, 460. *See also* ASA
Fiorinal-C*, 377. *See also* codeine
first-generation antipsychotics, 157, 276
Flagyl, 207, **217-219.** *See also* metronidazole
Flagystatin*, 207, **217-219.** *See also* metronidazole
flavoxate, 230
floctafenine, 384, **385-387**

Flomax, 87, 178, **180-181.** *See also* tamsulosin

Flomax CR, 178, **180-181.** *See also* tamsulosin

Flonase, 313. *See also* fluticasone

Florazole ER, 207, **217-219.** *See also* metronidazole

Florinef, 314. *See also* fludrocortisone

Flovent Diskus, 357, **363-364.** *See also* fluticasone

Flovent HFA, 357, **363-364.** *See also* fluticasone

Floxin, 206. *See also* ofloxacin

Fluanxol Depot, Fluanxol Tablets, 276. *See also* flupenthixol

fluconazole, 162, 167, 257, **258-259**

fludrocortisone, 97, 314

flumethasone, 314, 315

flunisolide, 313, 314

fluocinolone, 315

fluocinonide, 315

fluorometholone, 314

fluoroquinolones, 112, 113, 114, 119, 126, 128, 154, 163, 165, 166, 206, 211-213

fluoxetine, 148, 250

flupenthixol, 276

fluphenazine, 276

Fluphenazine Omega, 276

flurazepam, 195

flurbiprofen, 384, **385-387**

flutamide, 134, 225

fluticasone, 158, 313, 315, 357, **363-364**

fluvastatin, 413, **414-415**

fluvoxamine, 250

FML Forte, 314. *See also* fluorometholone

folic acid, 247, 355, 483

Foradil, 356. *See also* formoterol

formoterol, 356

Fortovase Roche, 283. *See also* saquinavir

Fosamax, **296-298.** *See also* alendronate

fosamprenavir, 283

fosinopril, 189, **190-191**

Fragmin, 233, **235-237.** *See also* dalteparin

framycetin, 205

Fraxiparine, Fraxiparine Forte, 233, **235-237.** *See also* nadroparin

Froben, Froben SR, 384, **385-387.** *See also* flurbiprofen

furosemide, 122, 131, 143, 327, **328-330,** 458

fusion inhibitor, 283

Fuzeon, 283. *See also* enfurvitide

FXT, 250. *See also* fluoxetine

• *G* •

gabapentin, 148, 156, 162, 238, **243-244**

galantamine, 184

ganciclovir, 288

Garamycin Ophthalmic Ointment, Garamycin Ophthalmic Optic Solution, Garamycin Opthalmic Drops, Garamycin Otic Drops, Garamycin Topical Preparations, 205. *See also* gentamicin

Garasone Ophthalmic* (solution and ointment), 314. *See also* betamethasone

Garasone Ophthalmic Ointment, 205. *See also* gentamicin

Garasone Otic*, 314. *See also* betamethasone

gemfibrozil, 347

Gen-Acebutolol (Type S), 290. *See also* acebutolol

Gen-Acebutolol, 290. *See also* acebutolol

Gen-Acyclovir, **288-290.** *See also* acyclovir

Gen-Alendronate, **296-298.** *See also* alendronate

Gen-Alprazolam, 194. *See also* alprazolam

Gen-Amantadine, 267. *See also* amantadine

Gen-Amilazide*, 327, **332-334.** *See also* amiloride; hydrochlorothiazide

Gen-Amiodarone, **200-202.** *See also* amiodarone

Gen-Amoxicillin, 207, **219-220.** *See also* amoxicillin

Gen-Atenolol, 290, **291-293.** *See also* atenolol

Gen-Baclofen, 411. *See also* baclofen

Gen-Beclo AQ, 313. *See also* beclomethasone

Gen-Bromazepam, 194. *See also* bromazepam

Gen-Budesonide AQ, 313. *See also* budenoside

Gen-Captopril, 189, **190-191.** *See also* captopril

Gen-Carbamazepine CR, 237, **238-240.** *See also* carbamazepine

Gen-Ciprofloxacin, 206, **212-213.** *See also* ciprofloxacin

Gen-Citalopram, 250, **253-254.** *See also* citalopram

Gen-Clindamycin, 206, **214-216.** *See also* clindamycin

Gen-Clobetasol, 315. *See also* clobetasol

Gen-Clomipramine, 424. *See also* clomipramine

Gen-Clonazepam, 195, 237, **240-242.** *See also* clonazepam

Gen-Clozapine, 277. *See also* clozapine

Gen-Combo Sterinebs*, 356, 357, **357-359,** **360-362.** *See also* ipratropium; salbutamol

Gen-Cyclobenzaprine, **411-413.** *See also* cyclobenzaprine

Gen-Diltiazem, Gen-Diltiazem CD, 300, **302-304.** *See also* diltiazem

Gen-Doxazosin, 178, **179-180.** *See also* doxazosin

Gen-Etidronate, 296, **298-299.** *See also* etidronate

Gen-Fenofibrate Micro, 347, **348-349.** *See also* fenofibrate

Gen-Fluconazole, 257, **258-259.** *See also* fluconazole

Gen-Fluoxetine, 250. *See also* fluoxetine

Gen-Fosinopril, 189, **190-191.** *See also* fosinopril

Gen-Gabapentin, 238, **243-244.** *See also* gabapentin

Gen-Gemfibrozil, 347. *See also* gemfibrozil

Gen-Gliclazide, **388.** *See also* gliclazide

Gen-Glybe, 388, **390-391.** *See also* glyburide

Gen-Hydroxychloroquine, 351. *See also* hydroxychloroquine

Gen-Indapamide, 327, 437. *See also* indapamide

Gen-Ipratropium, 357, **360-362.** *See also* ipratropium

Gen-Lamotrigine, 238, **244-246.** *See also* lamotrigine

Gen-Lovastatin, 413, **414-415.** *See also* lovastatin

Gen-Medroxy, **375-377.** *See also* medroxy-progesterone acetate

Gen-Meloxicam, **385-387.** *See also* meloxicam

Gen-Metformin, 388, **392-393.** *See also* metformin

Gen-Metoprolol (Type L), 290, **291-293.** *See also* metoprolol

Gen-Minocycline, 208. *See also* minocycline

Gen-Mirtazapine, Gen-Mirtazapine OD, 251. *See also* mirtazapine

Gen-Nabumetone, **385.** *See also* nabumetone

Gen-Naproxen EC, **385-387.** *See also* naproxen

Gen-Nitro, 381, **382-383.** *See also* nitroglycerin

Gen-Nortriptylene, 424. *See also* nortriptyline

Gen-Oxybutynin, **230-232.** *See also* oxybutynin

Gen-Paroxetine, 250. *See also* paroxetine

Gen-Pindolol, 291. *See also* pindolol

Gen-Piroxicam, **385-387.** *See also* piroxicam

Gen-Salbutamol Respirator Solution, Gen-Salbutamol Sterinebs P.F., 356, **357-360.** *See also* salbutamol

Gen-Selegiline, 267. *See also* selegiline

Gen-Sertraline, 250. *See also* sertraline

Gen-Simvastatin, 413, **414-415.** *See also* simvastatin

Gen-Sotalol, 291. *See also* sotalol

Gen-Sumatriptan, **408-410.** *See also* sumatriptan

gentamicin, 205

Gen-Temazepam, 195. *See also* temazepam

Gen-Terbinafine, 257, **259-261.** *See also* terbinafine

Gen-Ticlopodine, 272. *See also* ticlopidine

Gen-Timolol, 340, **342-343.** *See also* timolol

Gen-Topiramate, 238, **248-249.** *See also* topiramate

Gen-Trazodone, 251. *See also* trazodone

Gen-Triazolam, 195. *See also* triazolam

Gen-Valproic, 238, **242-243.** *See also* valproic acid

Gen-Verapamil, Gen-Verapamil SR, 300. *See also* verapamil

Gen-Warfarin, 232, **233-235.** *See also* warfarin

Gen-Zopiclone, 195, **198-199.** *See also* zopiclone

glargine, 117, 365, **367-369**

glatiramer, 149

gliclazide, 118, 388

glimepiride, 118, 388

glucagon, 118, 368

Glucobay, 388, **389-390.** *See also* acarbose

glucocorticoids, 97, 99, 313

GlucoNorm, 388, **396-397.** *See also* repaglinide

Glucophage, 388, **392-393.** *See also* metformin

glucorticoids. *See* corticosteroids

Glumetza, 388, **392-393.** *See also* metformin

glyburide, 118, 188, 292, 294, 295, 388, **390-391,** 396, 433, 443, 461

GnRH agonists, 111, 225. *See also* gonadotropin-releasing hormone agonists

gold, **351**

gonadropin-releasing hormone analogs, 134

goserelin, 225, **227-229**

Gravol, 120. *See also* dimenhydrinate

• *H* •

H2 receptor antagonists. *See* histamine-2 receptor antagonists

HAART, 135, 282

halcinonide, 315

Halcion 195. *See also* triazolam

Halog preparations, 315. *See also* halcinonide

haloperidol, 276

Haloperidol Injection USP, 276. *See also* haloperidol

Haloperidol LA, Haloperidol-LA Omega, 276. *See also* haloperidol

Handihaler, 80

HCT. *See* hydrochlorothiazide

heparin. *See* low molecular weight heparin

Heptovir, 282. *See also* lamivudine

Herplex-D, 288. *See also* idoxuridine

highly active antiretroviral therapy. *See* HAART

histamine-2 receptor antagonists, 126, 164

Hivid, 282. *See also* zalcitabine

hormone replacement therapy. *See* menopausal hormone therapy

Hp-PAC*, 206, 207, **219-220**, 400. *See also* amoxicillin; clarithromycin; lansoprazole
Humalog, 365, **366-369**. *See also* lispro
Humalog Mix25, Humalog Mix50, 365, **366-369**. *See also* premixed insulin
HumaPen Luxura, 82
Humatin, 205. *See also* paromomycin
Humulin 30/70, 365, **366-369**. *See also* premixed insulin
Humulin-N, 365, **366-369**. *See also* NPH
Humulin-R, 365, **366-369**. *See also* regular insulin
Hycodan, 377. *See also* hydrocodone
Hycomine*, Hycomine-S*, 377. *See also* hydrocodone
Hycort (enema), 315. *See also* hydrocortisone
Hyderm, 315, **325-326**. *See also* hydrocortisone
hydralazine, 132
hydrochlorothiazide, 19, 145, 458, 327, **332-334**
hydrocodone, 377
hydrocortisone, 97, 132, 314, 315, **325-326**
Hydromorph Contin, Hydromorph IR, 377. *See also* hydromorphone
hydromorphone, 377
Hydrosone, 315, **325-326**. *See also* hydrocortisone
HydroVal, 314, **325-326**. *See also* hydrocortisone
Hydroxychloroquine, 147, 351
hydroxyzine, 121, 261, **263-264**
hypoglycemic agents (oral), 118, 387-397
Hytrin, 178. *See also* terazosin
Hyzaar*, Hyzaar DS*, **192-194**, 327, **332-334**. *See also* hydrochlorothiazide; losartan

• *I* •

ibuprofen, 22, 152, 384, **385-387**
idoxuridine, 288
Imdur, 381. *See also* isosorbide-5-mononitrate
imipramine, 109, 424
imiquimod, 168
Imitrex, 46. *See also* sumatriptan
Imitrex DF Tablets, Imitrex Injection/Auto-Injector, Imitrex Nasal Spray, 46, **408-410**. *See also* sumatriptan
immunosuppressive drugs, 105, 121, 147, 156, 186, 351-355
Imovane, 195, **198-199**. *See also* zopiclone
Imuran, 351, **352-353**. *See also* azathioprine
indapamide, 327
Inderal-LA, 291, **293-295**. *See also* propranolol
indinavir, 283
indomethacin, 128, 129, 384, **385-387**
Inhibace, 189, **190-191**. *See also* cilazapril
Inhibace Plus*, 189, **190-191**, 327, **332-334**. *See also* cilazapril; hydrochlorothiazide
inhibitors, 124, 174
injectable contraceptive therapy, 307
Innohep, 233, **235-237**. *See also* tinzaparin
insulin, 24, 46, 82, 83, 84, 86, 117, 292, 294, 295, 365-369, 443, 461, 468
interferon beta, 149
interferon, 133
intermediate-acting insulins, 365, **366-369**
Invirase, 283. *See also* saquinavir
Iopidine, 340. *See also* apraclonidine
ipratropium, 107, 357, **360-362**
irbesartan, **192-194**

iron, 68, 92, 100, 144, 156, 174, 213, 423, 441. *See also* ferrous gluconate; ferrous sulphate
isoniazid, 163, 285, **286-287**
Isoptin SR, 300. *See also* verapamil
Isopto Carbachol, 341. *See also* carbachol
Isopto Carpine, 341, **345-346**. *See also* pilocarpine
isosorbide dintrate, 381
isosorbide-5-mononitrate, 381
Isotamine, 285, 286-287. *See also* isoniazid
isotretinoin, 97, 157, **402-404**
itraconazole, 162, 167, 257
IUDs, 115, 306, 307

• *K* •

Kadian, 378. *See also* morphine
Kaletra*, 283. *See also* lopinavir; ritonavir
Kenalog in Orabase, 314. *See also* triamcinolone
Keppra, 238. *See also* levetiracetam
ketoconazole, 257
Ketoderm, 257. *See also* ketoconazole
ketoprofen, 384, **385-387**
ketorolac, 384, **385-387**
ketotifin, 261
Kivexa*, 282. *See also* abacavir; lamivudine

• *L* •

labetalol, 291
Lamictal, 238, **244-246**. *See also* lamotrigine
Lamisil, 11, 246, 257, **259-261**. *See also* terbinafine
lamivudine, 133, 282
lamotrigine, 109, 123, 238, **244-246**
Lanoxin, 200, **202**. *See also* digoxin
lansoprazole, 400
Lantus, 365, **366-369**. *See also* glargine

Lasix, Lasix Special, 11, 327, **328-330.** *See also* furosemide
latanoprost, 341, **346-347**
L-dopa. *See* Levodopa
Lectopam, 194. *See also* bromazepam
leflunomide, 352
lente insulin, 365
Lescol, Lescol XL, 413, **414-415.** *See also* fluvastatin
letrozole, 140, 225
leukotriene antagonists, 106, 370-371
leuprolide, 225, 227
Levaquin, 206. *See also* levofloxacin
Levemir, 365, **366-369.** *See also* detemir
levetiracetam, 123, 238
Levitra, 397. *See also* vardenafil
levlofloxacin, 112. *See also* fluoroquinolones
levobunolol, 340
levocabastine, 261
Levodopa, 153, 156, 268
levodopa/benserazide*, 267
levodopa/carbidopa*, 267, **268-270**
levofloxacin, 112, 260
levonorgestrel, 115, 306, 307, **311-312.** *See also* morning-after pill
levothyroxine. *See* L-thyroxine
Librax, 194. *See also* chlordiazepoxide
lincosamines, 206, 213-216
Linessa 21*, Linessa 28*, 306, **307-309.** *See also* desogestrel; ethinyl estradiol
Liorisal Oral, 411. *See also* baclofen
liothyronine (T3), 139, 421
Lipidil EZ, Lipidil Supra, 347, **348-349.** *See also* fenofibrate
Lipitor, 413, **414-415,** 487. *See also* atorvastatin
lisinopril, 189, **190-191**
lispro, 117, 365, **366-369**
Lithane, **371.** *See also* lithium

lithium, 109, 371, **372-373**
Livostin Eye Drops, Livostin Nasal Spray, 261. *See also* levocabastine
LMW heparin. *See* low molecular weight heparin
Locacorten Vioform Cream*, 315, 257. *See also* clioquinol; flumethasone
Locacorten Vioform Ear Drops*, 314, 257. *See also* clioquinol; flumethasone
Lomotil, 11, 246, 261
long-acting anticholinergic agent, 357
long-acting beta-2 agonists, 356
long-acting insulins, 365, **366-369**
loop diuretics, 122, 332, 327
loperamide, 118, 141
Lopid, 347. *See also* gemfibrozil
lopinavir, 283
Lopressor, 64, 65, 290, **291-293.** *See also* metoprolol
Loprox, 257. *See also* ciclopirox
lorazepam, 194, **195-197,** 466, 467, 488
losartan, **192-194**
Losec, 11
Losec 1-2-3 A*, 206, **219-220,** 400. *See also* amoxicillin; clarithromycin; omeprazole
Losec 1-2-3 M*, 206, 207, **217-219,** 400. *See also* clarithromycin; metronidazole; omeprazole
Losec Capsules, Losec MUPS, Losec Tablets, 400. *See also* omeprazole
Lotensin, 189, **190-191.** *See also* benazepril
Lotriderm* 257, 315. *See also* betamethasone; clotrimazole
lovastatin, 413, **414-415**

Lovenox, Lovenox HP, 233, **235-237.** *See also* enoxaparin
low molecular weight heparin, 110, 232, 233, 235-237
lower gastrointestinal tract motility regulators, 338
Loxapac IM, 277. *See also* loxapine
loxapine, 277
Lozide, 327. *See also* indapamide
L-thyroxine (T4), 67, 92, 139, **421-423,** 484, 489
Lumigan, 341. *See also* bimatoprost
lumiracoxib, 384, **385-387**
Lupron, Lupron Depot, 225. *See also* leuprolide
Lyderm, 314. *See also* fluocinonide

• *M* •

M.O.S., M.O.S.-S.R., M.O.S.-Sulphate, 378. *See also* morphine
Maalox, 441. *See also* antacids
macrolides, 161, 206, 216-217
Manerix, 250. *See also* moclobemide
MAO inhibitors. *See* monoamine oxidase inhibitors
MAO-B inhibitors. *See* monoamine oxidase inhibitor-B
maprotiline, **424**
Marvelon*, 306, **307-309.** *See also* desogestrel; ethinyl estradiol
mast cell stabilizers, 107, 357
Mavik, 189, **190-191.** *See also* trandolapril
Maxalt, Maxalt RPD, 408. *See also* rizatriptan
Maxidex, 314. *See also* dexamethasone
Maxitrol*, 205, **208-210,** 314. *See also* dexamethasone; neomycin
Medrol, 314. *See also* methylprednisolone

Medrol Acne Lotion*, 207, 314. *See also* methyprednisolone; sulfur

medroxy-progesterone acetate, 307, **309-311, 375-377**

mefenamic acid, **385-387**

meloxicam, **385-387**

memantine, 184, **185-186**

menopausal hormone therapy, 139, 148, 166, 374-377

meperidine, 40

Meridia, 265. *See also* sibutramine

Mesalamine, 187. *See also* 5-aminosalicylic acid; 5-ASA

Mesasal, 187. *See also* 5-aminosalicylic acid

M-Eslon, 378. *See also* morphine

Metadol, 377. *See also* methadone

metformin, 100, 118, 140, 154, 388, **392-393**, 394, 484

methadone, 377

methimazole, **283-285**

methocarbamol, 411

methotrexate, 121, 352, **353-355**, 441

Methotrexate, Methotrexate Tablets USP, 352, **353-355**

methotrimeprazine, 277

methyldopa, **176-178**

methylphenidate, 108, **416-418**, 445, 450

methyprednisolone, 314, 315

methysergide, 129

metoclopramide, 150, 338

metolazone, 327, 458

metoprolol, 64, 131, 290, **291-293**, 466

Metrocream, **207, 217.** *See also* metronidazole

MetroGel, **207, 217.** *See also* metronidazole

MetroLotion, 207, **217-219.** *See also* metronidazole

metronidazole, 126, 157, 164, 166, 167, 207, **217-219**

Mevacor, 413, **414-415.** *See also* lovastatin

Micardis, **192-194**, **327.** *See also* telmisartan

Micardis Plus*, **192-194,** 327, **332-334.** *See also* hydrochlorothiazide; telmisartan

Micatin, 257. *See also* miconazole

miconazole, 257

Micozole, 257. *See also* miconazole

mineralocorticoid, 97

Minitran, 381, **382-383.** *See also* nitroglycerin

Minocin, 208. *See also* minocycline

minocycline, 97, 157, 208, 447

Min-Ovral 21*, Min-Ovral 28*, 306, **307-309.** *See also* ethinyl estradiol; levonorgestrel; norgestrel

minoxidil, 108

Miostat, 341. *See also* carbachol

Mirapex, 267, **270-271.** *See also* pramipexole

mirtazapine, 251

Mobicox, **385-387.** *See also* meloxicam

moclobemide, 250

modafinil, 416

Modecate Concentrate, 276. *See also* fluphenazine

Modulon, 338. *See also* trimebutine

Moduret*, 37, 327, **332-334.** *See also* amiloride; hydrochlorothiazide

Mogadon, 195. *See also* nitrazepam

mometasone, 158, 313, 315, **316-317**

Monistat 7 Dual-Pak, 257. *See also* miconazole

Monistat 7 Vaginal Cream, 257. *See also* miconazole

monoamine oxidase inhibitor-B, 153, 267

monoamine oxidase inhibitors, 116, 177, 239, 250, 252, 254, 256, 269, 342, 379, 409, 412, 417, 425, 443

Monocor, 290. *See also* bisoprolol

Monopril, 189, **190-191.** *See also* fosinopril

montelukast, 106, **370-371**

morniflumate, 87

morning-after pill, 24. *See also* oral contraceptives

morphine, 378

Motrin, 384, **385-387.** *See also* ibuprofen

moxifloxacin, 112, 206

MPA. *See* medroxy-progesterone acetate

MS Contin, 378. *See also* morphine

MS-IR, 378. *See also* morphine

Multipill*, 483-484

mycophenolate, 121, 352

Mycostatin Topical Powder, 257. *See also* nystatin

Myfortic, 352. *See also* mycophenolate

Myochrysine, 351. *See also* gold

• N •

nabumetone, **385-387**

nadolol, 291

nadroparin, 233, **235-237**

naltrexone, 98

Naprosyn, **385-387.** *See also* naproxen

naproxen, 21, 129, **385-387**

naratriptan, 408

narcotic analgesics, 116, 129, 152, 156, 457

Nardil, 250. *See also* phenelzine

Nasacort AQ, 313. *See also* triamcinolone

Nasonex, 313, **316-317.** *See also* mometasone

nateglinide, 388

Navane, 277. *See also* thiothixene

nelfinavir, 283

NeoMedrol*, 315. *See also* methyprednisolone

Neo-Medrol Acne Lotion*, 205, 207, **208-210.** *See also* neomycin; sulfur

neomycin, 205, **208-210**

Neoral, 351. *See also* cyclosporine

Neosporin Cream, 205, **208-210.** *See also* neomycin

Neosporin Eye and Ear Solution, 205, **208-210.** *See also* neomycin

Neosporin Irrigating Solution, 205, **208-210.** *See also* neomycin

Neosporin Ointment, 205, **208-210.** *See also* neomycin

Nerisalic*, 315. *See also* diflucortolone

Nerisone, 315. *See also* diflucortolone

Neurontin, 238, **243-244.** *See also* gabapentin

nevirapine, 283

Nexium, 400. *See also* esomeprazole

Nexium 1-2-3 A*, 206, 207, **219-220,** 400. *See also* amoxicillin; clarithromycin; esomeprazole

niacin, 147

Nicoumalone, 232. *See also* coumarins

NidaGel, 207, **217-219.** *See also* metronidazole

nifedepine, 300

nilutamide, 225

nitrates, **380-383**

nitrazepam, 195

Nitro-Dur, 381, **382-383.** *See also* nitroglycerin

nitrofurantoin, 165, 166

nitroglycerin, 101, 130, 132, 381, **382-383**

Nitroimidazoles, **217-219,** 207

Nitrol, 381, **382-383.** *See also* nitroglycerin

Nitrolingual Pump Spray, 381. *See also* nitroglycerin

Nitrostat, 381. *See also* nitroglycerin

Nizoral Cream, Nizoral Shampoo, 257. *See also* ketoconazole

NMDA receptor antagonists, **185,** 267. *See also* alzheimer's disease medications

N-methyl d-aspartate. *See* NMDA receptor antagonists

NNRTIs. *See* non-nucleoside reverse transcriptase inhibitors

non-dihydroyridine calcium channel blockers, 300, **302-304**

non-nucleoside reverse transcriptase inhibitors, 135

non-selective beta blockers, 291, **293-295**

non-sulfonylurea insulin secretagogues, 388, **396-397**

nonsteroidal anti-inflammatory drugs, 54, 105, 110, 123, 125, 128, 129, 147, 148, 152, 158, 164, 272, 273, 355

norelgestromin, 306

norethindrone, 306

norethindrone acetate, **375-377**

norfloxacin, 206

Norgesic, 460. *See also* ASA

norgestimate, 306, **307-309**

norgestrel, 306, **307-309**

Noritate, 207, **217-219.** *See also* metronidazole

Norpramin, 424. *See also* desipramine

Norvasc, 300, **301-302,** 487. *See also* amlodipine

Novahistex DH*, 377. *See also* hydrocodone

Novahistine DH*, 377. *See also* hydrocodone

Novamilor*, 327, **332-334.** *See also* amiloride; hydrochlorothiazide

Novamoxin, 207, **219-220.** *See also* amoxicillin

Novasen, **272-274,** 460. *See also* ASA

Novir, Novir SEC, 283. *See also* ritonavir

Novo-5 ASA, **187-188.** *See also* 5-aminosalicylic acid

Novo-Acebutolol, 290. *See also* acebutolol

Novo-Alendronate, **296-298.** *See also* alendronate

Novo-Alprazol, 194. *See also* alprazolam

Novo-Amiodarone **200-202.** *See also* amiodarone

Novo-Ampicillin, 207. *See also* ampicillin

Novo-Atenol, 290, **291-293.** *See also* atenolol

Novo-Azathioprine, 351, **352-353.** *See also* azathioprine

Novo-Azithromycin, 206, **216-217.** *See also* azithromycin

Novo-Betahistine, **349-351.** *See also* betahistine

Novo-Bicalutamide, 225, **226-227.** *See also* bicalutamide

Novo-Bisoprolol, 290. *See also* bisoprolol

Novo-Bromazepam, 194. *See also* bromazepam

Novo-Bupropion SR, 251, **255-257.** *See also* bupropion

Novo-Captopril, 189, **190-191.** *See also* captopril

Novo-Carbamaz, 237, **238-240.** *See also* carbamazepine

Novo-Cefaclor, 206. *See also* cefaclor

Novo-Chlorpromazine, 276. *See also* chlorpromazine

Novo-Cilazapril, 189, **190-191.** *See also* cilazapril

Novo-Ciprofloxacin, 206, **212-213.** *See also* ciprofloxacin

Novo-Citalopram, 250, **253-254.** *See also* citalopram

Novo-Clavamoxin 875*, 207, **219-220.** *See also* amoxicillin

Novo-Clindamycin, 206, **214-216.** *See also* clindamycin

Novo-Clobazam, 194, 237. *See also* clobazam

Novo-Clobetasol, 315. *See also* clobetasol

Novo-Clonazepam, 195, 237, **240-242.** *See also* clonazepam

Novo-Clonidine, 176. *See also* clonidine

Novo-Clopate, 195. *See also* clorazepate

Novo-Cloxin, 207. *See also* cloxacillin

Novo-Cyclobenzaprine, **411-413.** *See also* cyclobenzaprine

Novo-Difenac, Novo-Difenac-K, Novo-Difenac SR, 384, **385-387.** *See also* diclofenac

Novo-Diflusinal, 384, **385-387.** *See also* diflusinal

Novo-Diltiazem, Novo-Diltiazem HCl ER, Novo-Diltiazem CD, 300, **302-304.** *See also* diltiazem

Novo-Dipam 195. *See also* diazepam

Novo-Divalproex, 237, **242-243.** *See also* divalproex

Novo-Domperidone, 337, **338-339.** *See also* domperidone

Novo-Doxazosin, 178, **179-180.** *See also* doxazosin

Novo-Doxepin, 424. *See also* doxepin

Novo-Doxylin, 208. *See also* doxycycline

Novo-Fenofibrate Micronized, 347, **348-349.** *See also* fenofibrate

Novo-Fluconazole, 257, **258-259.** *See also* fluconazole

Novo-Fluoxetine, 250. *See also* fluoxetine

Novo-Flurprofen, 384, **385-387.** *See also* flurbiprofen

Novo-Flutamide, 225. *See also* flutamide

Novo-Fosinopril, 189, **190-191.** *See also* fosinopril

Novo-Gabapentin, 238, **243-244.** *See also* gabapentin

Novo-Gemfibrozil, 347. *See also* gemfibrozil

Novo-Gliclazide, 388. *See also* gliclazide

Novo-Glimepiride, 388. *See also* glimepiride

Novo-Glyburide, 388, **390-391.** *See also* glyburide

Novo-Hydrazide, 327, **332-334.** *See also* hydrochlorothiazide

Novo-Hydroxyzin, 261, **263-264.** *See also* hydroxyzine

Novo-Indapamide, 327. *See also* indapamide

Novo-Ipramide, 357, **360-362.** *See also* ipratropium

Novo-Ketoconazole, 257. *See also* ketoconazole

Novo-Ketorolac, 384, **385-387.** *See also* ketorolac

Novo-Ketotifen, 261. *See also* ketotifen

Novo-Lamotrigine, 238, **244-246.** *See also* lamotrigine

Novo-Leflunomide, 352. *See also* leflunomide

Novo-Levobunolol, 340. *See also* levobunolol

Novo-Levocarbidopa, 267, **268-270.** *See also* levodopa/carbidopa*

Novo-Levofloxacin, 206. *See also* levofloxacin

Novo-Lexin, 206, **210-211.** *See also* cephalexin

Novolin ge (30/70, 40/60, 50/50), **365**

Novolin ge NPH, 365, **366-369.** *See also* NPH

Novolin ge Toronto, 365, **366-369.** *See also* regular insulin

Novolin-Pen 4, 82

Novo-Lorazem, **195-197.** *See also* lorazepam

Novo-Lovastatin, 413, **414-415.** *See also* lovastatin

Novo-Medrone, **375-377.** *See also* medroxy-progesterone acetate

Novo-Meloxicam, **385-387.** *See also* meloxicam

Novo-Metformin, 388, **392-393.** *See also* metformin

Novo-Methacin, 384, **385-387.** *See also* indomethacin

Novo-Metoprolol, 290, **291-293.** *See also* metoprolol

Novo-Minocycline, 208. *See also* minocycline

Novo-Mirtazapine, Novo-Mirtazapine OD, 251. *See also* mirtazapine

NovoMix 30, 365, 369

Novo-Moclobemide, 250. *See also* moclobemide

Novo-Nabumetone, **385-387.** *See also* nabumetone

Novo-Nadolol, 291. *See also* nadolol

Novo-Naprox, Novo-Naprox-EC, Novo-Naprox Sodium, Novo-Naprox Sodium DS, Novo-Naprox SR, **385-387.** *See also* naproxen

Novo-Norfloxacin, 206. *See also* norfloxacin

Novo-Nortriptyline, 424. *See also* nortriptyline

Novo-Ofloxacin, 206. *See also* ofloxacin

Novo-Oxybutynin, **230-232.** *See also* oxybutynin

Novo-Paroxetine, 250. *See also* paroxetine

Novo-Pen VK, 207. *See also* penicillin V

Novo-Peridol, 276. *See also* haloperidol

Novo-Pindol, 291. *See also* pindolol

Novo-Pirocam, **385-387.** *See also* piroxicam

Novo-Pramine, 424. *See also* imipramine

Novo-Pranol, 291, **293-295.** *See also* propranolol

Novo-Pravastatin, 413, **414-415**

Novo-Prazin, 178. *See also* prazosin

Novo-Prednisone, 314, **319-322.** See also prednisone

Novo-Profen, 384, **385-387.** See also ibuprofen

Novo-Propamide, 388. See also chlorpropamide

Novo-Purol, 426, **427-428.** See also allopurinol

NovoRapid, 365, **366-369.** See also aspart

Novo-Risperidone, 277, **280-282.** See also risperidone

Novo-Rythro Estolate, 207. See also erythromycin

Novo-Rythro Ethylsuccinate, 207. See also erythromycin

Novo-Selegiline, 267. See also selegiline

Novo-Semide, 327, **328-330.** See also furosemide

Novo-Sertraline, 250. See also sertraline

Novo-Simvastatin, 413, **414-415.** See also simvastatin

Novo-Sotalol, 291. See also sotalol

Novo-Spiroton, 327, **330-332.** See also spironolactone

Novo-Spirozine*, 327, **330-332, 332-334.** See also hydrochlorothiazide; spironolactone

Novo-Sumatriptan, **408-410.** See also sumatriptan

Novo-Sundac, **385-387.** See also sulindac

Novo-Temazepam, 195. See also temazepam

Novo-Terazosin, 178. See also terazosin

Novo-Terbinafine, 257, **259-261.** See also terbinafine

Novo-Tiaprofenic, **385-387.** See also tiaprofenic acid

Novo-Ticlopodine, 272. See also ticlopidine

Novo-Timol, 291. See also timolol

Novo-Topiramate, 238, **248-249.** See also topiramate

Novo-Trazodone, 251. See also trazodone

Novo-Triamzide*, 327, **332-334.** See also hydrochlorothiazide; triamterene

Novo-Trimel*, Novo-Trimel DS*, Novo-Trimel Oral Suspension*, 207, **221-222.** See also sulfamethoxazole/trime-thoprim

Novo-Triptyn, **424-426.** See also amitriptyline

Novo-Valproic, 238, **242-243.** See also valproic acid

Novo-Verapamil SR, 300. See also verapamil

Novo-Warfarin, 232, **233-235.** See also warfarin

Novo-Zopiclone, 195, **198-199.** See also zopiclone

Nozinan Injectable, Nozinan Syrup, Nozinan Tablets, 277. See also methotrimeprazine

NPH, 117, 365, **366-369.** See also insulin

NRTIS. See nucleoside or nucleotide reverse transcriptase inhibitors

NSAIDS. See non-steroidal anti-inflammatory drugs

Nu-Acebutolol, 290. See also acebutolol

Nu-Acyclovir, **288-290.** See also acyclovir

Nu-Alpraz, 194. See also alprazolam

Nu-Amilzide*, 327, **332-334.** See also amiloride; hydrochlorothiazide

Nu-Amoxi, 207, **219-220.** See also amoxicillin

Nu-Ampi, 207. See also ampicillin

Nu-Atenol, 290, **291-293.** See also atenolol

Nu-Baclo, 411. See also baclofen

Nu-Beclomethasone, 313. See also beclomethasone

Nu-Bromazepam, 194. See also bromazepam

Nu-Capto, 189, **190-191.** See also captopril

Nu-Carbamazepine, 237, **238-240.** See also carbamazepine

Nu-Cefaclor, 206. See also cefaclor

Nu-Cephalex, 206, **210-211.** See also cephalexin

nucleoside reverse transcriptase inhibitors, 135, 282

Nu-Clonazepam, 195, 237, **240-242.** See also clonazepam

Nu-Clonidine, 176. See also clonidine

Nu-Cloxi, 207. See also cloxacillin

Nu-Cotrimox*, Nu-Cotrimox DS*, Nu-Cotrimox Oral Suspension*, 207, **221-222.** See also sulfamethoxazole/trimet hoprim

Nu-Cromolyn, 357

Nu-Cyclobenzaprine, **411-413.** See also cyclobenzaprine

Nu-Desipramine, 424. See also desipramine

Nu-Diclo, Nu-Diclo SR, 384, **385-387.** See also diclofenac

Nu-Diflunisal, 384, **385-387.** See also diflunisal

Nu-Diltiaz,Nu-Diltiaz-CD 300, **302-304.** See also diltiazem

Nu-Divalproex, 237, **242-243.** See also divalproex

Nu-Domperidone, 337, **338-339.** See also domperidone

Nu-Doxycycline. See also doxycycline

Nu-Erythromycin-S, 207. See also erythromycin

Nu-Fenofibrate, 347, **348-349.** See also fenofibrate

Nu-Fluoxetine, 250. *See also* fluoxetine

Nu-Flurbiprofen, 384, **385-387.** *See also* flurbiprofen

Nu-Gemfibrozil, 347. *See also* gemfibrozil

Nu-Glyburide, 388, **390-391.** *See also* glyburide

Nu-Ibuprofen 384, **385-387.** *See also* ibuprofen

Nu-Indapamide, 327. *See also* indapamide

Nu-Indo, 384, **385-387.** *See also* indomethacin

Nu-Ipratropium, 357, **360-362.** *See also* ipratropium

Nu-Ketoprofen-SR, 384, **385-387.** *See also* ketoprofen

Nu-Levocarb, 267, **268-270.** *See also* levodopa/carbidopa

Nu-Lovastatin, 413, **414-415.** *See also* lovastatin

Nu-Loxapine, 277. *See also* loxapine

Nu-Medopa, **176-178.** *See also* methyldopa

Nu-Mefenamic, **385-387.** *See also* mefenamic acid

Nu-Metformin, 388, **392-393.** *See also* metformin

Nu-Metoclopramide, 338. *See also* metoclopramide

Nu-Metop, 290, **291-293.** *See also* metoprolol

Nu-Moclobemide, 250. *See also* moclobemide

Nu-Naprox, **385-387.** *See also* naproxen

Nu-Nifed, 300. *See also* nifedipine

Nu-Nifedipine-PA, 300. *See also* nifedipine

Nu-Nortriptylene, 424. *See also* nortriptyline

Nu-Oxybutynin, **230-232.** *See also* oxybutynin

Nu-Pen-VK, 207. *See also* penicillin V

Nu-Pindol, 291. *See also* pindolol

Nu-Pirox, **385-387.** *See also* piroxicam

Nu-Pravastatin, 413, **414-415.** *See also* pravastatin

Nu-Prazo, 178. *See also* prazosin

Nu-Prochlor, 277. *See also* prochlorperazine

Nu-Propranolol, 291, **293-295.** *See also* propranolol

Nu-Salbutamol Solution, 356, **357-359.** *See also* salbutamol

Nu-Selegiline, 267. *See also* selegiline

Nu-Sertraline, 250. *See also* sertraline

Nu-Sotalol, 291. *See also* sotalol

Nu-Sulindac, **385-387.** *See also* sulindac

Nu-Temazepam 195. *See also* temazepam

Nu-Terazosin, 178. *See also* terazosin

Nu-Tetra, 208, **223-224.** *See also* tetracycline

Nu-Tiaprofenic, **385-387.** *See also* tiaprofenic acid

Nu-Ticlopodine, 272. *See also* ticlopidine

Nu-Timolol, 291. *See also* timolol

Nu-Trazodone, Nu-Trazodone-D, 251. *See also* trazodone

Nu-Triazide*, 327, **332-334.** *See also* hydrochlorothiazide; triamterene

Nu-Trimipramine, 424. *See also* trimipramine

Nu-Valproic, 238, **242-243.** *See also* valproic acid

NuvaRing*, 306. *See also* ethinyl estradiol; etonogestrel

Nu-Verap 300. *See also* verapamil

Nu-Zopiclone, 195, **198-199.** *See also* zopiclone

Nyaderm, 257. *See also* nystatin

nystatin, 257

• *O* •

OC, OCT. *See* oral contraceptive therapy

Ocufen, 384, **385-387.** *See also* flurbiprofen

Ocuflox, 206. *See also* ofloxacin

ofloxacin, 112, 206

Ogen, 374, **375-377.** *See also* estropipate

olanzapine, 11, **277-279,** 488

olopatadine, 261

olsalazine, 187

omeprazole, 400

ondansetron, 150

Optimine, 261. *See also* azatadine

Optimyxin Plus Solution, 205, **208-210.** *See also* neomycin

Oracort, 314. *See also* triamcinolone

oral contraceptive therapy, 306, **307-309**

oral contraceptives, 97, 115, 123, 134, 148, 153, 466, 467

Orap, 277. *See also* pimozide

orlistat, 150, **265-266**

Ortho 0.5/35*, 306, **307-309.** *See also* ethinyl estradiol; norethindrone

Ortho 1/35*, 306, **307-309.** *See also* ethinyl estradiol; norethindrone

Ortho 7/7/7 *, 306, **307-309.** *See also* ethinyl estradiol; norethindrone

Ortho-Cept*, 306, **307-309.** *See also* desogestrel; ethinyl estradiol

oseltamivir, 142, 288

Ostac, 296. *See also* clodronate

Otrivin, 317

oxaprozin, **385-387**

oxazepam, 195, 488

oxcarbazepine, 238

Oxeze Turbuhaler, 356. *See also* formoterol
oxprenolol, 291
oxybutynin, 139, **230-232**, 435
oxycodone, 129, **378-380**
OxyContin, **378-380**. *See also* oxycodone
Oxy-IR, **378-380**. *See also* oxycodone
Oxytrol, **230-232**. *See also* oxybutynin

• *p* •

Panectyl, 261. *See also* trimeprazine
Pantoloc, **400-401**, 487. *See also* pantoprazole
pantoprazole, **400-401**
papaverine, 124
Pariet, 400. *See also* rabeprazole
Parlodel, 267, **335-337**. *See also* bromocriptine
Parnate, 250. *See also* tranylcypromine
paromomycin, 205
paroxetine, 148, 250
Parsitan, 267. *See also* ethopropazine
Patanol, 261. *See also* olopatadine
Paxil, Paxil CR, 250. *See also* paroxetine
PCE, 207. *See also* erythromycin
PDE5 inhibitors. *See* phosphodiesterase type 5 inhibitors
Pediapred, 314. *See also* prednisolone
Pediazole*, 207. *See also* erythromycin; sulfisoxazole
Pegasys RBV*, 288. *See also* ribavirin
Pegetron*, 288. *See also* ribavirin
penicillamine, 145
penicillin V, 207
penicillins, 23, 161, 164, 207, 211, **219-220**, 432, 433, 482
Penlac, 257. *See also* ciclopirox

Pennsaid, 384, **385-387**. *See also* diclofenac
Pentasa, **187-188**. *See also* 5-aminosalicylic acid
pentazocine, 378
Pepcid, 23, 126, 164. *See also* famotidine
Percocet*, **378-380**. *See also* acetaminophen; oxycodone
Percocet-Demi*, **378-380**. *See also* acetaminophen; oxycodone
Percodan*, **378-380**, 460. *See also* ASA; oxycodone
pergolide, 267
perindopril, 189, **190-191**
Permax, 267. *See also* pergolide
perphenazine, 277
Persantine, 272. *See also* dipyridamole
phenelzine, 250
phenobarbital, 123, 238
phentolamine, 124
phenytoin, 40, 123, 238, **246-248**
phosphodiesterase type 5 (PDE5) inhibitors, 124, 147, 179, 181
pilocarpine, 341, **345-346**
Pilopine HS, 341, **345-346**. *See also* pilocarpine
pimecrolimus, 121, 156, 167, 352
pimozide, **277**
pinaverium, 143, 338
pindolol, 291
pioglitazone, 118, 388, **394-396**
piroxicam, **385-387**
pivampicillin, 207
Plan B. *See* morning-after pill
Plaquenil, 351. *See also* hydroxychloroquine
Plavix, 272, **274-276**. *See also* clopidogrel
Plendil, 300. *See also* felodipine
PMS-Alendronate, **296-298**. *See also* alendronate
PMS-Amiodarone, **200-202**. *See also* amiodarone

PMS-Atenolol, 290, **291-293**. *See also* atenolol
PMS-Azithromycin, 206, **216-217**. *See also* azithromycin
PMS-Baclofen, 411. *See also* baclofen
PMS-Bicalutamide, 225, **226-227**. *See also* bicalutamide
PMS-Brimonidine Tartrate, 340, **341-342**. *See also* brimonidine
PMS-Bromocriptine, 267, **335-337**. *See also* bromocriptine
PMS-Butorphanol, 377. *See also* butorphanol
PMS-Captopril, 189, **190-191**. *See also* captopril
PMS-Carbamazepine, 237, **238-240**. *See also* carbamazepine
PMS-Carvedilol, 291. *See also* carvedilol
PMS-Cholestyramine, 304. *See also* cholestyramine resin
PMS-Cilazapril, 189, **190-191**. *See also* cilazapril
PMS-Ciprofloxacin, 206, **212-213**. *See also* ciprofloxacin
PMS-Citalopram, 250, **253-254**. *See also* citalopram
PMS-Clonazepam, 195, 237, **240-242**. *See also* clonazepam
PMS-Cyclobenzaprine, **411-413**. *See also* cyclobenzaprine
PMS-Desipramine, 424. *See also* desipramine
PMS-Desonide, 315. *See also* desonide
PMS-Dexamethasone, drops, elixir, 314. *See also* dexamethasone
PMS-Diclofenac, PMS-Diclofenac SR, 384, **385-387**. *See also* diclofenac

PMS-Domperidone, 337,
338-339. *See also*
domperidone
PMS-Fenofibrate Micro,
347, **348-351.** *See also*
fenofibrate
PMS-Fluoxetine, 250. *See
also* fluoxetine
PMS-Gabapentin, 238,
243-244. *See also*
gabapentin
PMS-Gemfibrozil, 347. *See
also* gemfibrozil
PMS-Glyburide, 388,
390-391. *See also*
glyburide
PMS-Hydrochlorothiazide,
327, **332-334.** *See also*
hydrochlorothiazide
PMS-Hydromorphone, 377.
See also
hydromorphone
PMS-Indapamide, 327. *See
also* indapamide
PMS-Lamotrigine, 238,
244-246. *See also*
lamotrigine
PMS-Levobunolol, 340. *See
also* levobunolol
PMS-Lithium Carbonate,
371, **372-373.** *See also*
lithium
PMS-Lithium Citrate, 371,
372-373. *See also*
lithium
PMS-Lorazepam, **195-197.**
See also lorazepam
PMS-Lovastatin, 413,
414-415. *See also*
lovastatin
PMS-Loxapine, 277. *See
also* loxapine
PMS-Meloxicam, **385-387.**
See also meloxicam
PMS Metformin, 388,
392-393. *See also*
metformin
PMS-Methylphenidate,
416-418. *See also*
methylphenidate
PMS-Metoprolol-L, 290,
291-293. *See also*
metoprolol
PMS-Mirtazapine, 251. *See
also* mirtazapine
PMS-Moclobemide, 250. *See
also* moclobemide
PMS-Morphine Sulfate SR,
378. *See also* morphine

PMS-Oxybutynin, **230-232.**
See also oxybutynin
PMS-Oxycodone-
Acetaminophen*,
378-380. *See also*
oxycodone
PMS-Paroxetine, 250. *See
also* paroxetine
PMS-Phenobarbital, 238.
See also phenobarbital
PMS-Pravastatin, 413,
414-415. *See also*
pravastatin
PMS-Risperidone, 277,
280-282. *See also*
risperidone
PMS-Sertraline, 250. *See
also* sertraline
PMS-Simvastatin, 413,
414-415. *See also*
simvastatin
PMS-Sotalol, 291. *See also*
sotalol
PMS-Sumatriptan, **408-410.**
See also sumatriptan
PMS-Terazosin, 178. *See
also* terazosin
PMS-Terbinafine, 257,
259-261. *See also*
terbinafine
PMS-Timolol, 291, 340,
342-343. *See also*
timolol
PMS-Topiramate, 238,
248-249. *See also*
topiramate
PMS-Trazodone, 251. *See
also* trazodone
PMS-Valproic Acid, 238,
242-243. *See also*
valproic acid
PMS-Valproic Acid EC, 238,
242-243. *See also*
valproic acid
PMS-Zopiclone, 195,
198-199. *See also*
zopiclone
podofilox, 168
polymyxin-bacitracin, 114
Polypill*, 483
Pondocillin, 207. *See also*
pivampicillin
potassium-sparing
diuretics, 52, 122, 327,
330-332
PPIs. *See* proton pump
inhibitors
pramipexole, 156, 267,
270-271

Pravachol, 413, **414-415.**
See also pravastatin
pravastatin, 413, **414-415**
prazosin, 178
Pred Forte, 314, **317-319.**
See also prednisolone
Pred Mild, 314, **317-319.**
See also prednisolone
prednicarbate, 315
prednisolone, 314, **317-319**
prednisone, 97, 107, 141,
147, 314, **319-322**
Premarin Tablets, 374,
375-377. *See also*
conjugated estrogens
Premarin Vaginal Cream,
374, **375-377.** *See also*
conjugated estrogens
premixed insulin, 365, 369
Premplus Cycle Tablets,
375-377. *See also*
conjugated estrogen;
medroxy-progesterone
acetate
Premplus Tablets, **375-377.**
See also conjugated
estrogen; medroxy-
progesterone acetate
Prepulsid, 14. *See also*
cisapride
Preterax*, 189, **190-191,**
327. *See also*
indapamide; perindopril
Prevacid, 400. *See also*
lansoprazole
Prevacid Fas Tab, 400. *See
also* lansoprazole
Prevex HC, 315, **325-326.**
See also hydrocortisone
Prexige, 384, **385-387.** *See
also* lumiracoxib
primidone, 123, 162, 238
Prinivil, 189, **190-191.** *See
also* lisinopril
Prinzide*, 189, **190-191,**
327, **332-334.** *See also*
hydrochlorothiazide;
lisinopril
probenecid, 128
prochlorperazine, 150, 277
Prochlorperazine Mesylate
Injection, 277. *See also*
prochlorperazine
Proctodan HC*, 315. *See
also* hydrocortisone
Proctofoam HC*, 315. *See
also* hydrocortisone

Proctol*, 205, 315. *See also*
framycetin;
hydrocortisone
Proctosedyl*, 205, 315. *See also* framycetin;
hydrocortisone
Procytox, 351. *See also*
cyclophosphamide*
progesterone, **375-377**
progestin, 145, **375-377**
Prograf, 352. *See also*
tacrolimus
Prolopa, 267. *See also*
levodopa/benserazide*
Prometrium, **375-377**, 437.
See also progesterone
Propaderm, 315. *See also*
betamethasone
Propecia, **182-183**. *See also*
finasteride
propoxyphene, 378
propranolol, 129, 138, 162,
291, **293-295**, 435, 460
Propyl-Thyracil, 283,
284-285. *See also*
propylthiouracil
propylthiouracil, 21, 283,
284-285, 446
Proscar, **182-183**. *See also*
finasteride
prostaglandin analog eye
drops, 127
prostaglandin analogs, 341
protease inhibitors, 135,
283. *See also* HAART
proton pump inhibitors,
126, 164, **399-401**
Protopic, 352. *See also*
tacrolimus
Provera-Pak, **375-377**. *See*
also medroxy-
progesterone acetate
Provera Tablets, **375-377**.
See also medroxy-
progesterone acetate
Prozac, 250. *See also*
fluoxetine
psoralens, 167
Pulmicort Nebuamp, 357.
See also budesonide
Pulmicort Turbuhaler, 357.
See also budesonide
pyrazinamide, 163, 285
pyridoxine. *See* vitamin B6

• *Q* •

quetiapine, **277**, 488
quinapril, 189, **190-191**

quinine, 149
Qvar, 357. *See also*
beclomethasone

• *R* •

rabeprazole, 400
radioactive iodine, 138, 283
raloxifene, 152, 404,
405-406
ramipril, 189, **190-191**
RAN-Atenolol, 290, **291-293**.
See also atenolol
RAN-Carvedilol, 291. *See*
also carvedilol
RAN-Ciprofloxacin, 206,
212-213. *See also*
ciprofloxacin
RAN-Citalopram, 250,
253-254. *See also*
citalopram
RAN-Domperidone, 337,
338-339. *See also*
domperidone
RAN-Fentanyl Transdermal
System, 377. *See also*
fentanyl
RAN-Lovastatin, 413,
414-415. *See also*
lovastatin
RAN-Metformin, 388,
392-393. *See also*
metformin
RAN-Zopiclone, 195,
198-199. *See also*
zopiclone
Rapamune, 352. *See also*
sirolimus
rapid-acting insulins, 365,
366-369
rasagiline, 153, 267
ratio-Aclavulanate*, 207,
219-220. *See also*
amoxicillin; clavulanate
ratio-Acyclovir, **288-290**.
See also acyclovir
ratio-Amcinonide, 315. *See*
also amcinonide
ratio-Amiodarone, **200-202**.
See also amiodarone
ratio-Atenolol, 290,
291-293. *See also*
atenolol
ratio-Azithromycin, 206,
216-217. *See also*
azithromycin
ratio-Baclofen, 411. *See also*
baclofen

ratio-Beclomethasone AQ,
313. *See also*
beclomethasone
ratio-Bicalutamide, 225,
226-227. *See also*
bicalutamide
ratio-brimonidine, 340,
341-342. *See also*
brimonidine
ratio-Calmydone*, 377. *See*
also doxylamine;
hydrocodone
ratio-Carvedilol, 291. *See*
also carvedilol
ratio-Ciprofloxacin, 206,
212-213. *See also*
ciprofloxacin
ratio-Citalopram, 250,
253-254. *See also*
citalopram
ratio-Clindamycin, 206,
214-216. *See also*
clindamycin
ratio-Clobazam, 194, 237.
See also clobazam
ratio-Clobetasol, 315. *See*
also clobetasol
ratio-Clonazepam, 195, 237,
240-242. *See also*
clonazepam
ratio-Codeine, 377. *See also*
codeine
ratio-Coristex-DH*, 377. *See*
also hydrocodone
ratio-Cyclobenzaprine,
411-413. *See also*
cyclobenzaprine
ratio-Desipramine, 424. *See*
also desipramine
ratio-Dexamethasone, 314.
See also dexamethasone
ratio-Diltiazem CD, 300,
302-304. *See also*
diltiazem
ratio-Domperidone, 337,
338-339. *See also*
domperidone
ratio-Ectosone, 315. *See*
also betamethasone
ratio-Fenofibrate MC, 347,
348-351. *See also*
fenofibrate
ratio-Flunisolide, 313, 314.
See also flunisolide
ratio-Fluoxetine, 250. *See*
also fluoxetine

ratio-Gabapentin, 238, **243-244.** *See also* gabapentin

ratio-Gentamicin, 205. *See also* gentamicin

ratio-Glimepiride, 388. *See also* glimepiride

ratio-Glyburide, 388, **390-391.** *See also* glyburide

ratio-Ipratropium, ratio-Ipratropium UDV, 357, **360-362.** *See also* ipratropium

ratio-Ketorolac, 384, **385-387.** *See also* ketorolac

ratio-Lamotrigine, 238, **244-246.** *See also* lamotrigine

ratio-Levobunolol, 340. *See also* levobunolol

ratio-Lovastatin, 413, **414-415.** *See also* lovastatin

ratio-Meloxicam, **385-387.** *See also* meloxicam

ratio-Metformin, 388, **392-393.** *See also* metformin

ratio-Methotrexate, 352, **353-355.** *See also* methotrexate

ratio-Minocycline, 208. *See also* minocycline

ratio-Mirtazapine, 251. *See also* mirtazapine

ratio-Mometasone, 314. *See also* mometasone

ratio-Morphine, ratio-Morphine SR, 378. *See also* morphine

ratio-MPA, **375-377.** *See also* medroxy-progesterone acetate

ratio-Nortriptylene, 424. *See also* nortriptyline

ratio-Nystatin, 257. *See also* nystatin

ratio-Ocycocet*, **378-380.** *See also* acetaminophen; oxycodone

ratio-Oxycodan*, **378-380.** *See also* ASA; oxycodone

ratio-Paroxetine, 250. *See also* paroxetine

ratio-Pravachol, 413, **414-415.** *See also* pravastatin

ratio-Prednisolone, 314, **317-319.** *See also* prednisolone

ratio-Proctosone, 205. *See also* framycetin

ratio-Risperidone, 277, **280-282.** *See also* risperidone

ratio-Salbutamol HFA, 356, **357-359,** 487. *See also* salbutamol

ratio-Sertraline, 250. *See also* sertraline

ratio-Simvastatin, 413, **414-415.** *See also* simvastatin

ratio-Sotalol, 291. *See also* sotalol

ratio-Sumatriptan, **408-410.** *See also* sumatriptan

ratio-Temazepam, 195. *See also* temazepam

ratio-Terazosin, 178. *See also* terazosin

ratio-Topilene, 315. *See also* betamethasone

ratio-Topiramate, 238, **248-249.** *See also* topiramate

ratio-Topisalic*, 315. *See also* betamethasone; salicyclic acid

ratio-Toposone, 315. *See also* betamethasone

ratio-Trazadone, 251. *See also* trazadone

ratio-Triacomb*, 205, **208-210,** 257, 315. *See also* neomycin; nystatin; triamcinolone

ratio-Valproic, 238, **242-243.** *See also* valproic acid

ratio-Zopiclone, 195, **198-199.** *See also* zopiclone

regular insulin, 365, **366-369**

Rejuva-A, **402-404.** *See also* tretinoin

Relpax, 408. *See also* eletriptan

Remeron, Remeron RD, 251. *See also* mirtazapine

Reminyl, Reminyl ER, 184. *See also* galantamine

Renedil, 300. *See also* felodipine

Renova, **402-404.** *See also* tretinoin

repaglinide, 21, 118, 388, **396-397**

ReQuip, 267. *See also* ropinirole

Rescriptor, 283. *See also* delavirdine

Restoril, 195. *See also* temazepam

Retin-A, Retin-A Micro, **402-404.** *See also* tretinoin

retinoids, 96, 97, **401-404**

Retisol-A, **402-404.** *See also* tretinoin

Retrovir (AZT), 282. *See also* zidovudine

Revatio, 397, **398-399.** *See also* sildenafil

Reyataz, 283. *See also* atazanavir

Rhinalar, 313. *See also* flunisolide

Rhinocort Aqua, 313. *See also* budenoside

Rhinocort Turbuhaler, 357. *See also* budesonide

Rho-Nitro Pumpspray, 381. *See also* nitroglycerin

Rhotral, 290. *See also* acebutolol

Rhovane, 195, **198-199.** *See also* zopiclone

ribavirin, 133, 288

Rifadin, 285. *See also* rifampin

rifampin, 163, 285

Rifater*, 285, **286-287.** *See also* isoniazid; pyrazinamide; rifampin

rimexolone, 314

risedronate, **296-298**

Risperdal, Risperdal Consta, Risperdal M-Tab, Risperdal Oral Solution, 277, **280-282.** *See also* risperidone

risperidone, 277, **280-282,** 488

Ritalin, Ritalin SR, **416-418,** 445. *See also* methylphenidate

ritonavir, 283

rituximab, 147. *See also* biological response modifiers

Rivanase AQ, 313. *See also* beclomethasone

rivastigmine, 184

Rivotril, 195, 237, **240-242.** *See also* clonazepam
rizatriptan, 408
Robax Platinum*, 384, **385-387.** *See also* ibuprofen; methocarbamol
Rofact, 285. *See also* rifampin
rofecoxib, 14
ropinirole, 156, 267
Rosasol, 207, **217-219.** *See also* metronidazole
rosiglitazone, 118, 388, **394-396,** 484
rosuvastatin, 146, 413, **414-415**
Rovamycine, 207. *See also* spiramycin

• S •

SAB-Prochlorperazine Suppository, 277. *See also* prochlorperazine
SAB-Proctomyxin HC, 205. *See also* framycetin
Sabril, 238. *See also* vigabatrin
Salazopyrin, 187. *See also* sulfasalazine
Salazopyrin En-Tabs, 187, 352. *See also* sulfasalazine
salbutamol, 356, **357-359,** 360, 361, 363, 364, 371, 434
salicylic acid, 168
salmeterol, 106, 356, **359-360**
Salofalk, **187-188.** *See also* 5-aminosalicylic acid
Sandoz Acebutolol, 290. *See also* acebutolol
Sandoz Amiodarone, **200-202.** *See also* amiodarone
Sandoz Atenolol, 290, **291-293.** *See also* atenolol
Sandoz Azithromycin, 206, **216-217.** *See also* azithromycin
Sandoz Bicalutamide, 225, **226-227.** *See also* bicalutamide
Sandoz Bisoprolol, 290. *See also* bisoprolol

Sandoz Bupropion SR, 251, **255-257.** *See also* bupropion
Sandoz Carbamazepine, 237, **238-240.** *See also* carbamazepine
Sandoz Ciprofloxacin, 206, **212-213.** *See also* ciprofloxacin
Sandoz Citalopram, 250, **253-254.** *See also* citalopram
Sandoz Clonazepam, 195, 237, **240-242.** *See also* clonazepam
Sandoz Cortimyxin Ophthalmic Ointment*, 205, **208-210,** 314. *See also* hydrocortisone; neomycin
Sandoz Cortimyxin Otic Solution*, 205, **208-210,** 314. *See also* hydrocortisone; neomycin; polymyxin-bacitracin
Sandoz Cyclosporine, 351. *See also* cyclosporine*
Sandoz Diclofenac, Sandoz Diclofenac Rapide, Sandoz Diclofenac SR, 384, **385-387.** *See also* diclofenac
Sandoz Diltiazem CD, Sandoz Diltiazem D, 300, **302-304.** *See also* Diltiazem
Sandoz Famciclovir, 288. *See also* famciclovir
Sandoz Felodipine, 300. *See also* felodipine
Sandoz Fluoxetine, 250. *See also* fluoxetine
Sandoz Gliclazide, 388. *See also* gliclazide
Sandoz Glimepiride, 388. *See also* glimepiride
Sandoz Glyburide, 388, **390-391.** *See also* glyburide
Sandoz Leflunomide, 352. *See also* leflunomide
Sandoz Lovastatin, 413, **414-415.** *See also* lovastatin
Sandoz Metformin FC, 388, **392-393.** *See also* metformin

Sandoz Metoprolol (Type L), 290, **291-293.** *See also* metoprolol
Sandoz Minocycline, 208. *See also* minocycline
Sandoz Mirtazapine, Sandoz Mirtazapine FC, 251. *See also* mirtazapine
Sandoz Nabumetone, **385-387.** *See also* nabumetone
Sandoz Nitrazepam, 195. *See also* nitrazepam
Sandoz Opticort*, 205, 314. *See also* dexamethasone; framycetin
Sandoz Paroxetine, 250. *See also* paroxetine
Sandoz Pentasone*, 205, 315. *See also* betamethasone; gentamicin
Sandoz Pindolol, 291. *See also* pindolol
Sandoz Prednisolone, 314, **317-319.** *See also* prednisolone
Sandoz Proctomyxin*, 205, 315. *See also* framycetin; hydrocortisone
Sandoz Risperidone, 277, **280-282.** *See also* risperidone
Sandoz Salbutamol, 356, **357-359.** *See also* salbutamol
Sandoz Sertraline, 250. *See also* sertraline
Sandoz Simvastatin, 413, **414-415.** *See also* simvastasin
Sandoz Sotalol, 291. *See also* sotalol
Sandoz Sumatriptan, **408-410.** *See also* sumatriptan
Sandoz Terbinafine, 257, **259-261.** *See also* terbinafine
Sandoz Ticlopidine, 272. *See also* ticlopidine
Sandoz Timolol, 340, **342-343.** *See also* timolol

Sandoz Topiramate, 238, **248-249.** *See also* topiramate
Sandoz Valproic, Sandoz Valproic EC, 238, **242-243.** *See also* valproic acid
Sandoz Zopiclone, 195, **198-199.** *See also* zopiclone
saquinavir, 67, 283
Sarna HC, 315, **325-326.** *See also* hydrocortisone
second-generation antipsychotics, 109, 157, 277
Sectral, 290. *See also* acebutolol
Select 1/35*, 306, **307-309.** *See also* ethinyl estradiol; norethindrone
selective estrogen receptor modulators, 111
selective serotonin reuptake inhibitors, 102, 116, 125, 151, 250
selective-norepinephrine reuptake inhibitors, 125
selegiline 153, 267
Serc, **349-351.** *See also* betahistine
Serevent, Serevent Diskhaler Disk, Serevent Diskus, 356, **359-360.** *See also* salmeterol
SERMs. *See* selective estrogen receptor modulators
Seroquel, 277. *See also* quetiapine
serotonin antagonists, 150
serotonin receptor agonists, 129
serotonin receptor partial agonist, 338
serotonin-norepinephrine reuptake inhibitors, 102, 116, 250
sertraline, 250
short-acting anticholinergic agents, 357
short-acting beta-2 agonists, 356, 360, 361, 363, 364, 371
sibutramine, 150, 265
sildenafil, 65, 124, 179, 181, 382, 397, **398-399**

simvastatin, 62, 88, 413, **414-415,** 474
Sinemet, Sinemet CR, 267, **268-270.** *See also* levodopa/carbidopa
Sinequan, 424. *See also* doxepin
Singulair, **370-371.** *See also* montelukast
Sintrom, 232. *See also* nicoumalone*
sirolimus, 352
skeletal muscle relaxants, 125, **411-415**
SNRIs. *See* serotonin-norepinephrine reuptake inhibitors
Sodium Aurothiomalate, 351. *See also* gold
sodium bicarbonate, 144, 186
sodium cromoglycate, 99, 107, 357. *See also* mast cell stabilizers
Sofracort*, 205, 314, **323.** *See also* dexamethasone; framycetin
Soframycin Nasal Spray, 205. *See also* framycetin
Soframycin Skin Ointment, 205. *See also* framycetin
Soframycin Sterile Eye Drops, 205. *See also* framycetin
Soframycin Sterile Eye Ointment, 205. *See also* framycetin
Sofra-Tulle, 205. *See also* framycetin
Solangé, **402-404.** *See also* tretinoin
Soriatane, 402. *See also* acitretin
sotalol, 291
spiramycin, 207
Spiriva, 357, **362-363.** *See also* tiotropium
spironolactone, 52, 97, 122, 131, 134, 327, **330-332**
Sporanox Capsules, Sporanox Oral Solution, 257. *See also* itraconazole
SSRIs. *See* selective serotonin reuptake inhibitors

Starlix, 388. *See also* nateglinide
statins, 102, 113, 130, 144, 146, 160, 305, **413-415,** 483, 487
stavudine, 282
Stemetil, 277. *See also* prochlorperazine
steroids, 52, 79
steroid-sparing agents. *See* immunosuppressive drugs
Stieprox, 257. *See also* ciclopirox
Stieva-A, **402-404.** *See also* tretinoin
Stievamycin Preparations*, 207, **402-404.** *See also* erythromycin; tretinoin
stimulants, 108, **416-418**
Strattera, 250. *See also* atomoxetine
streptomycin, 163
sufinpyrazone, 128. *See also* uricosuric agents
sulfa drugs, 329, 331, 333, 391
sulfacetamide, 114, 207
Sulfacet-R*, 207. *See also* sulfacetamide; sulfur
sulfamethoxazole/ trimethoprim*, 97, 113, 154, 158, 165, 166, 207, **221-222,** 436, 441
sulfas, 38, 181, 207, **221-222**
sulfasalazine, 141, 186, 187, 352
sulfisoxazole, 207. *See also* sulfas
sulfonylurea drugs, 118, 188, 388
sulfur, 207. *See also* sulfas
sulindac, **385-387**
sumatriptan, 46, **408-410**
Supeudol, **378-380.** *See also* oxycodone
Suprefact, Suprefact Depot, 225. *See also* buserelin
Surgam, Surgam SR, **385-387.** *See also* tiaprofenic acid
Sustiva, 283. *See also* efavirenz
Symbicort Turbuhaler*, 107, 356, 357. *See also* budesonide; formoterol

Symmetrel, 267. *See also* amantadine
Synphasic*, **306**. *See also* ethinyl estradiol; norethindrone
Synthroid, **421-423,** 487. *See also* L-thyroxine (T4)

• *T* •

tacrolimus, 121, 156, 167, 352
tadalafil, 124, 397
Talwin Tablets, 378. *See also* pentazocine
Tamiflu, 288. *See also* oseltamivir
tamoxifen, 111, 224, 226
tamsulosin, 87, 155, 178, 178, **180-181**
Tapazole, 283, **284-285.** *See also* methimazole
taprimidone, 162
Tarka*, 189, **190-191,** 300. *See also* trandolapril; verapamil
Taro-Amcinonide, 315. *See also* amcinonide
Taro-Carbamazepine, 237, **238-240.** *See also* carbamazepine
Taro-Ciprofloxacin, 206, **212-213.** *See also* ciprofloxacin
Taro-Clindamycin, 206, **214-216.** *See also* clindamycin
Taro-Fluconazole, 257, **258-259.** *See also* fluconazole
Taro-Mometasone, 315, **316-317.** *See also* mometasone
Taro-Phenytoin, 238, **246-248.** *See also* phenytoin
Taro-Simvastatin, 413, **414-416.** *See also* simvastatin
Taro-Sone, 315. *See also* betamethasone
Taro-Terconazole, 258. *See also* terconazole
Taro-Warfarin, 232, **233-235.** *See also* warfarin
tazarotene, 96, 156, 402

Tazorac Cream, Tazorac Gel, 402. *See also* tazarotene
Tebrazid, 285. *See also* pyrazinamide
tegaserod, 143, 338
Tegretol, 237, **238-240.** *See also* carbamazepine
telmisartan, **192-194**
Telzir, 283. *See also* fosamprenavir
temazepam, 142, 195
Tenofovir, 282
Tenoretic*, 290, **291-293,** 327. *See also* atenolol; chlorthalidone
Tenormin, 290, **291-293.** *See also* atenolol
Tenoxicam, **385-387**
Tenuate, Tenuate Dospan, 265. *See also* diethylpropion
Terazol, 258. *See also* terconazole
terazosin, 155, 178
terbinafine, 162, 257, **259-261**
terbutaline, 356
teriparatide, 152
testosterone, 140, 145, 152, 418, **419-420**
tetracycline, 208, **223-224**
tetracyclines, 97, 126, 157, 161, 208, **222-224,** 444
Teveten, **192-194**
Teveten Plus*, **192-194,** 327, **332-334.** *See also* eprosartan; hydrochlorothiazide
thalidomide, 446
The Patch. *See* transdermal contraceptive patches
The Pill, 307. *See also* oral contraceptives
theophylline, 107, 112
thiazide diuretics, 122, 137, 327
thiazolidinediones, 118, 154, 388, **394-396**
thioridazine, 256
thiothixene, 277
Thyroid Hormone, 421. *See also* desiccated thyroid
Tiamol, 315. *See also* fluocinonide
tiaprofenic acid, **385-387**

Tiazac, Tiazac XC, 300, **302-304.** *See also* diltiazem
Ticlid, 272. *See also* ticlopidine
ticlopidine, 272
timolol, 291, 340, **342-343**
Timoptic, Timoptic-XE, 340, **342-343.** *See also* timolol
tinzaparin, 233, **235-237**
tiotropium, 357, **362-363**
tipranavir, 283
TOBI Tobramycin Inhalation Solution, 205. *See also* tobramycin
Tobradex*, 205, 314, **323.** *See also* dexamethasone; tobramycin
tobramycin, 205
Tobrex, 205. *See also* tobramycin
Tofranil, 424. *See also* imipramine
tolbutamide, 388
tolterodine, 139, 230
Topamax, 238, **248-249.** *See also* topiramate
Topicort, 315. *See also* desoximetasone
topiramate, 123, 129, 162, 238, **248-249**
Toradol, 384, **385-387.** *See also* ketorolac
tramadol, 152
Trandate, 291. *See also* labetalol
trandolapril, 189, **190-191**
tranquillizers, 488
transdermal contraceptive patch, 115, 306
Transderm-Nitro, 381, **382-383.** *See also* nitroglycerin
transvaginal contraceptive ring, 115, 306
tranylcypromine, 250
Trasicor, 291, 437. *See also* oxprenolol
Travatan, 341. *See also* travoprost
travoprost, 341
trazodone, 251
tretinoin, 96, 168, **402-404**
Triaderm, 315. *See also* triamcinolone
triamcinolone, 313, 314, 315

triamterene, 327
triazolam, 142, 195
Tri-Cyclen, 306, **307-309**
Tri-Cyclen LO*, 306,
   307-309. *See also*
   ethinyl estradiol;
   norgestimate
tricyclic antidepressants,
   102, 109, 116, 125, 129,
   143, 152, 239, 249, 489
trifluoperazine, 277
trifluridine, 288
trihexyphenidyl, 267
Trilafon, 277. *See also*
   perphenazine
Trileptal, 238. *See also*
   oxcarbazepine
trimebutine, 338
trimeprazine, 261
trimipramine, 424
Trimix*, 124, 125. *See also*
   alprostadil; papaverine;
   phentolamine
Trinalin*, 261. *See also*
   azatadine
Trinipatch, 381, **382-383.**
   See also nitroglycerin
Triphasil 21*, Triphasil 28*,
   306, **307-309.** *See also*
   ethinyl estradiol;
   levonorgestrel
triple therapy*, 164. *See*
   also clarithromycin;
   amoxicillin; proton
   pump inhibitors
Triquilar 21*, Triquilar 28*,
   306, **307-309.** *See also*
   ethinyl estradiol;
   levonorgestrel
Trizivir*, 282. *See also*
   abacavir; zidovudine
Trusopt, 341, **344-345.** *See*
   also dorzolamide
Truvada*, 282. *See also*
   emtricitabine; tenofovir
Turbuhaler, 80
Tussionex*, 377. *See also*
   hydrocodone
Twinject auto-injector, 99
Tylenol, 23. *See also*
   acetaminophen
Tylenol #3, 487
Tylenol with Codeine*, 377.
   See also codeine
type II 5 alpha-reductase
   inhibitors. *See* alpha-
   reductase inhibitors

typical antipsychotics. *See*
   first-generation
   antipsychotics
TZDs. *See*
   thiazolidinediones

• *U* •

upper gastrointestinal tract
   motility modifiers, 337,
   338-339. *See also*
   dopamine antagonists
uricosuric agents, 128
Uromax, **230-232.** *See also*
   oxybutynin

• *V* •

Vagifem Vaginal Cream,
   374-377. *See also* 17
   beta estradiol
valacyclovir, 114, 134, 158,
   288
valganciclovir, 288
Valisone Scalp Lotion, 315.
   See also betamethasone
Valisone-G*, 205, 315. *See*
   also betamethasone;
   gentamicin
Valium Roche Oral, 195. *See*
   also diazepam
valproate. *See* valproic acid
valproic acid, 109, 123, 238,
   242-243
valsartan, **192-194**
Valtrex, 288. *See also*
   valacyclovir
vardenafil, 124, 397
Vaseretic*, 189, **190-191,**
   327, **332-334.** *See also*
   enalapril;
   hydrochlorothiazide
Vasotec, 189, **190-191.** *See*
   also enalapril
venlafaxine, 148, 250,
   251-253
Ventodisk Diskhaler, 356,
   357-359. *See also*
   salbutamol
Ventolin Diskus, 356,
   357-359. *See also*
   salbutamol
Ventolin HFA, 356, **357-359.**
   See also salbutamol
Ventolin Nebules P.F., 356,
   357-359. *See also*
   salbutamol

Ventolin Oral Liquid, 356,
   357-359. *See also*
   salbutamol
Ventolin Respirator
   Solution, 356, **357-359.**
   See also salbutamol
verapamil, 103, 104, 144,
   300
Vesanoid, **402-404.** *See also*
   tretinoin
Vexol, 314. *See also*
   rimexolone
Vfend, 258. *See also*
   voriconazole
Viaderm-K.C., 205, **208-210.**
   See also neomycin
ViadermKC*, 315. *See also*
   hydrocortisone;
   triamcinolone
Viagra, 65, 180, 181, 382,
   397, **398-399.** *See also*
   sildenafil
Vibra-Tabs, 208. *See also*
   doxycycline
Videx, 282. *See also*
   didanosine
Videx EC, 282. *See also*
   didanosine
vigabatrin, 238
Vigamox, 206. *See also*
   moxifloxacin
Vioform Hydrocortisone*,
   257, 315, **325-326.** *See*
   also clioquinol;
   hydrocortisone
Vioxx, 14. *See also*
   rofecoxib
Viracept, 283. *See also*
   nelfinavir
Viramune, 283. *See also*
   nevirapine
Virazole, 288. *See also*
   ribavirin
Viread, 282. *See also*
   tenofovir
Viskazide*, 291, 327,
   332-334. *See also*
   hydrochlorothiazide;
   pindolol
Visken, 291. *See also*
   pindolol
Vitamin A, 266, 402
Vitamin A Acid, **402-404.**
   See also tretinoin
vitamin B6, 163, 262, 287
vitamin B12, 101, 392, 393,
   401

vitamin D, 144, 226, 229, 247, 266, 298, 322
vitamin E, 266
vitamin K, 233, 235, 266, 442
Voltaren, Voltaren Rapide, 384, **385-387.** *See also* diclofenac
Voltaren Ophtha, 384, **385-387.** *See also* diclofenac

• *W* •

warfarin, 68, 69, 104, 110, 160, 232, **233-235,** 442, 443, 460
Wellbutrin SR, Wellbutrin XL, 251, **255-257.** *See also* bupropion
Westcort Preparations, 315, **325-326.** *See also* hydrocortisone
Winpred, 314, **319-322.** *See also* prednisone

• *X* •

Xalacom*, 340, 341, **342-343, 346-347.** *See also* timolol; latanoprost
Xalatan, 341, **346-347.** *See also* latanoprost
Xanax, Xanax TS, 194. *See also* alprazolam
xanthine oxidase inhibitors, 128

Xatral, 178. *See also* alfuzosin
Xenical, **265-266.** *See also* orlistat

• *Y* •

Yasmin 21*, Yasmin 28*, 306, **307-309.** *See also* drospirenone; ethinyl estradiol

• *Z* •

zafirlukast, 370
Zalcitabine, 282
zaleplon, 142
zanamivir, 142, 288
Zarontin, 237. *See also* ethosuxamide
Zaroxolyn, 327. *See also* metolazone
Zatiden, 261. *See also* ketotifen
Zatidor, 261. *See also* ketotifen
Zelnorm, 338. *See also* tegaserod
Zerit, 282. *See also* staduvine
Zestoretic*, 189, **190-191,** 327, **332-334.** *See also* hydrochlorothiazide; lisinopril
Zestril, 189, **190-191.** *See also* lisinopril

Ziagen, 282. *See also* abacavir
zidovudine, 282
Zithromax, 206, **216-217.** *See also* azithromycin
Zocor, 413, **414-415,** 474. *See also* simvastasin
Zoladex 3.6mg, Zoladex LA, 225, **227-229.** *See also* goserelin
zolmitriptan, 408
Zoloft, 250. *See also* sertraline
Zomig, Zomig Nasal Spray, Zomig Rapimelt, 408. *See also* zolmitriptan
zopiclone, 142, 194, 195, **198-199**
Zovirax Cream, Zovirax Ointment, Zovirax Oral, **288-290.** *See also* acyclovir
Z-PAK, 206, **216-217.** *See also* azithromycin
zuclopenthixol, 277
Zyban, 251, **255-257.** *See also* bupropion
Zyloprim, 426, **427-428.** *See also* allopurinol
Zyprexa, Zyprexa IntraMuscular, Zyprexa Zydis, **277-279.** *See also* olanzapine

General Index

• A •

absorption of medication, 17–20, 91–92
acetylcholine, 99
acid-related diseases, 399
acne, 96–97, 223, 307, 401
active ingredient, 27
acute hepatitis, 133
acute labrynthitis, 120
Addison's disease, 97–98
ADHD. *See* attention-deficit/hyperactivity disorder
administering your medication. *See* taking your medication
adrenal glands, 97, 312–313
adrenaline, 83
adverse interactions. *See* drug interactions
adverse reactions. *See* side-effects
AeroChamber, 77
age, and drug choice, 38
agonist, 174
AIDS, 135, 282
ailments, common
   acne, 96–97
   Addison's disease, 97–98
   alcoholism, 98
   allergies, 98–99
   Alzheimer's disease, 99
   anemia, 100–101
   angina, 101–102
   anxiety disorders, 102–103
   arrhythmias, 103–104
   arthritis, 104–105
   asthma, 106–107
   athlete's foot, 107–108
   attention-deficit/hyperactivity disorder (ADHD), 108
   baldness, 108
   bedwetting, 109
   bipolar disorder, 109
   blood clots, 110
   cancer, 110–111
   chlamydia, 112
   chronic obstructive pulmonary disease (COPD), 112–113, 212
   claudication, 113
   cold sores, 114
   common cold, 114
   conjunctivitis, 114
   coronary artery disease, 101
   cough, 115–116
   depression, 116
   diabetes, 117–118
   diarrhea, 119
   dizziness, 119–120
   dyslipidemia, 146
   ear infections, 120–121
   eczema, 121
   edema, 121–122
   endocarditis prophylaxis, 122
   endometriosis, 123
   epilepsy, 123
   erectile dysfunction, 124–125
   essential tremor, 162
   fibromyalgia syndrome (FMS), 125
   flatulence, 125–126
   gastro-esophageal reflux disease (GERD), 126
   gastroenteritis, 126
   genital herpes, 133–134
   genital warts, 168
   glaucoma, 127
   gonorrhea, 127–128
   gout, 128
   headaches, 129
   heart attack, 130
   heart failure, 131–132
   hemorrhoids, 132
   hepatitis, viral, 132–133
   hirsutism, 134
   HIV/AIDS, 135
   hyperprolactinemia, 136
   hypertension, 136–138
   hyperthyroidism, 138
   hypothyroidism, 139
   infertility, 140
   inflammatory bowel disease (IBD), 140–141
   influenza, 141–142
   insomnia, 142
   irritable bowel syndrome (IBS), 143
   kidney failure, 143–144
   kidney stones, 144–145
   lipid disorders, 146–147
   lupus, 147
ailments, common
   menopause, 148
   menstrual cramps, 148
   multiple sclerosis (MS), 149
   muscle cramps, 149
   nausea, 150
   obesity, 150
   obsessive-compulsive disorder (OCD), 151
   osteoporosis, 151–152
   pain, 152
   Parkinson's disease, 152–153
   pneumonia, 153
   polycystic ovary syndrome (PCOS), 154
   prostatis, 154–155
   prostatism, 155
   psoriasis, 155–156
   reduced libido, 145
   restless legs syndrome (RLS), 156
   rosacea, 156–157
   schizophrenia, 157
   shingles, 157–158
   sinusitis, 158
   smoking cessation, 159
   stroke, 159–160
   syphilis, 160–161
   throat infections, 161
   toenail infections, 161–162
   tuberculosis (TB), 163
   ulcer, 163–165
   urinary incontinence, 139–140
   urinary tract infections, 165–166
   vaginal dryness, 166
   vaginal infections, 166–167
   vitiligo, 167
   vomiting, 150
   warts (skin), 168
alcohol
   and drug interactions, 47, 69, 442–443
   as non-medicinal ingredient, 29
alcoholism, 98

allergens, 98, 106
allergic reactions, 432–433
allergies
    anaphylactic reactions, 98
    drug allergies, 34, 38, 432–433
    information from your pharmacist, 48–49
    non-medicinal ingredients, 30
    severe allergic reactions, 460
    therapy, 98–99, 261–264
altered thinking, 457
Alzheimer's disease, 99, 183–186
ameba, 218
analog, 174
anaphylactic reactions, 98
anemia, 100–101, 174
angina, 101–102, 291, 293, 380–381, 382
anogenital warts, 168
antagonist, 174
anticholinergic side-effects, 457
anxiety disorders, 102–103, 194
aqueous humour, 127
arrhythmias, 103–104, 199
arthritis, 104–105, 128, 319, 352, 453
"as needed," 63
ascites, 330
asthma, 106–107, 319, 356, 370
atherosclerosis, 113, 124, 159, 190
athlete's foot, 107–108
atopic eczema (atopic dermatitis), 121
atrial fibrillation, 103, 291, 293
attention-deficit/hyperactivity disorder (ADHD), 108, 416, 450–451
autoantibodies, 97

• *B* •

back pocket, drug storage in, 84
bacterial meningitis, 33–34
bacterial vaginal infections, 166
bacterial vaginosis, 218

baldness, 108, 182
beaver fever, 218
bedwetting, 109, 424
behind-the-counter drugs, 24–25
benign prostatic hypertrophy, 155
best-selling prescription drug classes, 488
best-selling prescription drugs, 487
binding agents, 29
biohazard container, 85
bipolar disorder, 109, 278, 280, 371, 372
birth control pills, 64
bladder infections, 165
blister packs, 455
blocker, 174
blood clots, 110, 232, 271
blood counts, 174
blood pressure, drop in, 119
body mass index (BMI), 150
bone resorption, 296
brand-name drugs, 26, 27–29
brand names, 28
breast cancer, 111, 224–229, 405, 406
breast milk, 22
breastfeeding
    classification of drug safety, 447–448
    drug safety, 445–449
    infant, harm to, 447
    prescription drug use, 173, 446–448
    safety of medications, 39
    telling your doctor, 35
    telling your pharmacist, 44
breathing difficulties, 51
bronchitis, 153

• *C* •

C. difficile gastroenteritis, 218
CAMs, 25–26
Canadian Hypertension Education Program (CHEP), 137
Canadian International Pharmacy Association, 476
Canadian Verified Internet Pharmacy Practice Sites, 476

cancer, 110–111, 224–229
candida infections, 258
capsules, 66, 73. *See also* oral drugs
car, drug storage in, 84
cardiopulmonary resuscitation (CPR), 461
cardiovascular diseases, 300
cardioversion, 104
catastrophic drug plan, 479–480
celiac disease, 48, 92
cellular level, 20–21
cellulitis, 211, 216
cerebrovascular disease, 159
changing doses, 61
chicken-pox virus, 157, 289
"child-proof" pill bottles, 44, 453
children
    dosage, 449
    drug safety, 449–452
    inhalers and, 79
    and prescription drugs, 173
    side-effects, 450
    stimulant medicines, 450–451
    storage of medications, 84
    swallowing medicine, 452
children, and drugs, 38
chlamydia, 112, 219
cholesterol levels, 146–147, 304
chronic hepatitis, 133
chronic obstructive pulmonary disease (COPD), 112–113, 216, 219, 221, 223, 319, 356
classification of drugs, 25, 172, 447–448
claudication, 113
clinical practice guidelines, 12, 95
clotting factors, 235
coatings, 29
cold, common, 114
cold sores, 114
combination drugs, 37
common cold, 114
common warning labels, 51–52
compassionate care program, 475

Compendium of Pharmaceuticals and Specialties (CPS), 15, 447
complementary and alternative medicines (CAMs), 25–26, 443–444
complementary drugs, 36
conflicting medicines, 92
confusion, 44
congestive heart failure, 131, 192
conjunctivitis, 114, 209, 212
connective tissue diseases, 319
constipation, 457
consumption of prescription drugs
    list of drugs in wallet, 55
    package insert, understanding, 52–53
    taking all your prescribed drugs, 54–55
    understanding prescription label, 49–51
    warning labels, 51–52
    watching for drug interactions, 57
    watching for effectiveness, 53–54
    watching for safety, 54
contact lenses, 75
continuing your medication, 70–72
contraception, 64, 115, 306–312
convulsion, 123, 237
coronary artery disease, 101, 290, 300
corticosteroids, 97
cortisol, 312–313
costs. *See* drug costs
cough, 115–116
creams, 82
Crohn's disease, 140, 141
crushing medications, 52
cryptococcal meningitis, 258
cystitis, 211, 212, 219, 221
Cytochrome P-450, 21

• D •

daily dose, 62
deep vein thrombosis (DVT), 110, 232
dehydration, 458
dementia, 99, 280

depression, 116, 249–257, 270, 423
diabetes, 117–118, 365, 387
diabetes insipidus, 332
diabetic peripheral neuropathy, 152, 424
diarrhea, 119
diastolic value, 136
dilutents, 29
DIN (Drug Identification Number), 50
discarding leftover medication, 85
discharge from hospital, 468–469
discontinuing medication. *See* stopping your medication
disintegrating agents, 29
dispensing date, 51
dispensing errors, 90
dispensing prescription drugs. *See* pharmacists
dizziness, 119–120, 349
"do not crush" warning, 52
doctors
    choice of prescription drug, 35–39
    and drug costs, 471–472
    information from your doctor, 39–41
    and informed consumer, 41
    reasons for prescribing a drug, 33–34
    role of, 11–12, 33–41
    samples, 36
    side-effects, asking about, 438
    specific properties of a drug, 36–37
    taking your drugs to your appointments, 57, 90
    what to tell your doctor, 34–35
    your health, and drug choice, 38–39
dosage
    alternating between different doses, 63
    "as needed," 63
    changing doses, 61
    children, 449
    daily, 62
    and doctor's choice of drug, 36
    and effectiveness, 90–91

exceeding dosage, warning label, 51
extreme precision requirements, 66
four times daily, 62
frequency, in prescription, 42–43
information, 39
knowing your dosage, 60–61
missing a dose, 63–64
precise measurements, 61
on prescription label, 50
schedules, 62–63
for seniors, 455
specific number of hours apart, 63
stopping before prescription is finished, 69–70
three times daily, 62
twice daily, 62
dose-related side-effects, 433–434
dosettes, 455
downregulation, 20
drug allergies, 34, 38, 432–433
drug classifications, 25, 172, 447–448
drug costs
    alternative, less-expensive drugs, 35
    buying drugs over the Internet, 475–476
    and choice of medication, 36
    compassionate care program, 475
    coverage, 44
    government assistance, 474–475
    pricing of prescription drugs, 473
    private health insurance, 475
    splitting a pill or tablet, 65
    and your doctor, 471–472
    and your pharmacist, 472, 473–474
drug interactions
    alcohol, 47, 69, 442–443
    with another prescription drug, 47
    checking for, 174–175

with complementary and alternative medicine interactions, 443–444
described, 441
drug-drug interactions, 47, 441–442
drug-food interactions, 47, 442
drug-sunshine interactions, 444
information from your pharmacist, 47
with non-prescription drugs, 47
with over-the-counter drugs, 47
side-effects, 38
understanding, 441–444
watching for, 57
what to tell your doctor, 34–35
drug intolerances, 34, 38, 48–49, 436–437
drug overdose, 460, 461–462
drug patents, 26
drug plans, 24, 44, 472, 479–480
drug reactions. *See* drug interactions
drug safety
breastfeeding, 445–449
children, 449–452
pregnancy, 445–449
seniors, 453–458
drug samples, 36
drug studies, 486
drugs. *See also* prescription drugs
behind-the-counter drugs, 24–25
body's cells, effect on, 20–21
brand-name drugs, 26, 27–29
classification, 25
combination drugs, 37
defined, 15
entering the body, 16–17
generic drugs, 26–29
how drugs work, 16–22
leaving the body, 21–22
non-prescription drugs, 34–35, 47
over-the-counter drugs, 22–24, 47, 68
receptors, 20

route, in your body, 16–17
Schedule I drugs, 25
Schedule II drugs, 25
Schedule III drugs, 25
trade name, 50
unscheduled, 25
dry mouth, 457
dry powder inhalers, 80
duration of treatment, 40
dyes, 29
dyslipidemia, 146

• *E* •

ear drops, 75–76
ear infections, 120–121, 322–323
eczema, 121
edema, 121–122, 328, 330, 332
effectiveness of medication
absorption of medication, 91–92
certainty, need for, 482
determining if medicine is working, 88–89
and dosage, 90–91
as factor in drug choice, 36
non-response rates, 89
responsiveness, 89
the right diagnosis, 89
the right medicine, 89
taking medication properly, 91
watching for effectiveness, 53–54
the wrong medication, 89
the elderly. *See* seniors
emergencies
determining an emergency situation, 459–461
drug overdose, 460, 461–462
poison control centre phone numbers, 462
running out of prescription medicine, 463–464
emergency department, 464–466
empty stomach, 67–68
end stage renal disease, 144
endocarditis prophylaxis, 122
endometriosis, 123, 310
enemas, 81

enlarged prostate, 136, 155
enteric coating, 66
enzyme, 174
epilepsy, 123, 237
epinephrine, administering, 83
erectile dysfunction, 124–125, 397
errors, 11–12, 90
esophagus, 17, 18
essential tremor, 162
ethanol, 29
excess humidity, 84
expense of drugs. *See* drug costs
expiration dates, 46
exposure to sunlight, 52
extrasystoles, 103
eye drops, 74–75
eye ointments, 75

• *F* •

faintness upon standing, 457
fatigue, 457
FDA drug classification during pregnancy, 448
federal government, 474
fetus, harm to, 446–447
fibromyalgia syndrome (FMS), 125, 411
financial assistance, 474–475
finishing medication, 51
flatulence, 125–126
flavours, 29
"the flu," 142
foods
and absorption of medicine, 92
to avoid at any time, 68–69
drug-food interactions, 47, 442
grapefruit or grapefruit juice, 52, 68, 69
taking medication with food, 67
when not to take medication, 67–68
forgetting your medicine at home, 86–87
four times daily, 62
fungal infections, 257

• *G* •

gas, 125–126

gastro-esophageal reflux disease (GERD), 126, 338, 400

gastroenteritis, 126, 212, 221

gelatin, 29

generic drugs, 26–29, 474

generic names, 28, 50, 87, 96

genital herpes, 133–134, 288

genital warts, 168

GERD, 126

giardia, 218

gingivitis, 218

glaucoma, 127, 340

glucocorticoids, 97

gluten, 29, 48

gonorrhea, 127–128, 212, 216, 223

gout, 128, 427

government assistance, 474–475

grand mal epilepsy, 123

granulating agents, 29

grapefruit or grapefruit juice, 52, 68, 69

Graves' disease, 138, 283

green, leafy vegetables, 68–69

gum, 29

• H •

headaches, 33, 129

Health Canada, 25, 50

health problems, 34

heart attack, 101, 130, 291, 414

heart disease, 413. *See also* specific heart diseases

heart failure, 131–132

heart valve problem, 122, 219, 257

hemorrhoids, 132

hepatitis, viral, 132–133

hepatitis A, 133

hepatitis B, 133

hepatitis C, 133

herpes, genital, 133–134, 288

herpes simplex virus, 133

high blood pressure. *See* hypertension

hirsutism, 134, 330

HIV, 135, 282

holidays. *See* travelling

hormonal contraceptive therapy, 115

hormonal disorders, 124

hospitalizations
discharge from hospital, 468–469

emergency department, 464–466

inpatient wards, 466–468

things to do before leaving, 468

things to do immediately after leaving, 469

humidity, excess, 84

hyperprolactinemia, 136, 334

hypertension, 19, 32, 136–138, 176, 179, 192, 293, 300, 326, 328, 330, 332

hyperthyroidism, 138, 283

hypothyroidism, 99, 136, 139, 421

• I •

idiosyncratic reactions, 436

immunocompromised, 114

imprinted names, 480

improperly taking medications, 487

incontinence, urinary, 139–140

indigestion, 67

infertility, 140

inflammation, 353

inflammatory bowel disease (IBD), 140–141, 186, 351, 352

influenza, 141–142

information sheet, 52–53, 480–481

informed consumer, 41. *See also* consumption of prescription drugs

inhalers
and children, 79

compressor, 80

described, 77

determining amount of remaining medicine, 79

dry powder inhalers, 80

spacer devices, 77, 79

using without spacer device, 78

inhibitor, 174

injections
administering epinephrine, 83

administering insulin, 82–83

biohazard container, 85

inpatient wards, 466–468

insomnia, 142, 198

insulin, administering, 82–83

insulin resistance, 117

intermittent claudication, 113

Internet pharmacies, 475–476

intestines, 18

intolerances. *See* drug intolerances

iron-deficiency anemia, 100

irritable bowel syndrome (IBS), 143, 337

• K •

Kaposi's sarcoma, 135

keeping track of your medications, 60

kidney disorders, 49

kidney failure, 143–144

kidney infections, 165–166

kidney stones, 144–145, 427

kidneys, 21, 453

Kosher diet, 49

• L •

lactose, 29

lactose intolerance, 48

leftover medication, 85

libido, reduced, 145

lifestyle therapy, 32

lipid disorders, 146–147, 304, 347

liquid medicines, 74. *See also* oral drugs

liver, 21

liver damage, 453

liver disorders, 49

lotions, 82

lubricants, 29

lupus, 147, 319

Lyme disease, 219, 223

• M •

magnesium stearate, 29

medical news reporting, 481

medical terms, 174

medicine. *See* drugs; prescription drugs

memory problems, 453

Meniere's disease, 120, 349

menopause, 148, 374

menstrual cramps, 148

metered dose inhaler. *See* inhalers

middle ear infections, 120, 211, 216, 219
migraine headaches, 33, 129, 248, 301, 303, 408
mineralocorticoids, 97
mini-stroke, 159
missing a dose, 63–64
mistakes. *See* errors
mouth rinse, 52
"Multipills," 483–484
multiple doses, 35
multiple sclerosis (MS), 149
muscle cramps, 149
muscle weakness, 453
myasthenia gravis, 352
mycoplasma pneumonia, 223
myelin cells, 149
myocardial infarction, 101, 130

• *N* •

name of your medicine, 39
National Association of Pharmacy Regulatory Authorities (NAPRA), 25, 476
nausea, 150
neurotransmitter, 174
new drugs, 37, 480, 485–486
Nobel, Alfred, 380
non-medicinal ingredients, 28, 29–30, 48–49, 175, 437–438
non-prescription drugs, 34–35, 47
non-response rates, 89
nose drops, 76
nose sprays, 77

• *O* •

obesity, 150, 264
obsessive-compulsive disorder (OCD), 151
ointments, 82
online pharmaceutical drug purchases, 475–477
oral drugs
  in bloodstream, 18–20
  "child-proof" pill bottles, 44
  from intestines to your blood, 17–18
  molecules in, 17–18
  from mouth to intestines, 17

non-medicinal ingredients, 28, 29–30
pill swallowing difficulties, 35
route, in your body, 17–20
splitting a pill or tablet, 64–66
swallowing pills and capsules, 73
oral route, 42
organ transplantation, 352
osteoarthritis, 104–105
osteoblasts, 296
osteoclasts, 296
osteomyelitis, 211, 219
osteoporosis, 32, 151–152, 296, 375, 405
otitis externa, 120
otitis media, 120, 211, 216, 219
outer ear infections, 120, 209
over-the-counter drugs, 22–24, 47, 68
overactive bladder, 139, 229–232
overdose, 460, 461–462

• *P* •

package insert, 52–53, 480–481
packing your prescription medication, 86
Paget's disease of bone, 297, 298
pain, 152, 377, 384–385
pancreatitis, 146
parabens, 29, 49
Parkinson's disease, 152–153, 267
patches, 66, 82
Patented Medicine Prices Review Board, 473
patience, 31–32
patient assistance program, 475
peanut oil, 29, 48
pelvic inflammatory disease, 214
peptic ulcer, 163–165
perforation, 163
periodontitis, 218, 223
peripheral edema, 121, 131
peripheral vascular disease, 113
Peyronie's disease, 124
pharmaceutical industry, 475

pharmacies in Canada, 489
pharmacists
  allergies, information about, 48–49
  asking questions, 44–45
  counselling patients, 481
  and drug costs, 472, 473–474
  drug interactions, information about, 47
  drug intolerances, information about, 48–49
  expiration dates, 46
  fees, 474
  how to take your drug, 45–46
  information from your pharmacist, 45–49
  information in prescription, 42–43
  Internet pharmacies, 475–476
  non-medicinal ingredients, information about, 48–49
  number of licensed pharmacists, 489
  quality time with, 481
  role of, 11–12, 41–49
  side-effects, information about, 47, 439
  staying with one pharmacist, 45
  storage of drug, 46
  unused medicine, 46
  what to tell your pharmacist, 44–45
pharmacy contact information, 50
pharmacy technician, 42
pharyngitis, 161, 216, 219
phlebitis, 110
photosensitive skin rash, 444
photosensitivity, 147
physician. *See* doctors
pill splitter, 65
pills. *See also* oral drugs
  amount of medicine in, 489
  big pills, 65
  "child-proof" pill bottles, 44, 453
  enteric coating, 66
  "Multipills," 483–484

pill swallowing
  difficulties, 35
seven-day pill organizer,
  44, 455
splitting a pill or tablet,
  64–66
swallowing pills, 73
pits, 155
plaques, 155
platelets, 174, 271
pneumonia, 135, 153, 212,
  214, 216, 219, 221
poison control centre
  phone numbers, 462
polycystic ovary syndrome
  (PCOS), 134, 140, 154
potency, 84
pregnancy
  brief exposure to
    prescription drugs,
    449
  classification of drug
    safety, 447–448
  drug safety, 445–449
  FDA drug classification,
    448
  fetus, harm to, 446–447
  morning sickness, 150
  nausea and vomiting,
    262
  oral retinoids, 97
  prescription drug use,
    173, 446–448, 449
  safety of medications,
    39
  telling your doctor, 35
  telling your pharmacist,
    44
prescription drug
  emergencies. See
  emergencies
prescription drug facts
  amount of medicine in a
    pill, 489
  best-selling, in Canada,
    487
  best-selling drug classes,
    in Canada, 488
  Canadian expenditure
    on, 486
  expense of drug study,
    486
  improperly taking
    medications, 487
  new drug approvals,
    485–486
  number of licensed
    pharmacists, 489

pharmacies in Canada,
  489
unapproved indications,
  488–489
prescription drug label,
  49–51
prescription drugs. See
  also drugs; specific
  drugs in Drug Index
  adverse interactions.
    See drug interactions
  the basics, 9–10
  best-selling, in Canada,
    487
  best-selling drug classes,
    in Canada, 488
  body's cells, effect on,
    20–21
  brand-name drugs, 26,
    27–29
  breastfeeding, 173
  and children, 173
  choices, 175
  combination drugs, 37
  concerns, 13
  determining
    effectiveness, 40
  drug, defined, 15
  duration of treatment,
    40
  effectiveness, 36
  entering the body, 16–17
  expense, 35
  expiration dates, 46
  generic drugs, 26–29
  how doctor chooses,
    35–39
  how to take, 45–46
  imprinted names, 480
  interactions. See drug
    interactions
  leaving the body, 21–22
  name of your medicine,
    39
  new drugs, 37
  non-response rates, 89
  oral drugs. See oral
    drugs
  packing, for travel, 86
  precise amounts, 66
  pregnancy, 173
  as prevention, 33
  pricing of, 473
  reason for taking, 40
  receptors, 20
  repeats, 40
  route, in your body,
    17–20

running out of, 463–464
safe and effective use of,
  12–13
side-effects. See side-
  effects
specific properties of a
  drug, 36–37
speed of response, 40
storage, 46, 84
strength, 37
taking your medication.
  See taking your
  medication
track record, 14
travelling, 85–87
as treatment, 33–34
unused medicine, 46
vs. behind-the-counter
  drugs, 24–25
vs. complementary and
  alternative medicines
  (CAMs), 25–26
vs. over-the-counter
  drugs, 22–24
when prescription
  required, 24
when required, 12
prescription errors, 11–12
prescription number, 50
prescriptions
  components of, 42–43
  reasons for, 33–34
  Rx, meaning of, 43
preservatives, 29
prevention, 33
private drug plans, 24
private health insurance,
  475
prolactin, 136
proper use of medications.
  See taking your
  medication
propionibacterium acnes, 96
prostaglandins, 148
prostate cancer, 111,
  224–229
prostatis, 154–155
prostatism, 155, 182
prostatitis, 211, 212, 221
provincial/territorial
  government, 474
pseumomebranous colitis,
  218
psoriasis, 155–156
psoriatic arthritis, 155
psychoses, 157, 276
puffers. See inhalers

pulmonary artery hypertension, 398
pulmonary edema, 121, 131
pulmonary embolism, 110
pulmonary thromboembolism, 110, 232
pyelonephritis, 212, 219, 221

• Q •

quantity in prescription, 50
quitting smoking, 159, 255

• R •

race, and drug choice, 39
Rapoport, David, 51
Raynaud's phenomenon, 147, 301, 303, 398
receptors, 20, 174
red blood cells, 174
reduced libido, 145
refills, 40, 70–72
remembering multiple doses, 35
reminder systems, 483
renal failure, 143–144
renal osteodystrophy, 144
repeats. *See* refills
responsiveness, 89
restless legs syndrome (RLS), 156, 268
rheumatoid arthritis, 105, 351
rhinovirus, 114
rickettsiae, 223
"rinse mouth" warning, 52
RNA, 20
room temperature, 84
rosacea, 156–157, 218, 223
routine, 455
running out of prescription medicine, 463–464

• S •

safety, 54. *See also* drug safety
salt substitutes, 52
samples, 36
Schedule I drugs, 25
Schedule II drugs, 25
Schedule III drugs, 25
schizophrenia, 157, 278, 280
seizure, 123, 237
self-injected medications, 82–83
self-prescribing, 23
seniors

age, and drugs, 38
anticholinergic side-effects, 457
drug safety, 453–458
faintness upon standing, 457
government assistance, 474
side-effects, 457–458
sleepiness, fatigue and altered thinking, 457
special risks, 453
staying organized, 454–455
unused or outdated medications, 454
sensitivity, increased, 453
seven-day pill organizer, 44, 455
severe allergic reactions, 460
sexual function, 19
sexually transmitted diseases and infections
chlamydia, 112
genital warts, 168
gonorrhea, 127–128
HIV/AIDS, 135
syphilis, 160–161
shift workers, 63
shingles, 157–158, 289
side-effects. *See also* specific drugs in Drug Index
allergic reactions. *See* drug allergies
anticholinergic side-effects, 457
appropriate course of action, 41
avoidance of side-effects, 438–440
children, 450
common side-effects, information about, 40
context, 48
dehydration, 458
dose-related side-effects, 433–434
and drug families, 38
drug interactions, 38
drug intolerances. *See* drug intolerances
and erectile dysfunction, 124
experiencing a side-effect, what to do, 440

idiosyncratic reactions, 436
information from your pharmacist, 47
interference with other health issues, 434–436
from non-medicinal ingredients, 437–438
questions to ask your doctor, 438
questions to ask your pharmacist, 439
questions to ask yourself, 439–440
seniors, 457–458
serious side-effects, information about, 41
understanding side-effects, 432–438
sinusitis, 158, 211, 212, 219, 221, 316
skin warts, 168
sleepiness, 457
small intestine, 17
small intestine diseases, 92
smart technology, 482
smoking cessation, 159, 255
sodium bicarbonate, 29
soya lecithin, 29, 48
soybean oil, 29, 48
spacer devices, 77, 79
spastic colon, 143
splitting a pill or tablet, 64–66
stomach, 18, 67–68
stomach surgery, 92
stomach ulcer, 165
stopping your medication
chronic conditions, 71
before prescription is finished, 69–70
sudden stopping, 72
storage of drug, 46, 84
strength of drug, 37
strength per unit, 50
streptococcus bacteria, 161
stress incontinence, 139
stroke, 159–160, 414
subacute bacterial endocarditis (SBE), 122
sugar, 29
sulfites, 29
sulphites, 49
sunlight
drug-sunshine interactions, 444
exposure of medication to, 84

exposure while taking
    medication, 52
photosensitive skin
    rash, 444
suppositories, 80
supraventricular
    arrhythmias, 103
supraventricular
    tachycardia (SVT), 104
swallowing medicine
    children, 452
    liquid medicines, 74
    pills and capsules, 73
sweeteners, 29
swimmer's ear, 120, 209
syphilis, 160–161, 223
systemic lupus
    erythematosis (SLE), 147
systolic value, 136

• *T* •

tablets. *See* oral drugs
take on empty stomach, 52
take with food, 52
taking your medication
    changing doses, 61
    creams, 82
    dosage, 60–61
    ear drops, 75–76
    and effectiveness, 91
    in emergency
        department, 464–466
    enemas, 81
    eye drops, 74–75
    eye ointments, 75
    with food, 67–68
    foods to avoid at any
        time, 68–69
    improperly, 487
    inhalers, 77–80
    injections, 82–83
    in inpatient wards,
        466–468
    keeping track of your
        medications, 60
    lotions, 82
    missing a dose, 63–64
    nose drops, 76
    nose sprays, 77
    ointments, 82
    and over-the-counter
        drugs, 68
    patches, 82
    refills, 70–72
    reminder systems, 483
    schedules, 62–63
    splitting a pill or tablet,
        64–66

stopping before
    prescription is
    finished, 69–70
suppositories, 80
swallowing liquid
    medicines, 74
swallowing pills and
    capsules, 73
things to avoid taking
    with, 68–69
vaginal preparations, 81
tartrazine, 29, 49
tension headaches, 129
Therapeutic Products
    Directorate, 50
thinking problems, 453
three times daily, 62
throat infections, 161
throat swab, 161
thrombotic
    thrombocytopenic
    purpura (TTP), 275
thrombus, 110
thyroid hormone, 138
"time released" medication,
    66
tinnitus, 120
toenail infections, 161–162,
    257
tolerance for drug, 482
tonsillitis, 216
tophi, 427
track record, 14
trade name, 50, 87
transient ischemic attack
    (TIA), 159
transparent coverings, 29
traveller's diarrhea, 221
travelling
    forgetting your medicine
        at home, 86–87
    packing your
        prescription
        medication, 86
    preparing for your trip,
        86
tremor, essential, 162
trichomonas vaginal
    infections, 167, 218
triglyceride levels, 146–147,
    304, 347
trips. *See* travelling
tuberculosis (TB), 163, 285
twice daily dose, 62
type 1 diabetes, 117, 365
type 2 diabetes, 117, 387
typhoid fever, 219

• *U* •

ulcerative colitis, 140, 141,
    324
ulcers, 163–165, 218, 219,
    223, 400
unapproved indications,
    488–489
unscheduled, 25
unused medicine, 46, 454
upregulation, 20
urge incontinence, 139
uric acid crystals, 128
uric acid nephropathy, 427
urinary frequency, 165
urinary incontinence,
    139–140
urinary tract infections,
    165–166
urination difficulties, 457
urine, 21
used needles, 85

• *V* •

vacations. *See* travelling
vaginal dryness, 166
vaginal infections, 166–167
vaginal preparations, 81
vegan diet, 49
vegetables, green and leafy,
    68–69
ventricular arrhythmias, 103
ventricular tachycardia
    (VT), 104
vertigo, 120
vesicles, 157
viral hepatitis, 132–133
viruses, 287
vitamin B12 deficiency,
    100–101
vitamin K, 68–69
vitiligo, 167
vitreous humour, 127
vomiting, 150

• *W* •

warning labels, 51–52
warts
    genital warts, 168
    skin warts, 168
white blood cells, 174
writing down your
    medications, 60

• *Y* •

yeast infections, 167